# Understanding the Secrets
# of Human Perception

## Peter M. Vishton, Ph.D.

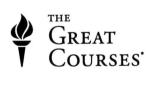

THE
GREAT
COURSES

PUBLISHED BY:

THE GREAT COURSES
Corporate Headquarters
4840 Westfields Boulevard, Suite 500
Chantilly, Virginia 20151-2299
Phone: 1-800-832-2412
Fax: 703-378-3819
www.thegreatcourses.com

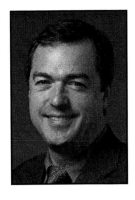

# Peter M. Vishton, Ph.D.
Associate Professor of Psychology
The College of William & Mary

Professor Peter M. Vishton is Associate Professor of Psychology at The College of William & Mary. He received his B.A. in Psychology and Computer Science from Swarthmore College in 1991 and his Ph.D. in Psychology and Cognitive Science from Cornell University in 1996. From 2000 to 2004, Professor Vishton served as an Assistant Professor in the Department of Psychology at Northwestern University. He has also served as the Program Director for Developmental and Learning Sciences at the U.S. National Science Foundation and is a Consulting Editor for the journal *Child Development*.

Professor Vishton has published articles in many of the top journals in the field of psychology, including *Science, Psychological Science, Experimental Brain Research, Teaching of Psychology*, and the *Journal of Experimental Child Psychology*. He is also the creator of the DVD *What Babies Can Do: An Activity-Based Guide to Infant Development*.

In addition to teaching, Professor Vishton studies the perception and action control of both infants and adults. His interests include cognitive, perceptual, and motor development; visually guided action; visual perception; computational vision and motor control; and human-computer interfaces. His research has been funded by the U.S. National Institute of Child Health and Development and the U.S. National Science Foundation.

Professor Vishton has presented his research at numerous conferences and invited talks throughout the United States. He has found a variety of evidence, among both children and adults, that the nature of sensory processing is altered by the actions we choose to perform. In essence, our intention to act on something changes how we perceive it. His ongoing work continues to explore how this aspect of the human senses develops and how the motor systems of the brain are involved in mediating the areas of the brain involved in perception.

When he isn't exploring the secret life of the human senses, Professor Vishton enjoys spending time with his family, reading, and distance running. He has completed 2 marathons and hopes to complete others in the future. He would very much like it if he could figure out how to change his perception of just how long 26.2 miles seems.

More information about Dr. Vishton and his research can be found at http://pmvish.people.wm.edu. ■

# Table of Contents

# Table of Contents

# Table of Contents

# Understanding the Secrets of Human Perception

**Scope:**

T his course aims to provide you with a better understanding and appreciation of your own senses. It explores all 5 of the traditionally defined senses—sight, hearing, touch, taste, and smell—and explains that human beings actually possess far more than these 5. By showing you how to consider the human senses through the lens of scientific inquiry and giving you a better understanding how the senses function, this course will help you experience the world around you more vividly and in more detail.

A sip of fine wine will taste good whether you have studied the human senses or not, but studying the senses has the capacity to greatly enrich your experience. After completing the course, therefore, you will be aware of how the sense of taste decodes different aspects of the wine, as well as how your senses of smell and vision contribute to that taste experience. You will also possess some understanding of how the emotion and memory systems of your brain respond to the glass of wine. A similar story can be told for our sensory experiences of colors, works of art, the faces of the people around us, and thousands of other elements of our world. We are surrounded by rich, complex, beautiful sensory experiences. This course aims to explain and enhance those sensory experiences.

This course takes an interdisciplinary approach to better understanding human sensation and perception. The 24 lectures are loosely organized into 5 sections. We begin with a physiological, neuroscientific approach to the senses. We consider the equipment the human sensory systems contain and how these components work individually and collectively to produce sensory perceptions. The next several lectures consider vision, building on our physiological knowledge to explore different aspects of this important modality to consider how we sense motion, depth, and color. In the third set of lectures, we will consider other modalities of sense perception—that is, we shift our focus to the senses of taste, smell, hearing, and touch. We discuss how these senses work in real-world situations as well—for instance, to mediate speech perception and pain. We next turn our attention to perception in context, continuing to build on these foundations by examining how the sensory systems work in complex, real-world situations. We consider, for instance, how our sensory experiences are influenced by attention, learning, and action behaviors.

Finally, we will be putting it all together. The last group of lectures will emphasize how all of the senses cooperate to produce our perceptions of the world around us. To name just a few examples, the course will explore magic, illusions, emotion perception, and how scientists have developed methods for fixing and replacing damaged sensory systems. ■

# Your Amazing, Intelligent Senses
## Lecture 1

In the 1970s, some of the world's first artificial intelligence researchers set out to program computers to think like people. One of their first ideas was to connect a computer to a video camera and program it to "see." They presumed this would be easy to do and planned this as a summer project. That was 40 years ago; that summer project is still incomplete.

- Computational vision researchers have made great advances: Computers can now interpret motion, print (although they still have trouble with handwriting), objects, and faces within reason.

- Yet even the fastest computers in existence with the best computational vision software are easily outperformed by the average 2-year-old child. We have a long way to go in fully understanding how human senses work.

- Tiny fluctuations in energy patterns impinge on our eyes, ears, skin, tongue, and nose, and within milliseconds, our brain produces a rich sensory experience of the world around us. Perception feels so easy and functions so automatically, yet the processes behind it are mind-bogglingly complex.

- By learning about your senses, you will come to better understand and appreciate the sensations and perceptions you experience and ultimately better understand yourself and the world around you.

- Humans are classically considered to have 5 senses: sight, hearing, touch, taste, and smell. We actually have many more than that. For instance, strictly speaking, we have one sense of touch dedicated to pressure, another for heat and cold, another for vibration and texture—the list could go on and on.

- You may notice this course focuses a lot of attention on the sense of vision. There are some historical and pragmatic reasons for this.

- The vast majority of perception research has been conducted—and continues to be conducted—on vision. It turns out to be the easiest sense to study.

- Vision research has also been predominant because humans and primates in general are extremely visual creatures. Some estimates indicate that as many as 80% of the neurons in the human cortex respond to visual stimuli.

- Thus, if we fully understand vision, we may be more than 20% of the way to understanding how our brain processes sensory information.

- It also turns out that many of the principles discovered by studying vision apply to the other senses as well; that is, the operating characteristics present in the neural networks that control vision seem to be present in the neural networks that control the other senses as well.

- Two themes will arise again and again as this course explores the different sensory systems. First, perception is simply amazing. Second, your sensory systems are inherently inferential, which is in large part how they achieve their amazing performance.

- Our first demonstration—a rapid serial visual presentation (RSVP) test—makes clear just how impressive human perception is.

- A test subject is shown a series of simple object pictures at a rate of about 10 per second (100 milliseconds per image). After several repetitions through the series, the subject is asked to write down what he or she saw. Most people can remember almost all of the images.

- In the second variation on RSVP, the subject is given a code word, such as "car." As the subject views the rapidly presented pictures, he or she must press a button every time a car appears. Most people find this task easy as well.

- Perhaps this does not surprise you. It should. The test subjects have never seen the pictures before. They see them for fractions of a second. The pictures lack any of the detail of real-world objects. Yet the visual system processes the information with ease.

- The RSVP task becomes more difficult at twice the speed—20 objects per second (50 milliseconds per picture). The visual system is not infinitely fast. It is possible to show a stimulus too quickly for a human to recognize something.

- Scientists have encountered no information-processing system capable of these speeds other than the human brain—no supercomputer, no other animals, nothing in the entire universe of scientific exploration.

- Auditory perception is just as precise, rapid, and generally amazing. When someone speaks, dozens of sound units reach your ears every second. You hear individual words, but they are embedded in a continuous, complex stream of sound.

- If you have ever listened to someone speaking a language that you do not know, you may have noticed that it seems like a continuous stream of unbroken sound. In a language you do know, however, your auditory system identifies words so quickly it does not need pauses.

- Computers have gotten better at parsing speech, but humans are still far better at this than even the best systems.

- As with vision, hearing feels so effortless, most people assume it is simple. But when scientists try to duplicate what the brain is doing, they quickly realize how amazing auditory perception is.

- We think of touch as registering pressure information through the skin, but much of the useful information comes through vibration. A smooth, hard surface produces a different pattern of vibration from a rough surface when you drag your fingertips across each.

- Our sensory systems gather a tremendous amount of information very quickly. Even more impressively, our brains almost instantly relate this incoming information to things we already know.

- Your sensory systems also take into account information about your immediate context in a flexible fashion. For instance, if you are in a grocery store looking for bananas, your attention will become attuned to the color yellow.

- This massive, complex, flexible, automatic, interactive, accurate perception process is going on all the time, every moment that you are awake, and to some extent even when you are not.

- How does human perception accomplish all of this? A full answer is beyond the scope of this lecture, but one of the keys is by being inherently inferential. Your brain makes educated guesses about the state of the world around you based on the sensory input it receives, and it is those educated guesses you perceive, not the input itself.

- These inferences occur automatically, rapidly, and outside of conscious awareness, based on extremely complex relationships between different sources of information, starting at the level of the sensory organs themselves.

- Try this blind spot test. Take a piece of paper with 2 X's on it, about 10 centimeters apart, and hold it an arm's length away from your eye. Cover your left eye and look at the left-hand X with your right eye, then slowly bring the paper toward you.

- At some point, the X on the right will seem to vanish, then reappear. The X is passing into a blind spot that occurs in your right eye where the axons of the retina converge at the optic nerve. There is one in your left eye as well.

- Ordinarily, you do not notice these black holes in your vision. Your visual system makes an educated guess about what is in that blind spot based on the nearby areas of the retina. In this case, you perceive something that is not even present—a blank spot on the paper!

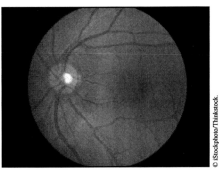

© iStockphoto/Thinkstock.

**The optic nerve (the light spot at left) is the biggest—but not the only—blind spot in the human retina.**

- Another demonstration: Make a grid of lines around the right-hand X, one substantially larger than the size of your blind spot so that your retina will be able to see it even after the X vanishes.

- Now make the X vanish again. What do you see in the blind spot? You should see the grid. Once again, your brain is making an educated guess about the missing information based on the context.

- These optic nerve regions are not the only blind spots in your eyes. A dense network of retinal arteries and veins is attached to the back of your eye, supplying the cells with oxygen and fuel but also creating tiny blind spots. It is as if we walk through the world looking through a lattice-work of vessels, yet we never notice them.

- Our brain fills in these gaps so well that some degenerative vision disorders such as macular degeneration and retinitis pigmentosa can go undetected for years.

- As we explore all of your senses over these 24 lectures, we will return frequently to the concept of inference. Understanding when and how these inferences are made is often the key to understanding perception.

- The visual system is not the only one that fills in missing stimuli. If someone were to cough while you were listening to this lecture, you would still experience what was said at that moment. Your brain would fill in the information based on the sounds you received before and after the cough.

- Hopefully, you are now convinced that perception is both amazing and inferential. The rest of this course will explore the operating characteristics of these sensory processes, starting with the hardware of sensation and perception.

- As we cover various topics, several themes will remain consistent. First, and most directly, all the material in this course is intended to help you better understand your own senses.

- As you become more aware of what you perceive and both how and why you perceive it, I believe that you will appreciate your senses—and the things you are sensing—more and more.

- All of the lectures will also be geared toward teaching you about the scientific process by which we have obtained our knowledge about the senses. A major goal of this course is to prepare you to be active consumers of new scientific results when you hear them.

- We know that information gathered from our senses is used to influence our actions; research suggests that the opposite is true as well. When you choose to perform a certain action, that choice influences your perception, often in fundamental ways.

- I will also talk more about my interest in perceptual development— that is, understanding adult sensory processes by looking at the perception of infants and newborns.

- In addition to my academic pursuits, I have worked as a human interface developer in an industrial setting. This course will also look at some very practical applications of perception research.

- Finally, I am, and will continue to be, a passionate user of my senses. The world is a beautiful place, and it is my senses that deliver that world to my mind. I hope that these lectures will help to spread some of that same enthusiasm to you.

## Suggested Reading

Goldstein, *Sensation and Perception.*

Gregory, *Eye and Brain.*

## Questions to Consider

1. In this lecture, I argue that perception is inherently inferential. Can you think of ways in which sensory inferences are different from inferences made in a more conscious, effortful fashion? Can you think of ways in which they are similar?

2. There is no question that perception is amazing. As you think back on your life, what were your top 10 sensory experiences? What made them the best?

# Your Amazing, Intelligent Senses
## Lecture 1—Transcript

In the 1970s, some of the earliest researchers in the field of artificial intelligence set out to program computers to think like people. As a first step, they connected a computer to a video camera and started to program it to "see" like we do. These researchers, like many, presumed that seeing is easy; so in their initial schedule of activities, these researchers planned to complete this vision part of their project over the course of just that first summer. Come the fall, then, once their computer could see, they would be able to tackle the hard problems of human cognition; things like problem solving, creativity, talking, and the like.

Well, it's about 40 years later now and that summer project still isn't finished. Computational vision researchers have made great advances, of course: Computers can interpret moving stimuli pretty well; they can interpret written text (although they still have a lot of trouble with natural handwriting); they can recognize some objects and even recognize faces pretty well, as long as the person hasn't recently purchased some new glasses or put on a lot of makeup. Actual humans, however, have no problems with any of these things. In general, even the fastest computers running the best computational vision software available are still easily outperformed by your average 2-year-old child. There is something almost miraculous about how richly detailed and accurate our perception is. We have a long way to go to really fully understand how our senses work.

My name is Peter Vishton. I am a Professor of Psychology at the College of William and Mary in Williamsburg, Virginia. For several decades now, I have been absolutely fascinated with human perception. Tiny fluctuations in energy patterns impinge on our eyes, ears, skin, tongue, and nose, and within milliseconds, our brain produces a rich sensory experience of the world around us. Perception feels so easy and functions so automatically that many people assume that there must not be much to it. Let me assure you that there is.

In this course, I want to tell you about the "Secret Life of the Senses"; about all of these amazingly complex and fascinating things that your senses are doing all the time, whether you are aware of it or not. I mentioned that we have a long way to go to completely understand our senses, but that's not to say that we don't already know a lot. By learning about these things, I hope that you'll come to better understand and appreciate the sensations and perceptions that you have, and ultimately to better understand yourself and the world around you.

We classically consider humans as having 5 senses: We see, hear, touch, taste, and smell. This course will consider all of these. Indeed, I'll explain that we actually have many more than 5 senses. For instance, our sense of touch arises from the activity of a wide range of different types of neurons, all of which function independently from one another. Strictly speaking, we have one sense of touch dedicated to pressure, another for heat and cold, another for vibration and texture; the list could go on and on. And that's just one of our senses.

While this course will include information about all of the senses, you may notice that I seem to focus a lot of my attention on the sense of vision. There are some historical and pragmatic reasons for this. Firstly, the vast majority of perception research has been conducted—and continues to be conducted—on vision. It turns out to be much easier to set up the materials required for a study of vision than for the other senses. For a study of the sense of smell, for instance, you need to have a variety of carefully produced and controlled chemical stimuli. You may also need specialized equipment to deliver a precise amount of this olfactory stimulus. It's also a little known fact that after the scent of something gets into your nose, it takes a long time—dozens of minutes—for the chemical to fully clear out of the nose again so that it's fresh and ready for the next trial. So if you run a smell experiment with a few dozen trials, you may need several hours of time with each one of your study participants. Contrast this with a simple vision experiment. You may only need some pictures or a simple computer-generated display. Within a few seconds, the visual system is reset and ready to go for the next trial, so you can run a study with hundreds or thousands of trials rather than just a dozen or so. Another reason that vision research has been predominant is that humans and primates in general are extremely visual creatures. Some estimates have indicated that as many as 80 percent of the neurons in the human cortex respond to visual stimuli. Thus, if we fully understand vision, we may be more than one-fifth of the way to understanding how our brain processes sensory information.

Reasons such as this have led to the predominance of vision research in our study of the senses. But there is some good news here: It turns out that many of the principles discovered by studying vision apply to the other senses as well; that is to say that the operating characteristics that are present in the neural networks that control vision seem to be present in the neural networks that control the other senses as well. So while I, like the researchers in this field, may tend to emphasize vision, when you're learning about vision, you're also learning about the other senses.

In this first lecture, I want to try to explain 2 different things that will come up again and again as we explore your different sensory systems. First, we'll talk about the simple fact that perception is amazing. Second, I want to convince you that your sensory systems are inherently inferential, and this is a big part of how they achieve their amazing performance.

Hopefully you already think perception is interesting and amazing; why else would you be listening to me? With this first demonstration, I want to make clear, however, just how impressive your perception is. I'm going to show you a series of simple object pictures. They're pictures that you haven't seen before, and I'm going to show you those pictures in a very rapid succession. Perception researchers call this "rapid serial visual presentation," or "RSVP" for short. This sequence of images that you're seeing is being presented at a rate of about 10 per second, about 100 milliseconds per image. As you view these objects, you might just notice that you can recognize them, even with this very brief viewing time for each one. If I stopped the RSVP images and then asked you to write down all of the objects you remember, you might be able to write out a list of many of them, but you probably wouldn't get them all.

But that's a harder task than the one I want to ask you to do right now. To write that list of objects out, you'd have to not only perceive and recognize the objects but encode them in your memory and then successfully retrieve the names as you wrote down what you'd seen. For the moment, all I want to establish is that you can do the recognition part of this task; that in a matter of 100 milliseconds, you can perceive the pattern of light in the image and associate it with some verbal label that you already have stored in your mind. To do this, I'll give you a probe word and ask you to respond when you see the object picture that goes with it. Let's try "car." Watch the images and imagine pressing a response button as soon as you see one. Okay, go ahead and do that now; press your "button" when you see a car. Let's try another one. This time, press your imaginary button when you see a computer.

If you're like most people, you'll find that you can do this rather easily. It will still work if I give you a broad category name instead of the name of a single item. This time, press your button whenever you see a vehicle. This time, press the button when you see something you would eat. I can even do it with an object feature: Press the button when you see something that flies. You're able to do all of these tasks with only 100 milliseconds of viewing time, and you can do it pretty easily at that.

I just want to stop for a moment and point out how amazing this is. You can do this with these very simple images; images that lack all of the fine texture, color, and detail that you'd encounter if you were looking at the actual objects in real life. Also, you've never seen these pictures before today. Particularly on that initial run-through of the images, your visual system was doing all of its processing inside this tiny 100 milliseconds window, working from scratch with a brand new stimulus.

Let's try this RSVP task at a rate of 20 objects per second, so now only 50 milliseconds per picture. So now I want you to hit your imaginary button when you see a musical instrument. Now hit the button if you see something that you might eat for breakfast. You'll notice that this is much harder. Your visual system is not infinitely fast. It's possible to show a stimulus too fast for you to recognize something. But this is really fast. As long as you have about 100 milliseconds, the task is easy. As easy as this is for you, we've encountered no other information processing system capable of this other than the human brain; no supercomputer, no other animals, nothing in the entire universe of scientific exploration. The human brain—your human brain—is just flat amazingly good at this task.

Auditory perception is just as precise, rapid, and generally amazing. Consider the seemingly simple task of listening to someone talk. As you're listening to me right now, literally dozens of sound units are reaching your ears every second. You hear the individual words that I'm saying, but they're embedded in a continuous stream of sound that's quite amazingly complex. If you've ever listened to someone speaking a language that you don't know, it will be easier to be aware of this. Here's a recording of someone speaking Aymara. This is a Native American language spoken by about a million people who live in Western Bolivia. (If you do speak Aymara you'll just have to trust me for the next few things I say.)

As you listen to it, notice that it sounds like a continuous stream of unbroken sound. It seems like there are no pauses between the words as there are in English. Actually, there are no pauses in between the words, either in this recording or in the English speech that you're hearing right now. This lack of pauses in between words is true for all languages that humans commonly use. When you listen to me, you hear individual words, but there are no auditory "spaces" in between them. If I talk with gaps in between words it sounds very stilted to say the least. Your auditory system identifies the words in the sound patterns so fast and well that it doesn't need those pauses.

Consider even the sounds "ba" and "pa." "I'm swinging the 'bat'" is very different from "swinging my friend 'Pat.'" Handing you a "pill" and a "bill" are totally different. How do you know which one I'm saying? For both sounds, you start by constricting your vocal tract and building up pressure behind your lips. Then you release that pressure and exhale slightly. As you do, you engage your vocal cords and make a vowel sound ("ah"). You do the same thing with both sounds, "ba" and "pa." How do you make one sound or the other? The only difference, it turns out, is a slight change in the timing of the onset of the vocal cords; the so-called voice onset time. If you start the voicing at the same time you release that built-up pressure, you hear "ba." If you wait about 15 extra milliseconds, it comes out as "pa." Just 15 extra milliseconds; a little extra time. Short voice onset time, "ba"; just a tiny delay and you get "pa." These very fine distinctions, on the order of a few milliseconds, are made by your auditory system dozens of times per second in order to understand speech.

Computers have gotten better at parsing speech, but if you've ever tried to deal with the automatic ticket agent on a cell phone with a noisy connection then you know that humans are still far better at this than even the best systems. As with vision, hearing feels so easy, so effortless, that most people assume there must not be much to it. But when we try to duplicate what our brain is doing, we quickly realize just how amazing perception is.

Our sense of touch is amazing, too. We think of touch as registering pressure information through the skin, but much of the really useful information comes through vibration. If I drag my fingers across a smooth, hard surface, there's one pattern of vibration produced at my fingertips. If I drag it across a rough surface, another pattern results. Our brain is masterful at interpreting these patterns. If you reach into a bag stuffed with clothing, you'll be able to pick out that particular old flannel shirt or the jeans or the spandex, all of it based on just a few milliseconds of vibration information delivered through the fingers.

In this course, as we explore the human senses, we'll see this sort of thing over and over again. Our sensory systems gather a tremendous amount of information very, very quickly. Even more impressively, we almost instantly relate this incoming information to things that we already know. Your sensory systems also take into account information about your immediate context in a very flexible fashion. For instance, if you're in a grocery store looking for bananas, your attention will become very attuned to the color yellow. As you drive, your eyes and ears become attuned to the information needed to drive and less sensitive to other sources of information that aren't relevant. This massive, complex, flexible, automatic, interactive, accurate perception process is going on all the time, every moment that you're awake; and to some extent even when you aren't. Perception is amazing.

So how does human perception accomplish all of this? How does our brain outperform everything else in the known universe in terms of sensory processing? A full answer to this question is certainly beyond the scope of this first lecture, but one of the key tricks that our senses use is to be inherently inferential. Our brain makes educated guesses about the state of the world around us based on our sensory inputs, and it's those educated guesses that you perceive; not the sensory inputs themselves, but the results of our perceptual inferences. It's precisely because our senses are so good at making those inferences, so perceptually intelligent, that our perception is so amazing.

Now, most people think of inferences as cognitive operations that we perform in classes on logic and math. If John is taller than Betty, and Mark is shorter than Betty, then we can infer than John must be taller than Mark; right? The inferences I'm talking about here are related to this, but they occur automatically and outside of our conscious awareness. They occur very quickly and based on some extremely complex relationships between different information sources. And they don't only happen at a higher, cognitive level; the inferences start right at the level of the sensory organs themselves. Let's consider one class of inferential process that happens in your retina.

For this demonstration, you'll need a pen and a piece of paper. Almost any piece of paper will do; I usually use an 8.5 by 11 sheet folded in half. What you should do here is make 2 small X's maybe about 4 inches apart from one another. You want to make them relatively small, maybe about a quarter inch at the most. What you should then do is set your pen down, hold the piece of paper with the 2 X's in your right hand, and hold it out at arm's length. With your left hand, cover your left eye. I want you to fixate on the X on the left and very slowly bring it toward yourself. As you're doing this, you want to make sure you keep your right eye looking directly at the X on the left, but pay attention to the X on the right. As you bring the X's slowly closer to you, somewhere around there, the X on the right will vanish. You can do that a few times just to make sure to yourself that the X has vanished. Rather, the X is still there, but it really does seem to vanish when you have it at just the right position.

The X is still there, of course; you know that. What has happened is that the X has passed into the blind spot on the back of your right eye. This blind spot is caused by a characteristic of the anatomy of the human eye—of your eyes. Light passes through the pupil and the lens of the eye and projects onto the retina, which covers the back interior surface of the eyeball. The retina itself consists of a dense mosaic of light-sensitive neurons called photoreceptors. About one million neuronal connectors, called "axons," extend from each particular location on the retina to the optic nerve, located in a particular spot a few millimeters away from the center of the retina. The optic nerve is a bundle of about a million neurons that extends from each eye back into the head and the rest of the brain. At that location on the retina where the optic nerve begins, where the million axons all come together, they pile up on top of one another and create a blind spot, a location on the back of the eye where you are blind.

There's a blind spot on each of the eyes where you just can't see. Now, as you look around the world, you don't notice these "black holes" in your visual fields. Even when you cover one eye, you still don't see it. Even when the X vanished into the blind spot, you probably noticed that it didn't move into some sort of a black hole; it moved into a space that was the same color as the paper. In essence, your visual system makes an educated guess about what's in that blind spot—an inference based on the nearby areas of the retina—and it's that inference that you perceive. You're perceiving something that's not present in the visual input; you're perceiving the result of an inference.

So back to our X's again. This time, what I want you to do is, around the X that you're going to make vanish, draw a grid of vertical and horizontal lines. You might want to stop the video to give yourself a chance to draw that grid. It's important; it doesn't need to be perfectly straight, it's important that it be big enough that it extends beyond where the blind spot is located. Once you've drawn that grid, make that X vanish again. Once again, you want to hold the piece of paper out at arm's length in your right hand, cover your left eye with your left hand, fixate the X on the left, and slowly bring it toward yourself. At just the right position, you will notice the X on the right vanish. Now what I want you to pay attention to here after you've made that X vanish is what's in the blind spot. What's located where that X used to be before it disappeared? Assuming that all of this has worked the right way, you should see a blind spot filled with that grid texture. Based on the texture surrounding the blind spot, your visual system infers that that texture is in the area of the blind spot as well; and again, it's that inference—or rather the result of that inference—that you perceive.

This inferential process shows up throughout the visual system and, indeed, in the other senses as well; and it's a good thing that it does. These optic nerve regions aren't the only blind spots. If you've ever taken a flash photo of someone in a relatively dim room, you've probably noticed the "red eye" phenomenon. Superman isn't turning on his heat vision here, the little witch isn't really possessed, and the dog isn't haunted; their eyes are glowing because their retinas are reflecting the light of the camera's flash bulb. What you're seeing at the red spots in this photo—white for the dog—is actually a small image of the backs of their eyes; a small image of their retinas. If I were to zoom all the way in on one of those red spots, I would see something like the following.

In this photo of the human retina, the most striking feature is the dense network of veins and arteries that supply the cells here with oxygen and fuel. They're essential to the survival and function of retinal cells, but they also do something else: They block the light, preventing it from reaching the light-sensitive layers of cells on the retina. Every place where you see a retinal vein in this image is another place where the eye is blind. It's as if we walk through the world looking through a lacey lattice-work of these veins; yet we're never aware of them. Our brain fills in all of these tiny blind regions in the same way that it fills in the large blind spots associated with the optic nerves.

This filling-in process works so well that some degenerative vision disorders can go undetected for years. Macular degeneration results in a slow reduction in the cells near the center of visual field. Eventually, a patient with this disorder will notice a loss of the ability to read or recognize faces, but not until the disease has progressed very far. Our brain does such a good job of filling in missing sensory input that we just don't notice it. Similarly, retinitis pigmentosa, a disorder in which peripheral vision deteriorates, will often go undetected for years unless you visit a doctor and undergo testing. It's a good idea to make sure you visit your eye doctor regularly. The earlier these types of problems are detected, the more can be done to slow or stop their progress.

These inferential processes are some of the biggest secrets in the secret life of the senses; and not just for vision, but for all of the senses. As we explore all of your senses over these 24 lectures, we'll return to this concept frequently. Understanding when and how these inferences are made is often the key to understanding perception.

The visual system is not the only one to fill in missing stimuli. If you hear someone cough in the middle of one of my sentences, you'll still experience what I said at that moment. In fact, even if I were to skip a particular ... in this second sentence, you might still hear it. Your brain would fill it in based on the sounds that you did receive before and after the cough sound.

Hopefully you've been convinced that perception is both amazing and inferential. The lectures in this course will explore the operating characteristics of these sensory processes. We'll start by exploring the hardware of sensation and perception. I'll present information about the sensory organs, the neurons that connect with them, and the brain systems that make sense of the world around you. We'll then turn to several fundamental topics in the domain of visual perception; discussing how you perceive motion, depth, and color. With that background in hand, we'll consider how your perceptual systems function in the context of your body and the real non-laboratory world around you. We'll consider action control, attention, and perception; subliminal perception, perceptual development, and perceptual learning. We'll then turn our attention specifically to the non-visual modalities of perception. I'll present material on taste and olfaction, hearing, speech and language perception, the active use of the sense of touch, kinesthetic perception, and the perception of pain. At this point, you'll know a lot about the senses. With a good understanding of the basics, we'll begin looking at how all of these different topics come together in real-world situations. We'll discuss magic and illusions, perception and emotion, perceiving the thoughts of others, a concept known as opponent process, synesthesia, and fixing or replacing damaged sensory systems.

As we cover these very different topics, I have several goals for this course that will remain consistent. First, and most directly, all of this material will help you better understand your own senses. As you make your way through your day and perceive the world around you, I want you to be able to think not only about what you're perceiving, but about how and why you perceive it. As you become more aware of these things, I think you'll find that you appreciate your senses—and the things you're sensing—more and more.

Along with understanding and appreciating your senses more, all of the lectures will be geared to teaching you about the scientific process that's led us to our knowledge about the senses. I don't want you to be satisfied with me just telling you how your senses function. Whenever possible, I'll accompany my description of the theories about perception with evidence that supports those theories. Our understanding of the human senses continues to develop. There are new experiments being performed somewhere right now. Those results always have the potential to change our theories of perception. A major goal of this course is to prepare you to be active consumers of those new scientific results when you hear them. After you finish the course, I hope you'll think of yourself as an active, critically thinking, perception researcher.

So who am I? I mentioned at the opening of this lecture that I'm a professor at the College of William and Mary, where I've been a member of the psychology faculty since 2004. I've been a professor when all is said and done for about 16 years. I'm not finished learning, myself, however; I'm still a student of perception and psychology in general, for 30 years now and counting. I started that process as a freshman at Swarthmore College where I took an intro psych course on a whim to fulfill a liberal arts distribution requirement. Within a few weeks of listening to the material presented in that class, the direction of my academic career had been set. About 8 years later, I'd completed my doctoral work at Cornell University.

In addition to teaching, I spend a lot of time working on research. I study how perception and action control influence each other. We know that information gathered from our senses is used to influence our actions (things like reaching and driving); my research suggests that the opposite is true as well. When you choose to perform a certain action, that choice influences your perception, often in some fundamental ways. We'll discuss that more in later lectures. I'll also talk more later about my other interest in perceptual development. We can better understand our own adult sensory processes by looking at the perception of tiny infants, even newborns.

In addition to my academic pursuits, I've also worked as a human interface developer in an industrial setting. I think research on the senses is fascinating, plain and simple, but it can also be useful. The course will mention several areas where that's the case.

Finally, I am, and will continue to be, a passionate user of my senses. The world is a beautiful place, and it's my senses that deliver that world to my mind. I hope that these lectures will help to spread some of that same enthusiasm to you.

This concludes my overview of the course; now it's time to get down to business. In the next lecture, we'll discuss some of the basic biology of the perceptual system. I'll describe the sensory organs, the neurons they're connected to, and the brain regions that interpret the sensory input. I hope you'll join me.

# The Physiological Hardware of Your Senses
## Lecture 2

E ntire books have been written—and Nobel Prizes awarded—based on discoveries about the hardware of human perception we will only have minutes to discuss in this lecture. Thus, this lecture will not be comprehensive, but it should provide you with enough working knowledge of sensory physiology to carry you through the rest of the course.

- First, we will look at neurons and how they function; then, we will learn about transduction, by which the senses translate energy from the environment into electrical signals that neurons can use.

- Next, we will see how these transduced patterns of energy are organized in the human brain. We will briefly talk about the idea of specific nerve energies and what it means for human sensory experience.

- Finally, we will ponder how we can mentally represent the infinite range of things in the world with the finite number of neurons in our bodies.

- Neurons are specialized cells that are the basic building blocks of all human sensation and other mental processes. In addition to a cell body and organelles, neurons have 2 different types of long, branching fibers extending away from the cell body: dendrites and axons.

- These are the wires that a neuron uses to communicate with sensory organs, muscles, and other neurons. The dendrites receive inputs and the axons transmit outputs. The axons from one neuron grow very close to the dendrites of other neurons, but they never quite touch. The gap between is called a synapse.

- Neurons transmit information to one another by means of an electrochemical reaction called an action potential. These signals travel as quickly as 200 miles per hour, causing the axon to release a chemical called a neurotransmitter.

- This neurotransmitter spreads across the synapse to the dendrite. The presence of the neurotransmitter affects the likelihood of an action potential in the second neuron.

- Excitatory neurotransmitters increase the rate of action potentials in the second neuron. Inhibitory neurotransmitters decrease the rate of action potentials in the second neuron. Neurons can exhibit 100 action potentials per second, or they may go several minutes between pulses.

- Neurons may seem too simple to calculate everything we think and feel. Their power comes from their numbers—about 100 billion neurons with hundreds of trillions of synapses (so many we cannot know the exact number) in every person's body.

- The brain consists of a giant, amazingly complex network of different types of neurons. The patterns of connection and activity between neurons give the brain its information-processing power.

- All the things you sense and perceive are processed in your brain in the form of action potentials, so the first job of any sensory system is to translate the physical and chemical energy of the environment into action potentials. This process is called transduction.

- Let's run through an example of a transduction process for the sense of touch.

  o One specialized type of touch receptor neuron is a Pacinian corpuscle. Vibration inspires it to emit action potentials.

  o When there is no vibration, the cell produces few action potentials. If the cell is just pressed, it does not emit much activity. Either way, neurons with dendrites close to its axons are similarly inactive.

o The right rate of vibration, however—such as running your finger across the bristles of a comb—causes a chemical change within the cell that produces a train of action potentials, releasing more and more neurotransmitter.

o This produces that train of action potentials in nearby neurons and in all the neurons in the chain of nerves that lead from it to the spine and ultimately to the brain.

• The start of transduction is different for every sense, but the end of the process is always the same: a signal about something in the environment being delivered to the brain.

• All sensory neurons exhibit adaptation; they respond when a new stimulus starts but slow down and stop if the stimulus remains constant.

• For example, Merkel cells produce action potentials in response to slow changes in pressure, such as the consistent push you feel when you sit down. You perceive pressure on your legs as you sit, but after a while, you no longer notice it unless you deliberately turn your attention to it.

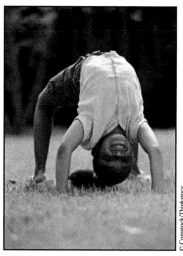

• Meissner corpuscles and Ruffini cells respond to different types of changes in physical force. Meissner corpuscles respond to abrupt

**Special nerves called Ruffini cells allow you to feel your skin stretch.**

© Comstock/Thinkstock.

onsets and removals of force. They are especially important in fine motor control, as in tool use. Ruffini cells send the signals that allow you to feel your skin stretching as you move. Many other receptors work to convey information about touch, such as information about temperature and pain.

- It is interesting that we perceive touch as a single modality given just how many different types of receptors are involved. Our brain combines them into a single perception, a single awareness of the world around us.

- The sense of smell has an even wider range of different transducers, located in the olfactory epithelium behind your nose. Molecules of particular chemicals have particular shapes, each of which fits a certain receptor. The neuron connected to that receptor then becomes active and delivers information to the brain.

- Taste works in much the same way, with particular receptors for bitter, sweet, sour, salty, and the recently discovered umami. There is a commonly held myth that these different types of receptors are only present in particular regions of the tongue, but all are found in all areas of the tongue.

- The senses of smell and taste connect through the mouth, nose, and throat. As you chew and swallow food, traces of it find its way up into the olfactory epithelium. Most of what you experience as taste is really orthonasal olfaction.

- Transduction for hearing takes place within the inner ear. Sound enters through the auditory canal, is amplified by the eardrum and some complex bony structures, and passes the snail-shaped cochlea.

- If you were to unroll the cochlea, you would have a long cone with a thin membrane stretched down its middle. Attached to the edges of this membrane are tiny hair-like cells connected to individual neurons. You hear something when these hair-like cells move.

- Low-frequency sounds cause the wider parts of the cochlear membrane to vibrate; high-frequency sounds cause the thinner parts of the cochlear membrane to vibrate.

- Most sounds are a mix of high-, middle-, and low-frequency sound waves. This mixed vibration is converted into a pattern of action potentials.

- The axons of the frequency-specific neurons are bundled into the auditory nerve, which then projects into the auditory cortex.

- Vision works in a similar manner. Light enters the eye through the cornea and the lens, which work together to focus a clear image on the retina. The lens thickens slightly when we look at something close up and relaxes to look at something far away.

- The retina contains a dense mosaic of light-sensitive cells, about a million in each eye. Each of these cone- or rod-shaped receptors contains a chemical that changes when light strikes it.

- When the concentration of light-modified chemical is high enough, it causes an action potential to be generated by the receptor cell. The action potential passes through a network of neurons, into the optic nerve, and into the primary visual cortex of the brain.

- The light-sensitive chemical is continually switched back to its initial form after this interaction with the light. In complete darkness, almost all this light-sensitive chemical is restored to the "ready" mode. If someone were to then turn on a light, the visual experience would be quite intense; a great burst of action potentials results.

- After you have a minute or so to adapt to the light, the intensity passes; the density of the light-sensitive chemical returns to a more typical state. This is one of several mechanisms that enable our visual system to deal with an enormous range of different lighting conditions.

- The region where sensory information arrives in the brain determines what will be perceived. For example, the light from different points on an object—say, a coffee mug—projects to different particular locations on the retina. The optic nerve carries these signals to specific points in a subcortical region called the lateral geniculate nucleus, where the spatial relationship between the points is maintained, at least in a very general fashion.

- The neurons in the lateral geniculate nucleus project to the back of the brain to a region called the primary visual cortex, where the majority of basic visual processing is accomplished. The spatial relations present on the retina and in the lateral geniculate nucleus are maintained in the visual cortex as well.

- This one-to-one relationship between the sensory input and the location of cortical activation is a principle that applies to all of the senses.

- Action potentials from touch-sensitive neurons in the skin are delivered to a region of the brain called the somatosensory cortex, which contains a virtual map of your body. The primary motor cortex, a region involved in coordinating actions, has a corresponding map that follows this same pattern.

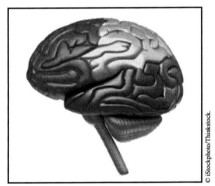

© iStockphoto/Thinkstock.

**Different regions of the brain correspond to different senses.**

- The relative sizes of the body parts in the brain's map do not correspond to their physical sizes. This reflects how certain areas of the body are more sensitive to touch than others.

- The sound map in the auditory cortex—located in the temporal lobes, near the sides of the head—is not arranged spatially like for the other senses but according to sound frequency (that is, pitch).

- The organization for taste and smell is actually quite a bit more complicated, but the principle is the same: Particular aromas and flavors produce certain patterns of activation.

- A general principle that applies to all of the senses is the law of specific nerve energies, first proposed by Johannes Müller in 1835, which states that all action potentials are the same except with regard to where they project in the brain.

- Imagine for a moment that we could unplug your optic nerve from the visual cortex and reconnect it to the auditory cortex. In principle, you would hear light.

- How can an infinite variety of stimuli be represented in our finite brains? Let's start with a very simple example: a single tilted line. This line could have any of an infinite number of orientations: 138.3456 degrees, 138.34566 degrees, and so on.

- It could be that a different neuron corresponds to the presence of each of these many, many orientations. Maybe when the line is vertical, your vertical-line neuron becomes active. Maybe another neuron is the horizontal-line neuron, and maybe there is one for a 45-degree line … on and on for every possible degree of arc.

- If we needed to devote a separate neuron to every single thing we could perceive, we would run out of neurons. Instead, the brain resolves this by encoding perceptions in terms of the pattern of response of several neurons rather than in terms of just one.

- In the visual cortex, a column of neurons encodes orientation. One cell prefers vertical lines, so when a vertical line is present, it exhibits a very high rate of action potentials. Other cells similarly respond best to 45- or 135-degree orientations, and so on.

- These cells respond most to their preferred orientation, but they also respond to similar orientations. By looking at the pattern of response across these 3 different cells, it is possible to infer any orientation across this range. This design principle shows up in all of our sensory processing.

- Similarly, there are cells in your retina that respond best to blue, green, and yellow light, but these cells also respond in a graded, predictable fashion to light that varies from their preferred color. By considering the relative rate of responses of these different types of receptors, we can perceive millions of different colors with only a few types of color receptors.

- Your brain makes its best guess about what is out there based on the pattern of incoming neural activation—from that spatial pattern of activation in your cortex—and that best guess is what you perceive.

## Suggested Reading

Hubel and Wiesel, *Brain and Visual Perception.*

Livingstone, *Vision and Art.*

## Questions to Consider

1. If Johannes Müller's doctrine of specific nerve energies states that what we perceive is a direct function of where the brain is activated, then what would our perception of the world be if we switched the optic nerve to project into the somatosensory cortex? What if we connected the olfactory bulb to project to the visual cortex?

2. If we developed an artificial neuron—a silicon computer chip that mimicked the processing of a neuron in every way—and if we took out one of your neurons and replaced it with one of these chips, what would your experience be? What if we replaced all of your neurons this way? Would we have created a perceiving, thinking, feeling machine?

# The Physiological Hardware of Your Senses
## Lecture 2—Transcript

Hello again, and welcome to the second lecture in this course about the senses. In this session, I'll present a broad physiological overview of human sensation and perception. Entire books have been written, and Nobel prizes awarded, based on some of the things that we'll only be able to consider for a few minutes in this lecture. What I want to convey won't be comprehensive, but it should provide you with a working knowledge of sensory physiology that will be important for the rest of the course. I also want to warn you that this will be a very biological lecture; actually, the next 3 will be. There are a lot of facts that I want to cover here, some of which are a little bit dry. I hope you'll stick with me, however. Once we have this under our belts, you'll have the tools to understand the secret life of the senses in much greater detail.

Okay, let's begin. First, I'll be telling you about neurons and how they function. Second, I'll describe transduction, the process by which each of your senses translates energy from the surrounding environment into the electrical signals that neurons use. Third, we'll consider how these transduced patterns of energy are organized in the human brain. I'll describe something called the Mueller Doctrine of Specific Nerve Energies and what it means for human sensory experience. Finally, I want to briefly ponder how we can mentally represent the infinite range of things that are out here in the world—infinite different shades of color, variations of shape and movement, different aromas—how we can represent an infinite number of different things given that our brain contains only a finite number of neurons.

Let's start at the microscopic level with the neuron. Neurons are the basic building blocks of all human sensation, perception, cognition, decision-making, and anything else that we might describe as "mental." Everything you've ever thought, felt, or remembered, even the thought that you just had a moment ago while listening to this sentence, all of that is the result of the activity of these neurons. A neuron is a specialized type of cell. It has a cell body and a nucleus, just like any other cell in the body; it takes oxygen and fuel from the bloodstream, just like any other cell; it also expels waste products and carbon dioxide back into the bloodstream, just like other cells.

The shape and function of neurons, however, are very distinctive. Neurons have 2 different types of long, branching fibers that extend away from the cell body. These are called dendrites and axons. These are the wires, if you will, that a neuron uses to communicate with the sensory organs, the muscles, and other neurons. The dendrites receive inputs and the axons transmit outputs. Here you can see a diagram of the axon of one neuron connecting to the dendrite of another. The ends of the axons from one neuron grow very close to the dendrites of other neurons, but they never quite touch. There's always a small gap in between these called a synapse. I'll come back to that synapse part in a moment.

Neurons transmit information to one another by means of a very particular electrochemical reaction called an action potential. Imagine for a moment that you could shrink yourself down to microscopic size and to sit next to an axon. Imagine that you're holding a tiny voltmeter; the same kind you would use to test to see if a battery still has any power left in it. Imagine putting one of the terminals of the voltmeter inside the axon while keeping the other just outside of it. Note, by the way, you would need microscopic scuba gear for this trip since you're swimming in the bloodstream here. When one of these action potentials occurs, you would notice the voltmeter's needle make a sudden jump. It would bounce from −70 millivolts to +40 millivolts and then back again over the course of about 30 milliseconds. If you had 2 of these voltmeters, one next to the other, you would notice that the needle would jump first at the spot closest to the neuron's cell body, and then just a few moments later at the site located further along the axon. These signals can travel very fast down the length of an axon; as fast as 200 miles per hour.

When the action potential reaches the end of one of the branches of an axon, it causes the neuron to release a chemical called a neurotransmitter from its end. This neurotransmitter spreads across the synapse to the dendrite on the other side. The presence of the neurotransmitter then affects the likelihood of an action potential in the second neuron. If this is an excitatory neurotransmitter connection, then the action potential from one neuron will increase the rate of action potentials in the second neuron. Sometimes the connections are inhibitory, however. The more active the first neuron is, the less active the second will become.

All of this happens very fast. Neurons can exhibit these action potentials as many as 100 times per second. At other times, however, they may go several minutes in between those pulses. These individual cells may seem too simple to calculate everything we think and feel. Their power, however, comes from how many there are: about 100 billion neurons with hundreds of trillions of synapses; so many that we don't know the exact number. We can only estimate it based on samples taken from small groups of neurons.

I should also note that there is a tremendous variety of different types of neurons located in different regions of the brain: Some have very long axons, as long as 2 meters; some have many, many short axons, hundreds of them; some look like baskets, some look like pyramids. Our brain consists of a giant, amazingly complex network of these neurons. The patterns of connection and activity form what is quite simply the most powerful information processing device in the known universe. How we get from these seemingly simple individual cells to a person that's conscious and capable of all of the things we do is one of the great mysteries in all of science.

All of the things you sense and perceive from the world around you are processed in your brain in the form of these action potentials. When you see something blue, there's nothing blue in your brain; there's a pattern of action potentials that corresponds to blue. When you smell some delicious chocolate cake in the oven, there's no chocolate in your brain; there's a pattern of action potentials that somehow means chocolate. Action potentials are the language, if you will, that your brain uses to represent and process sensory information, and all information as long as we're at it.

So the first job of any sensory system is to translate the physical and chemical energy of the environment around us into these action potentials. This process is called transduction. Let's run through an example of a transduction process for the sense of touch. There's a particular type of touch receptor called a Pacinian corpuscle. It's a specialized type of neuron that lives in the thin layer of fat cells under your skin. Like all neurons, it has axons and can produce trains of action potentials. This neuron doesn't have any dendrites, however. What inspires it to emit action potentials is vibration. When there's no vibration, the cell produces very few action potentials; so the neurons with dendrites close to its axons are similarly inactive. If the cell is pressed—just pushed—it similarly doesn't emit much activity. The physical construction of the cell is such that just the right rate of vibration—maybe what would be caused by running your finger across the bristles of a comb—causes a chemical change within the cell. That chemical change causes a train of action potentials to be produced.

As these action potentials reach the end of the cell's axons, neurotransmitter is released more and more. As it builds up in the synapse, it causes an action potential to be produced in the neuron connected to it, ultimately sending the signal to the spinal cord and the rest of the way up to the head. If you were sitting up in the brain watching these incoming signals, and if you knew which neurons were connected to that particular Pacinian corpuscle, then you could infer that something out there is vibrating. Transductions like this happen for all 5 of your senses. The start of transduction is different for every sense, but the end of the process is always the same, with a signal about the presence of something about the surrounding environment being delivered to the brain.

I've just described Pacinian corpuscles, one of the types of transducers that contribute to our sense of touch. There are many other types of receptors that work together to encode touch information. Merkel cells produce action potentials in response to slower changes in pressure, such as a consistent push that you might feel when press your hand against something and hold it there, or when you sit down. All of these cells exhibit some adaptation. That means that they respond when a new stimulus starts, but they slow down and stop if the stimulus remains constant. When you sat down just a few minutes ago, you probably perceived the pressure on your legs as you did; but you'll notice that you don't really feel it any more. That's in part because your Merkel receptors simply aren't responding any more. All transducers exhibit this adaptation response. If you walked into my grandmother's house, you would have smelled the unmistakable aroma of food, vanilla candles, and her dogs. As clear as this would be when you arrived, within a few minutes, you wouldn't be able to smell it anymore. That's because your olfactory transducers adapt as well.

Let's go back to touch for a minute. Along with Pacinian corpuscles and Merkel receptors, Meissner corpuscles and Ruffini cells respond to different types of changes in physical force. Meissner receptors respond to abrupt onsets of force, and again when the force is removed. It's believed that these receptors are especially important when you're using your hands to control the movements of tools, like pliers or a screwdriver. If you feel your skin stretching as you move, then it must be that there is some touch transducer that responds to that. Ruffini cells are the transducers in this case. There are many other receptors that work to convey information to use about touch; for instance, information about temperature and pain.

It's interesting that we perceive touch as a single modality given just how many different types of receptors are involved. There are many different types of mechanoreceptors located in different layers of the skin. All of these signal the presence of different properties of the environment. Our brain combines them into a single perception; a single awareness of the world around us.

Our sense of smell has an even wider range of different transducers. If you ever smell something, it's because at least a small bit of whatever that is—that chemical—has made its way through the air and landed on the receptor surfaces in your olfactory epithelium, located up behind your nose. Molecules of particular chemicals have particular shapes to them. If the shape is just right, then it will match up with the shape of one of those receptors. If it does, then the neuron connected to that receptor becomes active and delivers that information to the brain.

Taste works in much the same way, with particular receptors for bitter, sweet, sour, and salty. There's a commonly held myth that these different types of receptors are only present in particular regions of the tongue. There was a study published in 1901 by D. H. Hanig that identified different sensory thresholds for sweet, sour, salty, and bitter in different areas of the tongue. If something is only very, very, very slightly sweet, for instance, you might be able to sense that at the front of your tongue, but not the back. Most of our taste perception, however, involves things that have much stronger flavors than the ones used in that 1901 study. The Hanig result was vastly over-interpreted by readers of that paper as evidence that these different receptor types were only present in those areas of the tongue's surface. A few very well-drawn diagrams appeared in some textbooks and voilà, a myth was born. This has been very clearly shown to be incorrect. All of these different receptor types can be found in all areas of the tongue.

It's also been commonly believed that these 4 are the only types of taste receptors. This one isn't just a misconception of laypeople; actually, researchers believed this to be true until about the last 10 years or so. Recent studies have verified that there's a fifth class of receptors that can be found on the tongues of most people. It responds to something called "umami." I had a long conversation with a flavor researcher friend to try to get a description of what the umami flavor tastes like. She mentioned ripe tomatoes and the food additive MSG; that these items are things that activate these particular receptors. But that still didn't feel satisfactory to me. As I pressed her for a better description, she pointed out that it's really impossible to put many taste perceptions into words. How would you describe "salty" to someone who couldn't taste salt? How can you put "sweet" into words, except maybe to cite the foods we associate with it? I think the answer is that you can't; or at least that it's very hard, perhaps requiring the skills of poets rather than scientists.

There's something very profound here, I think. We have fundamental sensory, perceptual experiences and we can only relate some aspects of them to each other; other parts we just can't relate to each other, and only then in terms of how they relate to other perceptions that we have in common. Failing that, there's something inherently private about perception. It's something that we all do alone.

But enough philosophy for the moment; back to transduction. In the case of touch, I talked about how many different senses meld together into one. In the case of smell and taste, the same thing occurs. If we inhale a substance through the nostrils, we call that orthonasal olfaction. But it's all connected back there in our mouth, nose, and throat. As you chew and swallow food, traces of it will find its way up into the olfactory epithelium where the transducers are located. We don't often experience this as smell, but actually as taste; but most of the rich taste perceptions that we have are really just orthonasal olfaction.

Transduction for hearing takes place within the inner ear. Sound travels in through the auditory canal, where, after being amplified by the ear drum and some impressively complex bony structures, it's passed into a snail-shaped organ called the cochlea. If you were to unroll the cochlea, you would have a long, cone-shaped object with a thin membrane stretched down its middle. Attached to the edges of this membrane are tiny hair-like cells that are then connected to individual neurons. In order to hear something, you have to get these cells to move. The way you move them is by making a sound at just the right pitch. Low frequency sounds cause the wider parts of the cochlear membrane to vibrate, but do little to the thinner region. Conversely, high-pitched frequencies cause the thinner region to vibrate without having much impact on the wider part of the cochlea. Most sounds—most sounds we experience in the real world—are a complex mix of high-, middle-, and low-range sound frequencies. This mix of inputs causes a mix of vibration that is—you guessed it—converted into a pattern of action potentials. The axons of these frequency-specific neurons are bundled up into the auditory nerve, which then projects into the auditory cortex.

We've talked about vision a bit already, but it's worth reviewing just briefly in this context. Light enters the eye through the cornea and the lens, which work together to focus a clear image on the retina. The lens thickens slightly when we look at something close up to accomplish this. If we look off into the distance, the lens relaxes again for far accommodation. The retina contains a dense mosaic of light-sensitive cells, about a million on each eye. Each of these cone- or rod-shaped receptors contains a chemical that's changed from one form to another when light strikes it. This light-modified form of the chemical, when its concentration gets high enough, causes an action potential to be generated by the receptor cell. This is passed on through a network of neurons and into the optic nerve and then on to the primary visual cortex.

The light-sensitive chemical is continually switched back to its initial form after this interaction with the light, but it takes some time to happen. When you're in the dark, almost all of this light-sensitive chemical will be restored to its "ready" mode. After you've been in the dark for a while, if someone turns on a bright light, or even a not-so-bright light, the visual experience can be quite intense. That's because there's so much of that light-sensitive chemical ready to go that a great burst of action potentials results. After you've had a minute or so to adapt to the light, that intense feeling passes as the density of the light-sensitive chemical goes back to a more typical state. This is one of several mechanisms that enable our visual system to deal with such an enormous range of different lighting conditions; from a bright, sunny beach to a dark, moonless night.

So we've talked a lot today about transduction, the process by which your sensory systems take different kinds of energy and transform them into action potentials. Sound, light, chemical energy, physical pressure; they all turn into the same kinds of action potentials. How does your brain make sense of them? What happens when they get to the cortex? A general principle that applies here is that where the information projects into the cortex determines what will be perceived.

In the diagram, the viewer is looking at a mug. Three points on the mug are labeled as A, B, and C; this could be the rim, the handle, and a point on the saucer. The light from each of these points projects onto a particular location on the retina; that can also be labeled A, B, and C. The optic nerve makes its next synaptic connection with a subcortical region of the brain called the lateral geniculate nucleus. Again, there are particular points in that lateral geniculate nucleus labeled A, B, and C. Notice that B is still between A and C. The spatial relationship between the points is maintained, at least in a very general fashion. The neurons in the lateral geniculate nucleus project to the back of the brain; to the primary visual cortex. This is the region of the brain where the majority of our basic visual processing is accomplished. If you've ever been unfortunate enough to have something hit you on the head and afterwards you "saw stars," this is why. If the cells in this area are activated—usually by light, but sometimes by being damaged—we see things. The spatial relations present on the retina and in the lateral geniculate are maintained here in the visual cortex as well.

In the pattern of electrical, chemical activity here in the visual cortex, there is a retinotopic map of the visual input; a map that maintains the ordinal spatial relationships present on the retina and in the retinal input (that is, the things you're seeing). If I were to somehow reach in and electrically stimulate this person's visual cortex in a particular location, maybe right next to the neuron that we have labeled point B, he would see a flash of light at this location in the environment. Conversely, if there were a flash of light at that location in the world it would cause that neuron to become active.

This one-to-one relationship between the sensory input and a location of cortical activation is a principle that shows up for all of the senses. Action potentials from those touch-sensitive neurons in the skin are delivered to a region of the cortex called the somatosensory cortex. Now take a look at the map of your body as it's laid out on the surface of the cortex. If I were to reach into your brain and stimulate a particular spot on your somatosensory cortex—say, around the middle; just a little to the right of the top of your head—you would feel something touching you on the left arm. Conversely, if something touched you in that particular spot on the left arm, it would cause activity in that same region of the cortex. The primary motor cortex, a region involved in coordinating actions, has a corresponding map that follows this same pattern.

Notice that the relative sizes of the body parts in the diagram don't correspond to their typical physical sizes. That's not a mistake. It reflects how certain areas of the body are much more sensitive to touch than others. Very little brain space is devoted to sensing touch on the lower back. There are as many cortical neurons devoted to touch for your thumb as for your entire leg. These correspond very directly in a one-to-one fashion with how well we can perceive touch in these regions. "Cortex man" is a sculpture designed to represent the relative cortical space and sensitivity for different areas of the human body. Cortex man's hands, tongue, and mouth are enormous, but his legs, torso and arms are tiny by comparison. This alien-looking creature is actually quite human. His relative body part sizes are altered to reflect the brain space devoted to sensing touch in these regions.

The sound map in the auditory cortex—located in the temporal lobe, near the side of the head—is not arranged spatially like it is for these other senses we've talked about, but according to the frequency (that is, the pitch) of the sound. If I stimulated a particular location, you would hear a particular sound. Conversely, if I made that same sound, then this same region would be activated.

The organization for taste and smell is actually quite a bit more complicated, but the principle is the same: Particular aromas and flavors produce certain patterns of activation. If we were to activate those locations in the same way then the aromas and flavors would be experienced.

A general principle that applies to all of the senses is the "Law of Specific Nerve Energies," first proposed by Johannes Muller in 1835. The basic idea here is that all of the action potentials are the same except in regards to where they project in the brain. Our sensory experience for all of the senses corresponds to the spatial pattern of activity here in the cortex. Imagine for a moment that we could unplug your optic nerve (the one connected to the eyes) and reconnect it to the auditory cortex. In principle, when the light was projected onto your eyes, you would hear the light. Imagine that we took the nerves that project to your touch-specific somatosensory cortex and plugged them into your visual cortex. If we did, then when pressure was applied to your skin, you would see it rather than feel it.

I should note that the information processing that takes place in these regions of the cortex is very specialized. That is, for the case of hearing light, you would hear something, but you would probably not be able to actually make a whole lot of sense of the thing that you were seeing. This is all a little bizarre to ponder and technically not really feasible, but it illustrates the specific nerve energies idea. What we sense all comes down to where the action potentials are located in the brain.

The last topic that I want to consider from this physiological perspective today is how we can represent an infinite variety of stimuli with this finite brain. I want to start with a very simple example: a single tilted line. The first thing to note is that there are an infinite number of different orientations for a line—138.3456 degrees is just one; 138.34566 is another—and we're good at perceiving orientation. If the tilt of a line were changed by a tiny, tiny fraction of a degree you would be able to tell. It could be that there's a different neuron that corresponds to the presence of each of these many, many orientations. Maybe when the line is vertical, the "vertical line neuron" becomes active. Maybe there's another neuron that corresponds to horizontal orientation, and another for 45 degrees. Do we need one for every orientation that we can perceive; one for 45.56 degrees of tilt and one for 45.57 degrees?

We have many neurons in our brain, but if we needed to devote a separate neuron to every single thing that we could perceive, we would run out. We would need thousands to account for every orientation here, and this is just one line at one location on the retina.

Neurons are finite. The range of perception is seemingly infinite. How can both of these things be true? The brain accomplishes this by encoding percepts in terms of the pattern of response of several neurons rather than in terms of just one. In the visual cortex, at every location on that retinotopic map that we discussed, a column of neurons encodes orientation. There's a cell that prefers vertical lines. When a vertical line is present, it exhibits a very high rate of action potentials; maybe about 10 per second. There are also cells that similarly respond best to 45 and 135 degree orientations. Actually there are many more, but for our purposes, we can focus just on these 3. These cells respond most to their preferred orientation, but they also respond to similar orientations. For instance, the 45 degree cell responds, albeit with a slow rate of action potentials, to 75 degree tilts; maybe about 5 spikes per second for that 75 degree line. By looking at the pattern of response across these 3 different cells, it's possible to infer any orientation across this range. Imagine, for instance, that the 45 degree cell is quiet, the 90 degree cell is responding at 6 spikes per second, and the 135 degree cell at 3 spikes per second. If you scan this graph and find the position where all 3 of these things are true, you can infer that the line must be about 110 degrees of tilt. For any set of 3 response rates, you could calculate the best guess as to the line orientation. Even 38.4567 degrees of tilt will produce a particular pattern of response.

So here's our answer to our question of infinite perceptions with finite cells: The neurons are discrete and finite, but the range of average response rates is continuous and essentially infinite, just like the things that we perceive. This design principle shows up in all of our sensory processing. Color perception works just like this. There are cells in your retina that respond best to blue, green, and yellow light; but these cells also respond in a graded, predictable fashion to light that varies from their preferred color. By considering the relative rate of responses of these different types of receptors, we can perceive millions of different colors with only a few types of color receptors.

By that I mean we can infer the presence of millions of colors based on the responses of just a few cells.

Our sense of taste and smell make inferences like this as well. If the umami receptors on your tongue are activated by some piece of food, and if the food is warm and watery in texture and your olfactory system tells you there's a salty and peppery smell around, if all of those sensations are delivered to your brain at the same time, then you're likely to perceive tomato soup in your mouth. There's no need for a tomato soup neuron in order for you to perceive tomato soup. You recognize the sound of your friend's voice based on the distribution of sound frequencies that are produced in your cochlea. There doesn't need to be a specific neuron devoted to the voices of each of your particular friends. And this is how your senses work. Your brain makes its best guess about what's out there based on the pattern of incoming neural activation—from that spatial pattern of activation in your cortex—and that best guess is what you perceive.

In the next lecture, we'll take a further look at how your brain processes sensory and perceptual information. In particular, I'll describe how relatively new neuroimaging technologies have enabled researchers to look at the activity of a whole functioning brain at work. We're about to take a look under the hood of the sensory machine. I hope you'll join me.

# Neuroimaging—The Sensory Brain at Work
## Lecture 3

Some of the most exciting recent research on human sensation and perception has come from new techniques that enable us to see the patterns of brain activation that occur when people engage in particular mental tasks. Looking at the brain will not answer all our questions, but combining cognitive neuroscience with more traditional behavior-based measures of human performance offers us an ever more detailed understanding of the human senses.

- Even before the advent of these neuroimaging technologies, researchers had figured out a lot about the organization of the brain, such as which parts of the brain seem to mediate information relative to the particular senses.

- Most of that knowledge has been around for hundreds of years based not on data from high-tech equipment but on doctors' observations of patients who had suffered certain types of brain injury. Patients who had suffered severe trauma to the back of the head, for example, often lost their sight.

- Stroke survivors also often exhibit specific losses of function; posthumous autopsies, even years after the stroke, allowed researchers to make inferences about which areas of the brain were responsible for which functions.

- Neurologists used postmortem examinations to identify some strikingly specific deficits in brain-injured patients—such as Broca's aphasia, or productive aphasia (the ability to understand but not produce speech), and its opposite, Wernicke's aphasia, or receptive aphasia (the ability to produce but not understand speech)—that were later backed up by neuroimaging in living patients.

- One very famous patient was identified by the neurologist Oliver Sacks, a man who seemed fine in every way except that he could no longer recognize faces. Sacks recounts a story of this patient eating at a restaurant one night and complaining to his waiter about another customer who was staring at him. The confused waiter had to explain to this patient that there was no other customer—he was seated across from a mirror.

- This patient, after suffering an injury to his inferotemporal cortex on the right side, had lost the ability to recognize faces. Based on evidence like this, many researchers believe that this area of the human brain is specifically responsible for recognizing faces. A more general claim suggested by this type of finding is that the human brain contains separate subsystems for processing many different types of information.

- As fascinating as these studies of brain-injured patients are, and as much as they really do provide clues about how our brain makes sense of the world around us, they are very limited in a way.

- First, the damage from impact or stroke is often widespread and follows the constraints of the circulatory system, not the functional boundaries of individual brain systems. Multiple functional regions may be damaged to varying degrees by any injury.

- Second, the brain is good at compensating after it has been damaged. Patients often discover ways around their limitations, both consciously and unconsciously, masking the changes researchers seek to interpret.

- The advantage of functional neuroimaging over previous techniques is that it allows researchers to view whole, uninjured brains at work under more normal circumstances. It allows them to see which brain areas are active when study participants are listening to speech, looking at familiar faces, or doing other perceptual tasks.

- Functional magnetic resonance imaging (fMRI), which measures the rate of blood flow within the brain, has been used more and more frequently in recent years as it has become increasingly available and less expensive for researchers.

- The neurons that make up your central nervous system are specialized cells, but they are similar to the other cells in your body in many ways. They need oxygen and fuel from the bloodstream to function and survive, and they create waste, including carbon dioxide, which must be expelled.

- When any group of cells in your body becomes more active and starts using stored supplies, it signals your circulatory system that it will need more, and soon. If the demands grow large enough, your heart pumps faster to speed fresh blood to the places that it is needed.

- As early as the 1950s, medical researchers found that if a person was simply sitting still in the lab, staring at the wall, not really doing anything, a certain amount of blood was pumped into the brain.

- If that participant began performing mental arithmetic, the blood flow increased. The increase in mental activity generated an increase in the volume of blood pumped into the head.

- An fMRI, in a way, performs this same sort of measurement in a much more precise way. It can be tuned to measure the amount of blood flowing not just to the brain as a whole but to different regions of the brain.

- When some region of the brain becomes active, it calls out for more oxygenated blood to be sent to it. About 6 seconds later, the blood vessels are dilated, and the blood flow increases.

- A participant might be asked, for instance, to recall a visual memory from childhood. The resulting blood flow pattern would be recorded and would indicate which regions are involved in visual sensory memory functions.

- Many fMRI studies have been performed using faces as stimuli, inspired in part by that patient of Sacks's. Sure enough, if you show someone a series of faces, you get activations in the right inferotemporal cortex.

- Interestingly, you do not get those same activations if you flip the faces upside-down. This corresponded to a previous finding that people are not nearly as good at recognizing upside-down faces as upright faces.

- It also corresponds to the Thatcher illusion, where the face remains upright but each feature is flipped.

- A series of related fMRI studies has found that this face-processing area of the brain is not just a face-processing area but can be activated by a much wider range of stimuli. When birders looked at images of birds and car experts looked at images of cars, this area became active as well.

- However, as with upside-down faces for us face experts, when the bird and car images are flipped 2 things happen: The experts become much less accurate at recognizing the stimuli, and right inferotemporal cortex activation drops significantly.

- Many researchers have therefore taken to describing the right inferotemporal cortex as the expert visual pattern recognition region. Additional studies have reinforced this idea by noting how brain activation patterns change in this region as people progress from being novices to experts in some category.

- Whenever you hear about the discovery of a region of the brain that does $x$, whatever that is, you should interpret that cautiously. The brain is a very complex organ; understanding it will require thought that is just as careful and complex. Therefore, I want to present some reasons to be cautious in our reasoning about neuroimaging.

- Imagine that you are reading some text about someone flying an airplane across the ocean, and you are doing this while lying in an fMRI scanner. Which part of the brain processes reading?

- Your eyes would receive light from the viewing screen, pass that information along your optic nerves to your lateral geniculate nucleus and visual cortex. You would move your eyes, so your motor cortex would be active. You might find yourself remembering the time you flew on an airplane, and so memory regions of your brain would also become active.

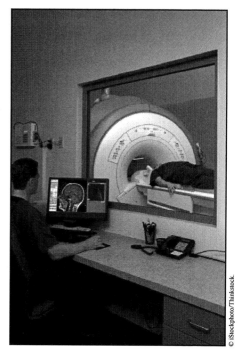

© iStockphoto/Thinkstock.

**A magnetic resonance imaging (MRI) scanner produces a map of brain blood flow using high-powered magnets.**

- If we were to look at the pattern of activity produced by your reading, we would find that almost your whole brain would light up. Neuroscientists talk about particular areas of the brain being responsible for particular functions, but the simple truth is that most of your brain is active most of the time.

- Say the perception researchers are interested in which areas of the brain are important for word reading. Therefore, they have their participants perform 2 different tasks: an experimental task and a control task.

- In the experimental task, participants read. In the control task, everything about the task is as identical as possible (the light, the eye movement, the memories, and so forth), except the participants do not read.

- The researchers then subtract the control pattern of activity from the experimental pattern and see what is left. The remaining activity is considered to be specifically responsible for the reading component of the activation.

- This type of study has been run many times. Reading typically causes increases in blood flow to particular regions in the left hemisphere where language processing usually occurs; this is especially true for right-handed people.

- It is therefore tempting to look at these results and presume that the rest of the brain is not involved in reading, but now you know this would be a mistake. Neuroimaging can show us which areas of the brain are more active in one task or another, but you should never conclude that the other areas of the brain are not involved.

- Some area may be equally involved in both the experimental and control tasks. If so, then neuroimaging cannot tell us about it.

## Suggested Reading

Hurley and Taber, *Windows to the Brain.*

Joyce, *Magnetic Appeal.*

## Questions to Consider

1. Imagine an fMRI experiment conducted to study the brain areas involved in listening to speech. The experimenters scan participants' brains while they listen to recordings of speech ($A$) and scrambled speech sounds ($B$). They subtract $B$ from $A$ and identify several brain areas that are more active for speech. If there is some brain area $X$ that is very active and

absolutely critical for processing both types of sounds, what will the researchers' conclusions about this area be after using this method?

2. Imagine that I show participants in an fMRI study pictures of my grandmother and also pictures of your grandmother. I subtract the activations for your grandmother from the activations for mine and identify a region that is more active for my grandmother. Have I identified the Grandmother Vishton region of the brain? How should I describe these findings? What would be a better way to proceed with my research?

# Neuroimaging—The Sensory Brain at Work
## Lecture 3—Transcript

Hello. In this third lecture, we're going to take a look under the hood of the human brain. Some of the most exciting recent research on human sensation and perception has come using new techniques that enable us to see the patterns of brain activation that occur when people engage in particular mental tasks.

What does your brain "do" when you recognize a face? What happens when you smell your favorite food? What's happening inside your head when you are perceiving things? Neuroimaging lets us take a peek inside without having to open the skull. Looking at the brain won't answer all of the questions that we have, but by combining cognitive neuroscience methods with more traditional behavior-based measures of human performance, a more detailed understanding of the human senses can emerge.

For many decades, brain researchers have sought to figure out how the functions of sensation and perception map onto particular brain regions. Neuroimaging has provided a terrific new set of tools for this, but it's worth noting that this enterprise of brain mapping is actually much older. I want to start today by talking about how neurologists have studied brain-injured patients for clues to how the brain implements human perception. We'll then focus on one particular neuroimaging technique that's been used very frequently over the past decade: functional magnetic resonance imagery, fMRI for short. I'll describe the metabolic processes behind this technique and some details about how it works. I'll then present some examples of studies that have used this method to advance our understanding of perception. As compelling as neuroimaging studies can be, I think many people have a tendency to over-interpret their results. I'll end today's lecture by providing some reasons to be cautious about how we interpret and rely upon fMRI results.

Let's start with some neurology. Neuroimaging techniques have provided us with the ability to see how the brain organizes the process of sensation and perception as never before. But even before the advent of these neuroimaging technologies—long before—researchers had figured out a lot about the organization of the brain. In the last lecture, I referred to which parts of the brain seem to mediate information relative to the particular senses. These 4 lobes—temporal, occipital, parietal, and frontal—are defined by anatomical landmarks and deep folds found on the cortical surface. Vision tends to be processed on the back of your brain, hearing in the temporal cortex, touch in the somatosensory cortex, and so on.

Most of that knowledge has been around for hundreds of years, based not on high tech equipment, but on doctors' observations of their patients after they'd suffered certain types of brain injuries. If a patient has suffered damage to the back of the head in which the skull was fractured, or even if someone suffers a severe closed-head injury, the ability to see is sometimes lost; the patient may become blind. Years later, after the patient has died, a doctor might examine the brain and discover that, indeed, there was significant damage to the occipital cortex. Strokes are another common source of brain injury, in which the blood vessels that supply the brain rupture or become blocked. In many cases a stroke results in death, but often the patient survives. Some survivors, however, exhibit specific loss of function after the stroke. Again, a posthumous autopsy may eventually reveal what areas of the brain were damaged.

The general reasoning here is that if a particular mental capacity is lost and a particular brain region is found to have been damaged, then the damaged brain region is likely associated with that mental capacity; not just for the brain-injured patient, but for regular, normal-functioning brains as well. Neurologists who use this approach have identified some strikingly specific deficits in brain-injured patients. For instance, patients have been identified who can still understand speech just fine, but who can no longer speak themselves. Patients with this type of "productive aphasia" are often found to have suffered damage to a region in their frontal cortex on the left side, called Broca's area. The area is named after Dr. Paul Broca, who was the first to identify this brain-behavior relation. Other patients can still speak perfectly, but have great difficulty understanding the speech of others. A different region of the brain, located just behind Broca's area, is often damaged in these "receptive aphasia" patients. Wernicke's area, as it's called, is similarly named after its discoverer, Carl Wernicke. Both of these areas are usually located on the left side of the brain, especially for right-handed people.

Neuroimaging studies have provided a great deal of evidence that this is how the brain implements language processing, with one area for perception and another area for production. But the theory was around for a long time before neuroimaging came along based on a consideration of where patients' heads were injured or by posthumously examining the brains of people who'd suffered strokes.

The effects of strokes can be even more specific than this, however. One very famous patient was identified by the neurologist Oliver Sacks. The patient seemed fine in every way except that he could no longer recognize faces. Sacks tells the story of this man having a meal in a local restaurant. He was enjoying his food and having a very nice time, but he was very distracted by this other man who kept looking at him. Every time he glanced up at this guy, he was still looking at him. He finally worked up the courage to stare back, but the man just continued to fixedly glare at him. Finally, when he could stand it no longer, he called his waiter over and asked him to please speak to this rude man who was ruining his meal. The waiter was very confused, and with some trepidation had to explain to this man that he wasn't looking at a rude patron of the restaurant but rather at a wall with a floor-to-ceiling mirror on it.

This patient, after suffering an injury to his inferotemporal cortex on the right side, had lost the ability to recognize faces. He couldn't recognize his friends, his wife; he couldn't even recognize his own face in the mirror. Based on evidence like this, many researchers believe that this area of the brain is specifically responsible for visually recognizing faces. This is interesting in terms of knowing where face processing takes place in the brain, but there's a more general claim that's certainly suggested by this type of finding. It may very well be that our brain contains separate subsystems for processing many different types of information; not just a separate subsystem for vision, but maybe one for vision of faces, vision of objects, vision of (fill in the blank). Perhaps the other senses have this type of organization as well—hearing for speech, hearing for music, hearing for animal sounds—who knows? By studying brain-injured patients and the types of deficits that emerge, it's hoped that we can identify just what this organization of the brain is, just how it's structured, and ultimately, how our perception takes place.

For instance, there's evidence, based on the study of brain-injured patients, that we have one visual system for recognizing objects and a separate visual system for controlling visually-guided actions, things like reaching. Other studies have suggested that a particular region of the brain is responsible for sensing the posture of your body, especially the parts you can't see. For instance, I know that my left arm is behind me and to the left, even though I can't see it. Even if I'm in complete darkness, I still know the posture of my body. If the proprioceptive system in my brain were damaged, I would have to see my body parts in order to know where they are. This is the everyday experience of stroke survivors who have suffered the loss of their sense of "proprioception," it's called. The ability to encode what we see into long-term memories is associated with a particular brain region; the ability to then recover those memories is associated with another. Patients have been studied who've lost all of these specific abilities while seeming to retain almost all other mental functions. I could go on and on here; there's a rich tradition of research in the domain of neurology.

As fascinating as these studies of brain-injured patients are, and as much as they really do provide clues about how our brain makes sense of the world around us, they're very limited in a way. For one thing, the damage that occurs from impact and stroke is often widespread, and often follows the constraints of the circulatory system rather than the functional boundaries of these individual brain systems. It may be that multiple functional regions are damaged to varying degrees by any single specific injury. Also, the brain is very good at compensating after it's damaged. Patients often figure out ways around their mental limitations—both consciously and, in many cases, unconsciously—such that the actual changes in brain function caused by the damage might be masked or at least difficult to interpret.

For instance, consider the man I described with the face recognition deficit. My claim—indeed, the claim of many who've studied him—is that he was completely fine in every other way except for the loss of his ability to recognize faces. That might be true, but he might have just found ways to compensate for all of those other problems except for recognizing faces. Maybe recognizing faces is just really hard in terms of perceptual discriminations. Faces are all quite similar to one another. Thus, what looks like a face-specific problem might actually be more general.

Problems like these have led some researchers to complain that studying the brain in this way—by studying individual brain-injured patients—is sort of like trying to figure out how televisions work by taking televisions and dropping them and then examining them to see how they've malfunctioned. Ideally, we'd like to be able to see the whole, uninjured brain at work under more normal circumstances. We'd like to be able to see what brain areas are active when a study participant is listening to speech, or looking at familiar faces, or doing other perceptual tasks. We would like to be able to see under the hood of this amazing brain, the whole thing, while it's doing what it normally does.

Thanks to several remarkable technologies, we can do just that. These techniques are generally referred to as "functional neuroimaging." There are a lot of different methods that have been developed to look at patterns of brain activity. Some rely on the electrical activity produced by the neurons when they exhibit those action potentials we've discussed. Others, such as the one I want to focus on now—fMRI, or functional magnetic resonance imagery—rely on an analysis of the flow of blood in the brain. This method has been used very frequently in recent years; it's become increasingly available and less expensive for researchers.

Before I get to the fancy gadgets, however, let's start by talking a little bit about brain metabolism. The neurons that make up your central nervous system are very specialized cells, but they're still similar to the other cells in your body in many ways. Neurons need oxygen and fuel from the bloodstream to function and survive. As they perform the processing associated with those action potentials, they create waste products, including carbon dioxide, which must be expelled in order for the cells to continue to function. When any group of cells in your body becomes active and starts using up its stored supplies, it signals your circulatory system that it will be needing more, and soon. Your arteries and veins have an impressive method of dealing with this. Some blood vessels dilate while others constrict, altering the flow of blood to keep all of the different subsystems in your body functioning. If the demands grow large enough, your heart begins pumping faster in order to speed the fresh blood to the places that it's needed.

Notice that I haven't mentioned the brain specifically yet. This resource allocation system works for your digestive system, your muscles; any part of your body. As early as the 1950s, medical researchers developed a technique for measuring the amount of blood flowing to the brain that's actually quite simple. The basic idea is to measure heart rate and blood pressure at the location of the carotid arteries. All of the blood that goes to your brain goes through these 2 large arteries located in the neck. These researchers found that if a person was simply sitting still in the lab, staring at the wall, not really doing anything, that a certain amount of blood was pumped into the brain. If the study participant remained just as still but began performing mental arithmetic, the blood flow increased. The experimenter would start saying math problems out loud: 3 times 4 plus 12 divided by 2 plus the square root of 16, and so on. The study participant wouldn't do anything, not even say the answer; the instructions were just to begin thinking about what the answer would be. Even though the physical activity of the participant was identical, the increase in mental activity was enough to generate an increase in the volume of blood pumped into the head.

fMRI is a wonder of modern science and engineering, but in many respects, it's just repeating this same kind of study with more precise measures; much more precise. An fMRI scanner can be tuned to measure the amount of blood flowing not just to the brain as a whole, but to different regions of the brain. An fMRI scanner consists of a large, very powerful magnet and a large set of magnetic detectors. Blood cells have magnetic properties to them. They're very weak magnetic properties, but when the cells move through this powerful magnetic field, they generate a tiny amount—a detectable amount—of electrical force. When some region of the brain becomes active, it calls out for more oxygenated blood to be sent to it. About 6 seconds later, the blood vessels are dilated and the blood flow increases. This tool enables us to ask what parts of the brain are responsible for a sensory function. For instance, if participants are asked to remember visual experiences, blood flow will increase to certain areas of the brain; if they're asked to remember an auditory experience, blood will increase its flow to other areas. This blood flow pattern indicates to us that these regions are involved in these sensory memory functions.

To use an example from the last lecture: If you were lying in an fMRI scanner and touched your arm in a particular location, then the cells in your somatosensory cortex that process that information would become active. About 6 seconds later, you would see an increase in the blood flow to the specific part of the somatosensory cortex that's performing that sensory process. If we repeated this while you received tactile stimulation on different parts of your arm and hand, we would be able to map out that region of your brain for you. This is really cool. You can watch the brain doing its work in real time using this fMRI technique.

Many fMRI studies have been done using face stimuli, inspired in part by that man with the brain injury to his right inferotemporal cortex; that man who seemed to only have lost his ability to recognize faces. Sure enough, if you show someone a series of faces, you get activations in this area of the brain, the right inferotemporal cortex. Interestingly, you don't get those same activations if you flip the faces upside down. This matches a finding that we aren't nearly as good at recognizing upside down faces as upright faces. It also fits with a particular visual display called the "Thatcher illusion," so-called because it was first produced using a photograph of former British Prime Minister Margaret Thatcher. The image on the left is just an upside down photo of a face. On the right, the photo has been inverted, but then the eyes and the mouth have been flipped again so that they are upright. The photo looks a bit strange, but not as strange as it will in a moment. These faces are upside down. You are looking at them, and seeing them, but you aren't seeing them with your inferotemporal cortex, which is the area of the brain that seems responsible for our expert face recognition abilities.

In a moment, I'm going to flip the pictures over and turn on your face processing brain regions. Before I do, I want you to take a moment to mentally rotate these images. If I showed you a picture of an upside down car or cup, you could certainly imagine what it would look like if it were right side up. That's what I want you to do with these faces. I hope you have it in mind now; that you have a clear expectation of what these faces will look like when they're right side up again. For the "regular" face, your intuitions about what the face would look like were probably not too far off, but most people say that the picture on the right just looks bizarre. There's a good reason that it looks so different, so much more unusual when the face is right side up. Our brain processes the upright faces using these very particular brain systems, and we're experts at using those systems.

We aren't nearly as expert when it comes to perceiving upside down faces. For the upside down faces, it's like we're inexperienced folks having a sip of some decent red wine. For the right side up faces, it's like we are expert connoisseurs of 20th century pinot noir wines of northern France being forced to endure a 2010 Vinny's Vino served over crushed ice. It just doesn't look right, and it's very, very salient.

There's one other aspect of inverting a face that was recently discovered by Peter Thompson at York University. He found that upside down faces often look thinner. You can see a bit of that with the Thatcher image that we just looked at, if you go back to that. It's not an enormously salient effect, but you can see if you look at it that the eyes in particular seem to be closer together in the inverted face. Indeed, it seems to be the cause of the effect (the inversion, that is). When we look at a right-side-up face, our brain takes a much closer, more detailed look at the internal features than when it's upside down. Ultimately, that's the cause of the Thatcher illusion I showed you as well. So if you, like me, would like to look thinner in the pictures people take of you, this course has a clear, scientifically supported tip: Stand on your head; it will make you look thinner.

I mentioned that when we look at faces, we're using a very expert area of the brain; we're very experienced when it comes to recognizing other human faces. This description is more relevant than you might think. A series of related fMRI studies has found that this face processing area of the brain is not really just a face processing area at all, but can be activated by a much wider range of stimuli. In some early studies, it was found that when bird experts looked at images of birds, their face processing regions became active. When car experts looked at car pictures, the area became active as well. Now if you looked at the same pictures that the bird and car experts looked at, your brains would become active, but not the right inferotemporal cortex. To get that, you have to be an expert with the particular types of stimuli that are being used. Any guess what happens if you present the bird and car images to the bird and car experts but flip the images upside down? Just like with the upside down faces for us face experts, when the bird and car images are flipped 2 things happen: One, the experts become much less accurate at recognizing the stimuli. Two, the right inferotemporal cortex activation drops far, far down.

So what should we call this face recognition region? It's used for face recognition, but it's also used for other things. Many have taken to describing this region of the right inferotemporal cortex as a region of the brain devoted to expert visual pattern recognition. Some additional studies have reinforced this idea by watching how brain activation patterns change as people progress from being novices with some category of objects to being experts with it. Several researchers developed a "made up" class of objects called "Greebles." These objects all have a central, vertically oriented part and subparts that protrude from their sides and fronts. Researchers interested in categorical perception have run a variety of studies in which people are taught to identify Greeble families and individuals.

For the particular study I'm interested in today, the 2 sets of Greebles were described as being from 2 different families; let's call them the Datwick family and the Blicket family. Greebles from these 2 families differed in general in terms of the shape of a large central part that was attached to them. Within each family, there were also individuals that differed in terms of the size and shape of other characteristics. They were actually given names; for instance, Mason and George. If you saw these labeled with their names enough times, you would be able to use those subtle differences in the size, shapes, and angles of their "ear" and "nose" parts, things like that—their different protrusions—to tell which one is "Mason" and which one is "George." Study participants learned to identify different families and individuals within these made-up families. It's presumably similar to the process by which we learn to identify different species and breeds of dogs, or maybe even families and individual faces of people.

The nice thing about using the artificial stimuli—these Greebles—is that they're totally novel; until a participant came into the lab to do this study, they would have had zero experience with Greebles. The researchers could thus watch the perceptual learning process right from the beginning. Participants would have weeks of experience with these things; they would quite literally become Greeble experts. As they were gaining this experience, the researchers would periodically put the participants into an fMRI scanner and see how their brains were processing the Greebles when they looked at them. At first, the participants' brains responded to Greebles the way they would respond to any object: A wide range of visual processing was seen. As they became Greeble experts, a strange thing happened: They started using smaller and more focused regions of their brain to process these Greebles, and they started to engage their inferotemporal cortex, around the same regions that are used to recognize faces. And I bet you can guess what happened if they turned the Greebles upside down: The participants' ability to recognize the Greebles greatly declined, as did the activity in these inferotemporal face recognition regions. This inversion-based recognition deficit is only present, however, after the participants become experts at Greeble identification.

This is a really nice set of studies, I think. It exhibits all of the best things that can happen when studies of human perception are combined with these neuroimaging techniques. We started with a basic set of perceptual phenomena: human face recognition, the effect of inverted faces, and the effects of experience and expertise. Then we added in the neuroscience approach: some compelling results from the study of a few brain injured patients, some scans of brains while people are recognizing faces. A particular area of the brain seems to be implicated.

It might be tempting to have stopped there: Aha! We have discovered where face recognition happens in the brain; this is the face recognizer part of the cortex; okay, on to the next topic. But the researchers thought deeply about their findings. Is this really about faces or just about recognizing individuals within a category of largely similar stimuli? The Greeble study—and there are a lot of experiments that were done there that I've glossed over—makes it clear that this region of inferotemporal cortex isn't a face area at all. Faces are only a part of what it does. Whenever you hear about the discovery of a region of the brain that does X, whatever that is—music perception, reading, math, etc.—you should interpret that cautiously. The brain is a very complex organ, perhaps the most complex organ we've ever studied. Understanding it will require thought that is just as careful and complex.

So, I've presented some reasons to be excited. I next want to present some reasons to be cautious in our reasoning about neuroimaging. Let's think about reading. What part of the brain processes that? When we view a set of images that correspond to letters and words, we instantly, effortlessly convert that into an understanding of the sounds and meanings associated with those words; we read them. How does the brain accomplish this? Imagine that you're reading some text, maybe a story about someone flying an airplane across the ocean, but you're doing this while you're lying in an fMRI scanner. Your eyes will be receiving light from the viewing screen, passing it along your optic nerves to your lateral geniculate nucleus and visual cortex, so all of those cells are going to be active; you'll be moving your eyes around as you're reading, so your motor cortex will be active; you might find yourself remembering the time that you yourself flew on an airplane, and so the parts of your brain involved in memory will become active. If we were to look at the pattern of activity produced by your reading, we would find that almost your whole brain would light up.

Neuroscientists talk about particular areas of the brain being responsible for particular sensory and mental functions, but the simple truth is that most of your brain is active most of the time. What perception researchers are really interested in, however, is which areas of the brain are important for computing a particular aspect of the reading function. How could I isolate that part of the brain? If I'm interested in word reading, then I want to have my scanning participants perform 2 different tasks; I'll call them the experimental task and the control task. In the experimental task, participants will read. In the control task, everything about the task will be as identical as possible, except the participants will not read. For studying this reading process, the experimental task will involve reading some words. In the control task, the participants will have all of the same sensory inputs, but they won't read. I'll then subtract the control pattern of activity from the experimental pattern and see what's left. That part that's left is what we'll conclude is specifically responsible for that reading component of the activation.

For instance, for the reading experimental task, I would have the participant lie in the scanner and look up at a computer screen. On the computer screen I would project a series of words; just a random mix of single words for the moment, nothing about airplanes and oceans. I would scan the brains of the participants while they read these words for several minutes. Now the control task: I would present strings of letters that were the same length as the words they had just read, but the letters would be chosen randomly, such that they were not words and thus unreadable. The participants would look at the words, receiving the same visual input in both the experimental and control tasks; so, in principle, the visual cortex would be just as active as for both. The eye movements would be pretty much the same for the 2 tasks; so while the motor cortex would be active in the experimental reading task, it would be just as active in the control task. So when I subtract the control out of the experimental scan, I should show about the same level of activity.

If I do this right, I should end up with a dark brain image everywhere except in the regions where there's an increase in the activity caused by the reading task. This type of study has been run many times, enabling the identification of areas in the brain associated with reading. Reading typically causes increases in blood flow to particular regions in the left hemisphere where language processing usually occurs; this is especially true for right-handed people. It's tempting to look at these results and presume that the rest of the brain is not involved in reading, but now you know that this would be a mistake. While people were performing this reading task, most of their brain was active.

To think about this, I often ask people to imagine doing neuroimaging on something simpler than a brain, something we understand very well; not the brain, but something simple like a kitchen appliance. My favorite kitchen appliance to ponder, actually, is a kitchen blender. Imagine that you have a standard kitchen blender; the kind you could use to make milkshakes, margaritas, Orange Julius, almost anything. You could also use the blender to grind walnuts. You're not supposed to grind walnuts in a blender, but I can tell you from experience that it's possible to do so. Imagine that I put my blender into some sort of activity scanner. I could measure the activity while made a milkshake; I'll call that the control task. I could also scan the activity while grinding walnuts; I'll call that the experimental task. If I subtract the control activity from the experimental activity, I would find that the motor is more active when grinding the walnuts. Aha! A new discovery: I have identified the region of the blender that grinds walnuts!

Hopefully it's clear why this isn't right. The whole blender is needed to grind walnuts. The whole blender is needed to make milkshakes, or mix much of anything. Neuroimaging can show us what areas of the brain are more active in one task or another, but you should never conclude based on this that the other areas of the brain aren't involved. Some area may be equally involved in both the experimental and control tasks. If it is, then neuroimaging can't tell us about it. Neuroimaging is fantastic as a tool for improving our knowledge of human thinking, but it isn't ever going to provide a simple answer key for our understanding of the human senses. We'll need to be more clever than that.

We're going to spend one more lecture pondering the nature of human brain organization before we begin digging more deeply into visual perception. I'll still talk about the brain from time to time throughout the rest of the course, but the next lecture will be the last in which it's front and center in our exploration of the senses. In this last brain lecture, I want you to think about a brain constructed from separate, independent "modules." There's some good evidence to support the idea that our senses work this way. Even though we only have a unitary, single perceptual experience, it seems to be produced by the interaction of a wide range of different, independent subsystems. I'll discuss evidence for this organization, talk about some of the modules that seem to be there in our brain, and then consider how our mind succeeds in putting all of those separate modules together again to give us the rich, combined sensory experience that we have. I look forward to talking with you then.

# Brain Modules—Subcomponents of the Senses
## Lecture 4

Perceptual processing may arise from many separate, independent modules, each of which consists of thousands or tens of thousands of neurons, interconnected with each other and the rest of the brain in very particular ways. They take in certain sources of information and ignore all others. They perform very specific processing, produce very specific outputs, and then send those outputs on to other modules.

- Even though we have a unitary, single perceptual experience of the world around us, our perceptions seem to arise from the interaction of a wide range of these different, independent, modular subsystems.

- Let's start by talking about retinotopic maps—how light gathered from the retina maintains its relative spatial organization in the visual cortex.

- There are many different retinotopic maps. Some represent edges, some colors, still others motion. These different maps are organized according to a modular framework and continue beyond the visual cortex into other regions of the brain.

- One of those modules processes information about the identities of objects; we call that the "what" pathway. Another processes information about objects' locations and movements; we call that the "where" pathway.

- The human brain contains 2 hemispheres, one on the left and one on the right. Each of these hemispheres contains a lateral geniculate nucleus and a visual cortex of its own.

- If there were 3 tiny spots of light out in the world at locations labeled *A*, *B*, and *C* and total darkness everywhere else, then inside the brain would be 3 spots of electrical activation in the lateral geniculate nucleus and nowhere else.

- In this situation, there are only 3 visual inputs out there in the world, but there are dozens of different retinotopic maps in the cortex. If I were to take a recording electrode and place it at different points in the lateral geniculate nucleus, I would find activity in some locations and not in others.

- In fact, alternating maps in the lateral geniculate nucleus are stimulated by input to the left and right eyes, making stereopsis— that is, 3-dimensional vision—possible.

- One group of neurons processes inputs from one eye and only one eye. Another set of neurons is similarly specialized for processing information from the other eye. Yet another set of neurons is specifically responsible for comparing the outputs of these separate eye modules.

- This divide-and-conquer organization shows up for many aspects of visual processing and sensory processing in general.

- Deeper in the lateral geniculate nucleus, I would find more of this left- versus right-eye organization, but the properties of the neurons would change. These magnocellular neurons have thicker axons, and they respond more quickly to input.

- Magnocellular neurons also respond to changes in brightness, but not so much to changes in color. They tend to project their axons into the dorsal or occipital cortex, roughly the top and back of the brain. Studies of patients with injuries to this area indicate that they have difficulty with the location and scale of objects.

- The parvocellular neurons, which do recognize color, tend to project more ventrally, toward the temporal regions on the side of the brain. If the brain is damaged in this area, patients have difficulty recognizing objects.

- Neuroimaging of undamaged brains supports these observations. All of this suggests that when you look at the world around you, you are actually looking at it with 2 very different visual systems.

- It is easy to imagine what the world would look like without a functioning "what" system. You have probably seen some novel object before, maybe an unusual kitchen gadget. It is significantly less common to experience a malfunction of the "where" system.

- Many stroke victims have this exact issue. One famous patient, referred to as DF, developed this disorder as the result of diffuse brain damage caused by carbon monoxide poisoning. If an object is placed within a certain large blind spot in the lower half of her visual field, she cannot identify it, nor even tell whether there is an object there at all.

- Yet if you ask her to, DF can reach out and pick up the object perfectly. Just like if you or I performed the task, DF's hand smoothly accelerates during the first half of the reach, forms into a configuration that matches the size and shape of the target, and smoothly decelerates until it makes contact with the target.

- Clearly, DF's blind spot is not blind. This visually guided grasping behavior makes it absolutely clear that visual processing is taking place. The pathway that processes "what" information is offline, but the pathway that processes "where" information is still very much functioning.

- Other patients have been identified who have damage to the dorsal pathway and seem to exhibit the opposite types of deficits—patients such as a man called RV. RV first visited doctors complaining of difficulty picking things up, namely making visually guided reaches. Yet once holding an object, he could manipulate it just fine.

- RV tended to open his hand fully and then move slowly and irregularly until he made contact with his target, like controlling an unfamiliar piece of construction equipment: You pull on the controls, wait to see what happens, and then pull on the controls again to correct the action.

- His ventral stream seemed to be intact, enabling him to perceive the world just fine, but his dorsal stream was damaged, making it difficult to gather information about where things were and use that to control smooth, efficient actions.

- In Lecture 3, I urged you to be cautious about overinterpreting subtraction-based fMRI studies. I want to urge similar caution here, even with this double-dissociation evidence. It may be that the complex interplay of all of the components is necessary for successful function.

- That does not mean that we should disregard the double-dissociation evidence completely. It inspires not just theories but also follow-up experiments. Work with normally functioning brains is needed to begin to nail down what is really happening.

- That research has been and is being done; we will consider it in more detail when we get to perception and action control. For the moment, I urge you to remain skeptical and wary of overinterpreting any individual source of data.

- Many people who study the brain and the mind have come to think of these types of modules as the basic building blocks of perception, action, and thought in general.

- The idea of these modules itself is quite old, dating back to the 18th-century concept of phrenology, developed by German physiologist Franz Joseph Gall.

- Dr. Gall spent a lot of time examining the shapes of his patients' heads. He presumed that the size of the skull indicates how big the underlying region of brain tissue is. (That is incorrect, by the way.)

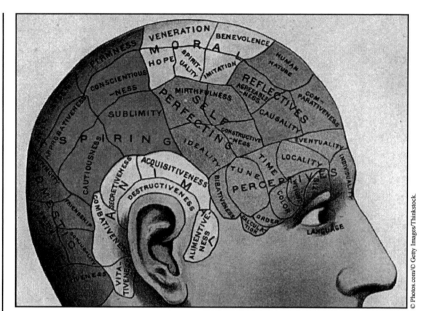

© Photos.com/© Getty Images/Thinkstock.

**The phrenologists were right about one thing: The brain is modular.**

- He had also developed his own map of how different mental perceptual faculties corresponded to particular regions of the brain. His map was largely incorrect as well, although the general idea of modular organization is correct.

- The philosopher Jerry Fodor published an extremely influential book titled the *Modularity of Mind* in the 1980s. In it, he laid out the notion of what a module must be from a very philosophical perspective:

  o A module, any module, is inherently informationally encapsulated. It considers certain sources of information but does not consider others.

  o A module is automatic. It does what it does all the time, without our choosing to engage it.

  o A module is localized to a particular segment of brain tissue.

- I have discussed a few brain modules in this lecture, but there are reasons to suspect that there are many others. Vision is an ideal example.

- Vision takes in a lot of information, but it does not take in everything. It is clearly encapsulated away from our conscious reasoning. It is also automatic: When you open your eyes, you do not have to choose to see; you just do. Finally, vision takes place in very particular parts of your brain.

- Within our visual system, however, there seem to be many submodules. In fact, there is some reason to believe that we create modules all the time as we learn about the world around us.

- Reading, for example, is a submodule of the visual system. When a word is placed in front of you, you do not choose to read it; the meaning of the word simply comes to mind.

- In addition to laying out the concept of modules, Fodor also made an interesting and compelling observation: Given the way science works, modules are the only parts of the brain we can ever hope to understand fully.

- Science progresses by making observations, developing theories, and generating hypotheses that enable those theories to be tested and refined. For that method to work, something about the topic of study must be consistent and repeatable.

- To the extent that the brain is able to consider any source of information, it is capable of performing differently every single time. This is part of what makes the brain so wonderful and flexible, but it means that no specific, detailed scientific theory can ever fully explain and test the brain's workings.

- Fodor acknowledged that the human mind is capable of much more than these modules he hypothesized, but he made a concrete prediction that has not yet been disproven: Any nonmodular things our minds can do can never be captured within a scientific theory.

## Suggested Reading

Sacks, *The Man Who Mistook His Wife for a Hat.*

Uttal, *The New Phrenology.*

## Questions to Consider

1. If the human brain consists of independent modules, how do we have a unitary, seamless perception of the world around us? What puts it all together?

2. Modules function in an informationally encapsulated fashion. That is, we do not have access to their inner workings, only the outputs. If one of our modules malfunctioned, how would we know it?

# Brain Modules—Subcomponents of the Senses
## Lecture 4—Transcript

In the second and third lectures of the course, we discussed some of the biology—the neuroscience—of human sensory processing. In Lecture 2, we considered transduction; the process by which energy from the environment is converted into patterns of neural impulses, the signals that are used by the brain to make sense of the world around us. I talked about what individual neurons do and about what neurons associated with particular sensory modalities do. In the third lecture, we started talking about not just individual neurons, but larger groups of neurons that perform particular functions. I talked in depth about the right inferotemporal cortex and its role in the perception of faces. I suggested the idea that there may be many regions of the brain that perform specialized processing of this type.

In this fourth lecture, I want to further develop this idea. I want to urge you to think about your brain and your perceptual processing as arising from many separate, independent modules. Each of these modules consists of thousands or tens of thousands of neurons, interconnected with each other and the rest of the brain in very particular ways. They take in certain sources of information and ignore all others. They perform very specific processing, produce very specific outputs, and then send those outputs on to other modules. There's a lot of evidence to support the idea that our senses and our brain in general is organized in this way. Even though we only have a unitary, single perceptual experience of the world around us, our perceptions seem to be produced to arise from the interaction of a wide range of these different, independent, modular subsystems. In this lecture, I'll discuss evidence for this organization, and talk about some of the modules that seem to be there in our brain.

Let's start by talking some more about retinotopic maps. In Lecture 2, I discussed retinotopic organization for visual transduction. Remember, that's the process by which light projects onto the retina, which then projects to the lateral geniculate nucleus, and then onto visual cortex. Remember also that these projections maintain a retinotopic map with the same relative spatial organization as on the retina itself. I talked about our retinotopic map in a general sense. In this lecture, I'll describe the fact that there are actually many different retinotopic maps: some represent edges, some colors, still others motion. These different maps are organized according to this modular framework.

These spatially organized projections continue beyond the visual cortex into other regions of the brain. These groups of projections are often referred to as pathways within the brain. In this lecture, I'll talk about 2 of these pathways that form 2 very big modules, maybe the biggest: One of those modules processes information about the identities of objects (we call that the "what" pathway); another processes information about objects' locations and movements (we call that the "where" pathway). Having explored this sampling of different modules, I'll finish this lecture by considering some of the consequences of having a brain that's organized in this way. If we accept the notion that the human brain is organized around these independent modules, what can that reveal about how sensation and perception function in general?

Okay, let's talk about retinotopic maps. Light travels in straight lines between surfaces in the environment and the eyes. The light then passes through the pupil and projects onto the back of the eye on the retina. Here, those locations in space and the positions on the retina are labeled as A, B, and C. The optic nerve axons project from particular places on the retina to particular places within the lateral geniculate nucleus. Axons from the lateral geniculate then project to particular locations in the primary visual cortex, located here on the back of the brain.

The human brain contains 2 hemispheres, one on the left and one on the right. Each of these hemispheres contains a lateral geniculate and a visual cortex of its own. The visual cortex is often referred to as V1, since it's the first place that visual information reaches the cortex. The lateral geniculate is just as important, but it sits below the cortical layers of the brain. It's referred to as a sub-cortical structure. There is no light in these areas of the brain, but the pattern of electrical activation there is sort of like a picture in the head. If there were 3 tiny spots of light out there in the world at those locations that we labeled A, B, and C, and if there were total darkness everywhere else, then inside the brain there would be 3 spots of electrical activation right there in the lateral geniculate.

If I were to probe the lateral geniculate with a recording electrode, I could sense the electrical activity in these regions. Exactly this technique has been used to study the nature of visual processing. Stimuli are presented to anaesthetized animals—usually cats or rats—while a tiny electrode is pushed into the brain tissue to probe the patterns of electrical activity there. Normally, of course, there isn't darkness and 3 spots of light; there's a very complex pattern of light from the world around us, and a correspondingly complex pattern of electrical activity there in the brain. But the principle is the same: The light information is transduced into a retinotopic map of electrical activation.

Okay. Hopefully this seems straightforward to you so far, because it's a dramatic oversimplification. There's only one cup, only one visual input, out there in the world, but there are dozens of different retinotopic maps back here in the lateral geniculate and the primary visual cortex. If I were to take a recording electrode and place it near the surface of the LGN in the right hemisphere, and if I recorded the outputs of that electrode here in the right hemisphere, I would find bursts of electrical activity only when I presented stimuli to one particular location in the right eye. If I pushed the electrode just a little deeper—less than a millimeter down—now the right eye stimuli would do nothing to activate it; now I would only find activity when stimuli were presented to a very precise location on the left eye. A little deeper and it would go back to the right eye. Still deeper, it would go back to the left again.

When we reach the unit on depth perception, we'll talk about something called stereopsis. This will be familiar if you've ever been to a 3D movie and worn special glasses that enable you to see things jump off the screen at you. Slightly different views of the world are projected onto your left and right eyes because your left and right eyes are in slightly different locations. In general, the closer some object is to your eyes, the greater the difference in that projection. By comparing the inputs of the 2 eyes, and by identifying locations in those inputs where there are differences, your brain can very precisely figure out the 3-dimensional structure of nearby surfaces. This alternating representation of the left and right eye inputs in the lateral geniculate is directly responsible for this stereopsis ability. Interconnections between these separate layers make it possible.

There's actually a very large percentage of people who don't possess this stereopsis ability; about 10 percent of the general population. If one of your eyes is injured at a particular phase of childhood and you have to wear a patch over one eye for a period of time, this left- versus right-eye modular organization can be greatly reduced or even vanish. I've talked with many students over the years who hear this and are actually a little relieved. They describe attending those 3D movies for years and wondering what everyone was oohing and ahhing about. One particular guy I talked with said that he'd learned to actually fake it pretty well; he could tell when something was supposed to be sticking out of the screen. He actually believed that everyone else in the theater was faking it, too.

Regardless, here we have one of the simplest modular organizations within the human visual system. A group of neurons processes inputs from one eye, and only one eye. There's other information in the visual input, but it ignores that completely. Another set of neurons is similarly specialized for processing information from the other eye. Yet another set of neurons is specifically responsible for comparing the outputs of these 2 separate eye modules. Putting it all together, we perceive a 3D visual world, but only after these separate subsystems are put together.

This divide-and-conquer organization shows up for many aspects of visual processing, and sensory processing in general. In fact, there's another modular separation shown here as well that's present in that lateral geniculate. If I were to push that electrode that we were putting into the lateral geniculate down deep enough, I would find more of this left- versus right-eye organization, but the properties of the neurons would change again. The cell bodies and axons of the neurons themselves in this area are bigger; the axons in particular are thicker than the ones near the top. For this reason, they're called "magnocellular" neurons. The smaller cells, located at the shallower depth, are referred to as "parvocellular." The functional properties of these neurons are also different. They respond sooner than the ones in the upper layer because those thicker axons convey the sensory signals faster. If I varied the type of stimuli that I presented to this animal's eyes, I would also find out that these cells respond to changes in brightness, but not so much to changes in color. These layers of the lateral geniculate are essentially color-blind.

Another big difference is in how these neurons project into the visual cortex; how they make that shift from the lateral geniculate and into the visual cortex. The magnocellular neurons tend to project their axons into the dorsal or occipital regions of the cortex, located roughly on the top and back areas of the brain. The parvocellular neurons tend to project in temporal regions of the brain, located on the side of the brain and the head. These 2 pathways are often referred to as "ventral" and "dorsal" based on spatial terminology developed by neuroscientists. Dorsal—like a dorsal fin on a fish—refers to the top region of the brain; ventral refers to the side.

Studies of brain injured patients have suggested that these 2 pathways form 2 more of these perceptual modules that I'm talking about. If the brain is damaged in the ventral pathway—the temporal lobe of the brain—deficits emerge in the ability to recognize objects. If the brain is damaged in that dorsal pathway, objects can still be recognized, but it's difficult to localize just where they are or how big they are. Neuroimaging of undamaged brains supports this theory as well. When a participant views some display and makes judgment about what objects it contains, more activation is seen in the ventral pathway. Conversely, if a participant views the same display while making judgments about where the objects are located—for instance, which of 2 objects is farther away than the other—then the dorsal region is activated more. All of this suggests that when you look at the world around you, you're actually looking at it with 2 very different visual systems. They work together and they're very interconnected, but they're separate just the same.

It's easy to imagine what the world would look like without a functioning "what" system. You've probably seen some novel object that you can't recognize before, maybe an unusual new kitchen gadget. You can see where the thing is and how big it is without actually being able to recognize what it is. Without a functioning "what" pathway in your brain, you would simply have this experience with all of the objects that you could see. It's much harder, I think, to imagine the experience of having a functioning "what" system without a functioning "where" system. You'd be able to know what objects were present in your immediate surroundings, but unable to know where they're located or how big they are. Sadly, there are many stroke victims who have this exact disorder.

One very famous patient—referred to as DF—had a heating system installed improperly in her house. When it turned on the first time, the house filled with carbon monoxide (an odorless, toxic gas) and she passed out. Fortunately, she was found before she died, but not before the oxygen deprivation had led to diffuse damage around the ventral, or "what," pathway of her brain. Since that time, she's had a large blind spot in the lower half of her visual field. If an object is placed within this blind spot, she can't identify it; not what it is or even if there's an object there in the blind spot at all. Even if you ask her to just guess, she performs essentially at chance on these types of tasks.

A strange thing happens, however, if you ask her to reach out and pick up the object in her blind spot: she does. I have to presume that the first time someone asked her to pick up the object in her blind spot that she said, "What object?" But I've never gotten a straight answer to that question from the people who've worked with her. Regardless, DF will certainly reach out and pick the object up. Even more compelling is the way in which she does so. Her hand moves in a straight line from wherever it is initially out to where the target is located. Just like you or I would, her hand smoothly accelerates during the first half of the reach, and then smoothly decelerates until it makes contact with the target. As she makes the reach, DF also forms her hand into a configuration that matches the size and shape of the target. This is one of those things that we very much take for granted when we reach out to pick up some object. If you ever reach for something and stop yourself right before your hand gets there, you'll notice that your fingers are shaped into a configuration that very precisely matches the size and shape of the target for which you're reaching. This process is so automatic that we think of it as being easy, but it's very precisely controlled. For what it's worth, you can't just grab any 2 points along the edge of an object and expect to produce a good, efficient grasp. The placement of your hand has to take into account the size and shape of the object for which you're reaching to pick out easily graspable points along its edges. DF does just that. She reaches out and grasps objects just like you or I would. Her grasping shows all of these same operating characteristics.

I described DF as having a large blind spot, but it's clearly not blind. This visually-guided grasping behavior makes it absolutely clear that there's a lot of visual processing taking place within that so-called blind spot. With DF, the ventral stream seems to be offline—the pathway that processes "what" information—robbing her of the ability to identify and consciously perceive the target object. However, her dorsal system—the pathway that processes "where" information—is still very much seeing things and using that vision to control her reaching actions.

Other patients have been identified who have damage to the dorsal stream and seem to exhibit the opposite types of deficits. One patient who's been studied extensively is referred to as RV. (Brain-injured patients, by the way, have historically been referred to by their initials. In recent decades, in order to protect their confidentiality, researchers have switched to arbitrarily picking letters; so R and V aren't actually his initials, but we'll refer to him as patient RV.) RV first visited doctors complaining not of a vision problem at all, but of a motor control problem. He had difficulty picking things up. His real problem, however, is making visually-guided reaches; something that makes sense given this "what" versus "where" modular organization we've been studying. His hand and arm control are, by themselves, just fine. Once RV is holding an object, he can manipulate it just as well as you or I could. (Although, you should note that we can usually manipulate things even with our eyes closed, without looking at an object. We can get the haptic information once we're actually grasping it.)

RV's deficits become apparent only when he is making a visually-guided reach to pick up some target. He tends to open his hand fully and then move slowly and irregularly until he makes contact with that target for which he's reaching. I've always likened this motor control aspect of RV to trying to control an unfamiliar piece of construction equipment like, say, a crane: You pull on the controls, wait to see what happens, and then pull on the controls again to correct the action. The same seems to happen with RV's reaching movements. His ventral stream seems to be intact, enabling him to perceive the world around him just fine; but his dorsal stream is damaged, making it difficult to gather information about where things are and use that to control smooth, efficient actions. Based on these types of findings, many researchers have taken to relabeling these "what" and "where" streams as "perception" and "action" streams.

With these 2 patients, DF and RV, we have what neurologists refer to as a "double dissociation": Two different areas are damaged and 2 different patterns of deficits are produced. In Lecture 3 on neuroimaging, I urged you to be cautious about over-interpreting subtraction-based fMRI studies. I made it analogous to an erroneous conclusion that, due to greater activity in the motor of a blender during walnut grinding, this motor component must be the "walnut grinding area" of the blender. I want to urge similar caution here, even with this double dissociation evidence that we have to work with.

Consider something simpler than 2 brain-injured patients (again, for the moment); let's go with 2 blenders this time. Imagine that the 2 blenders are initially identical, capable of doing all the things that blenders do, including making milkshakes and grinding walnuts. Imagine that I grind too many walnuts in blender A, so many that the motor begins to break down such that it can no longer grind walnuts; it's no longer strong enough. It can still make milkshakes with this weakened motor and do all of the other things that blenders do, but it can't grind walnuts. Blender A has a particular area of damage (the motor) and a particular pattern of deficit (it has a walnut-grinding deficit).

Now consider blender B. It's doing just fine until I drop the pitcher one day. In so doing, when it falls to the floor I make a thin crack in the side of the blender's pitcher. If I try to grind walnuts in this one, it's still fine; it's just a hairline crack. If I try to make milkshakes, however, I'm in trouble; the milkshake will leak all over the counter. Blender B now has a particular area of damage (the pitcher) and a particular pattern of deficit (a milkshake deficit).

Taken together, then, the 2 blenders exhibit a double-dissociation, just like DF and RV. In the case of DF and RV, you might be tempted to confidently conclude that the ventral stream does perception while the dorsal stream does action. With these blenders, however, I hope you can see the concern. I would clearly be wrong to say that the pitcher is responsible for making milkshakes while the motor is responsible for grinding walnuts. The whole blender, of course, is necessary to do any of these tasks. It's the complex interplay of all of the components that leads to successful blending.

So where does that leave us? What can we do with the DF and RV's double dissociation? Does it mean that we have to disregard it completely? No. I don't think it does. The patient work is compelling and inspiring, frankly; it's fascinating that it comes out the way it does. It inspires not just theories, but also follow-up experiments. Good research in this area often uses work with brain-injured patients as a starting point, but work with normally functioning brains is needed to begin to nail down what's really happening. That research has been and is being done. We'll consider it in more detail when we get to the unit on perception and action control. For the moment, I just want to urge you to remain skeptical and wary of over-interpreting any individual source of data.

Today, I've discussed left- versus right-eye processing modules at a very basic level of sensory processing. I've also just discussed "what" versus "where" modules—or perception versus action modules—at a higher, more cortical level of processing. Many people who study the brain and the mind have come to think of these types of modules as the basic building blocks of perception, action, and thought in general. The idea of these modules itself is quite old, dating back to an 18th century concept called "phrenology." If you had visited the office of Dr. Franz Joseph Gall in the late 1700s, he would have sat you down and spent a lot of time examining the shape of your head. Gall presumed 2 things. First, the size of the skull in different places can tell you how big the underlying region of brain tissue is. (That's incorrect, by the way.) Second, Gall had developed a map of how different mental perceptual faculties correspond to particular regions of the brain. His map, especially in terms of its details, has been largely shown to be incorrect as well. For instance, Gall's idea that your ability to perceive and reason about time is based on brain regions located over your eye seems very clearly wrong.

While Gall seems to have gotten pretty much all of the details wrong, his big concept of modular organization of the brain seems to have stuck. Most of the important advances in our understanding of how the brain implements perception and cognition have come from exactly this sort of discovery of how different brain areas perform specific tasks. The philosopher Jerry Fodor published an extremely influential book entitled the *Modularity of Mind* in the 1980s. In it, he laid out the notion of what a module must be from a very philosophical perspective. First, a module, any module, is inherently informationally encapsulated. That is, it considers certain sources of information but does not consider others. A module takes in only certain types of information and that's it. Remember, for instance, those layers of the LGN that only consider information from one eye and ignore the input from the other. Second, a module is automatic. It does what it does all the time, without our choosing to engage it. Here you can think of the dorsal action system that controls the visual processing that mediates how our fingers move during a reach without our ever being aware of it. Third, a module is typically localized to a particular segment of brain tissue. This is presumably the reason that we're able to discover these modules after people suffer particular brain injuries.

I've discussed a few modules in this lecture, but there are reasons to suspect that there are many others that fit this definition. Visual size perception in general seems to be one such module. Consider the horizontal-vertical illusion. This illusion is constructed with an upside-down "T" shape in which the horizontal and vertical lines are equal in length. The vertical line is set up so that it bisects the horizontal line. Even though the vertical and horizontal lines are equal in length, they don't look that way to most people who view them. Most report that the vertical line looks longer, much longer, by about 20 percent. If you slide that vertical line over to the side of the horizontal line—say over to the left edge—the illusion vanishes. When the vertical line is no longer in the middle of that horizontal line, the 2 lines look approximately equal in length. (For what it's worth, this horizontal-vertical illusion seems to be misnamed. It's the placement of the vertical in the middle of the horizontal that matters. You could actually rotate it 90 degrees and it would still appear that the line that was doing the bisecting is substantially longer than the line that's being bisected; but that's a story for another day.)

This illusion is very salient, even if you've seen it many times. It's even salient to me, and I made the figure. You can try this yourself if you'd like—you could draw your own upside down T-shape, using a ruler to be absolutely sure—to completely convince yourself that the vertical and horizontal extents of the figure are identical. Even if you've drawn the lines yourself with a very accurate ruler, when you step away from that drawing and look at the figure again, the vertical will still look longer, still by about 20 percent.

Vision, especially vision for size perception it seems, is informationally encapsulated. No matter how much information you get into your head that the 2 lines are identical in length, no matter how convinced you are that that's true, when you look at the figure again, your visual system will still tell you that the vertical line looks longer. Vision, like our other senses, takes in a lot of information, but it doesn't take in everything. It's clearly encapsulated away from our conscious reasoning. It's also automatic. When you open your eyes, you don't have to choose to see; you just do. Finally, and you know this already, vision takes place in a very particular part of your brain; many particular parts of your brain, actually. From Fodor's perspective, the ideal example of a module is, in fact, visual perception as a whole.

Within our visual system, however, there seem to be many other sub-modules. In fact, there's some reason to believe that we create modules all the time as we learn about the world around us. My favorite example of this is reading. When a word's placed in front of you, you don't choose to read it; the meaning of the word simply comes to mind. In fact, you can't even choose not to read something. Think of the logo of a well-known overnight delivery service (FedEx). You've probably seen it a hundred times. Think of the name of the company on the side of the truck, the big letters that make up that logo. You have, hopefully, a clear vision in mind of what that logo looks like; where's the arrow? It's there, it's right in front of you. It's hard to see because your reading "module" is dominating your visual processing; it's reading the letters that are there and not thinking of them just in terms of shapes. If you haven't found that arrow yet, it's between the E and the X at the end of the name. If you were a non-reader, say a 3-year-old who was just starting out with alphabet books, it would be easy to find that arrow; it would jump right off the page at you. It's only because you've formed that reading module that it's such a challenge.

In addition to laying out the concept of modules, and in so doing inspiring many perceptual and cognitive scientists to look for them, Fodor also made an interesting and compelling observation. From a brain science perspective, it's a good thing that these modules exist because given the way science works, they're the only parts of the brain that we can ever hope to really fully understand. For science to work, a few things are necessary. Science progresses by making observations, developing theories, and then generating hypotheses that enable those theories to be tested and refined. My 10th grade biology teacher taught me that this is called the hypothetico-deductive method. (Thank you, Mrs. Spitzer.) In order for that method to work, it has to be that there's something consistent and repeatable about the topic of study; in this case, the brain and our behavior.

To the extent that the brain is able to consider any source of information—any of the infinite range of information out there—then it's capable of performing differently every single time. This is a wonderful and important thing, actually. Picasso, Bach, Einstein, and Michael Jordan were so amazing because they found ways to think, create, and do things in ways that no one before them had found before. As wonderful and important as it is, however, it means that no specific, detailed scientific theory can ever fully explain and test it. Fodor acknowledged that the human mind is capable of much more than these modules he hypothesized, but he made a very concrete prediction; it's a prediction that hasn't been proven wrong yet, and it's been a good 30 years now: Those non-modular things that our minds do can never be captured within a scientific theory.

This is the last of the lectures in this course that will focus specifically on the brain. I'll still talk about the brain a fair amount, of course, but only as that brain research bears on the topic of sensation and perception that we're covering at the time. I hope that you feel comfortable with the basic equipment that we have at our disposal as we sense and perceive the world around us. I also hope that you have some familiarity with the strengths and limitations of how researchers in this area study and reason about the function of the brain.

In the next unit of the course, the next 3 lectures, I'll be telling you about 3 of the mainstays of human vision: how we perceive motion, color, and depth. Until then, I hope you enjoy your senses and feel some awareness of all of the automatic, usually unconscious, very modular things that your sensory systems do for you.

# Perceiving a World in Motion
## Lecture 5

Our visual system is very good at making sense of still pictures, but we live in a world of motion. Many studies have examined how we perceive stationary things, but modern perception researchers have realized that the thing our visual system is best at—perhaps the very thing it evolved to do—is perceive motion.

- Motion information is important for perceiving the location, shape, and identity of objects. It is arguably the foundation of almost everything else we perceive about the world.

- It turns out that we perceive motion—or rather infer motion—only after it has taken place, thanks not only to the way our brains our built but because of the way the universe functions.

- There is a very famous display called the Ames Room illusion. In it, 2 people of about the same height enter and stand in the back corners, one on the left and one on the right. A third person views them from the front through a small window.

- To the viewer, the person on the right might look about 6 feet tall, while the person on the left might look about 4 feet tall. The illusion is created by the fact that the person who appears to be small is significantly farther away than the person who looks tall, due to how the room is constructed.

- There are certain inferences that your visual system makes when it views any room. For instance, almost every room you have ever seen is approximately rectangular, as are most windows and floor tiles. The Ames Room is constructed of trapezoids instead, but from the viewer's angle (usually tightly restricted), they appear rectangular.

- If the viewer were allowed to move, the illusion would vanish almost instantly. As soon as relative motion information is available, the impression that the room is constructed of rectangular shapes goes away.

- Studies of illusions such as this have identified many sources of information that influence our perception of size, distance, color, and so forth. We make many inferences, great and small, about the world around us in this way.

- Sometimes these inferences come into conflict with one another; one aspect of an image says one thing while another aspect says the opposite, which is what produces most illusions.

- As many different sources of information as there are, motion information seems to be the most salient, powerful, and relied on by our brains.

- There are good reasons for this reliance on motion, including evolutionary ones. In the ongoing battle for survival among predators and prey, motion is a major weapon against camouflage.

- Motion also provides us with information about shapes, distances, and depth. Consider the kinetic depth effect, which allows you to infer a 3-dimensional shape from a series of 2-dimensional images, as well as telling you how that 3-dimensional shape is moving in space.

- One of the most interesting things about motion perception is that it is inferred after it has finished happening.

- Consider a still image in which a single square is present, motionless. Now consider another image with another identical motionless square located in a different position on the screen.

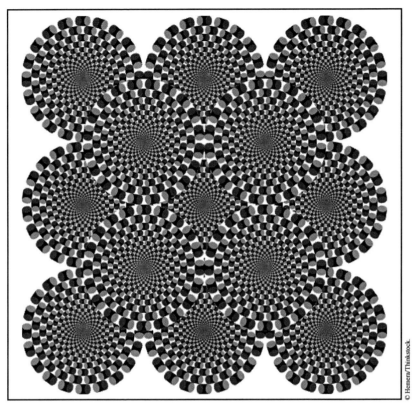

**The information in this image is so complex that, as you glance around it, your visual system makes its best guess and interprets it as motion.**

- If I were to rapidly alternate between these pictures, suddenly you would perceive them as a single square moving back and forth. This phenomenon is known as apparent motion because motion is perceived but nothing is actually moving. Your sensory system infers something that is not occurring and fills in the motion between them.

- Every time you watch a movie, you are seeing apparent motion. Movies are many still images presented in rapid sequence.

- You may have also had a flip book when you were a child, where flipping quickly through the pages made a figure appear in motion but flipping too slowly destroyed the illusion.

- A slightly more complex example consists of 2 stationary images. In one, a black square sits in the upper left and another in the lower right, while in the second there is a square in the lower left and one in the upper right.

- If I were to rapidly alternate between these images, there are at least 4 things you might see.

    ○ You might perceive it as 2 images without any motion at all—unlikely, but possible, and it is what is actually present.

    ○ You might see 2 squares alternately moving up and down.

    ○ You might see 2 squares alternately moving from side to side.

    ○ Your perception might switch back and forth between the latter 2 alternatives about every 30 seconds or so.

- By blocking certain portions of the image, you might force yourself to see other things.

- Even given all of these possibilities, your visual system makes its best guess—an inference—about what event would produce the sensory inputs you are receiving, and it is that inference you perceive, not the sensory inputs per se. Here, the inference is essentially always motion.

- Returning to the example in which a single square seems to move from one position to another, ponder with me the timing of the stimulus presentation and how it relates to the timing of your perception of the event.

- During the alternation, you perceived 3 things: the square at the starting location, the square in motion, and the square's arrival. Note, this perception does not match the order in which the events actually occur. The "arrival" occurred before the "motion," which never occurred at all.

- Your brain, as we will see with many aspects of perception, seems to construct the world that you experience. It fills things in spatially—as with blind spots—and with motion, it also seems to fill things in temporally and even to shift the order of events when it makes sense to do so.

- How does the visual system parse and interpret all this complex motion information? Let's begin to answer this question by considering 3 different situations that produce 3 different inputs on the retina.

- First, consider a stationary viewer looking at a stationary environment in which one object is moving—for instance, a person walking across your field of view. Your perception is obvious: The world is stationary; the man is moving.

- Next, consider a second situation, in which the entire background seems to move left across the retina. Two things could produce this situation: Perhaps the whole room is moving to the left, or perhaps you are moving your head to the right. In most situations, the movement of images projected onto our retinas is caused by a combination of these factors.

- Finally, consider a third situation in which a man is walking, but he remains stationary in the middle of the retina; meanwhile, the entire background drifts leftward across that retina. You produce such inputs whenever you follow a moving target with your eyes.

- The point here is that just because something is moving across your retina does not mean it is in motion. Conversely, just because something is stationary on your retina does not mean it is stationary.

- How do we figure out what is moving and what is not? At least part of the answer has to do with a close linkage between the motor systems that move our eyes and the sensory systems that process visual information.

- When your brain sends a command to your eyes telling them to move, it sends a copy of that command to your visual cortex. This copy is referred to as a corollary discharge. By subtracting the motion caused by your eye movements, your visual cortex is able to figure out what is moving and what is not.

- There are at least 2 good sources of evidence for corollary discharge, 1 of which you can see for yourself. Close one eye and gently press on the lower eyelid of your open eye with your index finger. This will cause your eye to jiggle slightly.

- Since you are controlling this movement with your finger and not your eye muscle, there is no corollary discharge to the visual cortex, and therefore the visual system does not subtract the motion. Thus the whole world will seem to move up and down.

- A famous lab experiment further supported the existence of corollary discharge. Some early behaviorist psychologists, seeking to prove that no thought, perception, or learning can take place without involving the body, put a test subject on a ventilator and paralyzed his entire motor system.

- The man disproved the theory; he remembered his time in paralysis quite clearly. But he reported another unexpected phenomenon. As soon as he became paralyzed, he noticed that the world seemed to jump around wildly, up and down and side to side.

- Eventually, he figured out that this happened whenever he tried to move his eyes. His eye muscles were paralyzed, but the corollary discharge system within the central nervous system was still active.

- When he tried to move his eyes, a signal was sent to his visual cortex telling it to expect a particular eye movement. When it did not take place, the visual cortex inferred that his whole environment had moved.

- Your visual system uses other information to make inferences about motions as well. One simple assumption is that any motion will follow the shortest possible path. But this rule is not followed blindly.

- Consider 2 still images of a person with a bent, raised knee. In one, the person's hand is held behind the knee; in the second, the hand is in front of the knee. If the images are presented in alternation, most people see the hand moving around the knee, rather than through.

- Now consider an image of a ball rolling across a stage from front left to back right. If we add shadows and shading consistent with that motion, the perception remains about the same.

- But if we add a shadow that moves from left to right across the surface, the ball seems to float into the air without changing its position in depth. A bouncing shadow can even make the ball seem to bounce up and down as it moves across the stage. In all of these situations, the motions of the actual ball remain constant. Only the shadows are changing.

- In Lecture 4, I talked about how your brain contains a large set of retinotopic maps—neurons with spatial organization that matches the organization of the retina. Many of these maps represent information about motion.

- One map encodes upward motion. Another set encodes downward motion. Another pair encodes leftward motion and rightward motion and so on. These layers function somewhat independently, but they are also connected in some interesting ways.

- For opposite directions, they are connected in an inhibitory fashion. That is, whenever the upward-sensitive neurons are active, they send signals that inhibit the activity of the corresponding downward-sensitive neurons and vice versa. This is called the opponent process.

- This system of organization is present for many aspects of sensory processing—not just motion but color, orientation, and even more complex combinations of stimuli.

- Interestingly, as you gaze at something that stimulates your downward-sensitive neurons, such as a waterfall, they are receiving a lot of their favorite input, but they are also growing fatigued; meanwhile, the upward-sensitive neurons are resting.

- After fatiguing the downward-sensitive neurons, if you look at something stationary, you are giving your downward- and upward-sensitive neurons the same amount of input. The downward-sensitive neurons will start losing the tug-of-war.

- Your visual system will infer from the upward-sensitive neurons' victory that there is upward motion present, and the stationary stimulus will appear to have upward motion.

## Suggested Reading

Nijhawan, "Motion Extrapolation in Catching."

Watanabe, *High-Level Motion Processing.*

## Questions to Consider

1.  If you gently push on your lower eyelid (and the eyeball beneath it), the world appears to move. The normal process of corollary discharge is bypassed. If I look out the window of a moving car, however, you do not perceive most of the world as moving. You correctly perceive that the world is stationary and you are moving through it. Even without corollary discharge, you can tell external motion from your own motion. How could an experimenter bypass this process?

**2.** Motion cannot be perceived until it has already happened. If I am trying to catch a ball as it flies through the air, I cannot perceive its motion until it has already moved. If that is so, then how can I catch it?

# Perceiving a World in Motion
## Lecture 5—Transcript

Hello again. In this lecture, I'd like to talk with you about motion perception. We can and often do look at still pictures, and our visual system is very good at making sense of them. Most of the time, however, we live in a world of motion; a world in which objects move from place to place, and in which we ourselves move. Our eyes move as we scan the environment and our whole bodies move as we walk or drive through it. There've been many studies of how we perceive stationary things, but modern perception researchers have realized that the thing our visual system is best at—perhaps the very thing that it evolved to do—is to perceive motion.

In this lecture, I want to talk with you about 3 aspects of how we sense motion. First, I'll explain how motion information is important for perceiving the location, shape, and identity of objects. I'll argue that it's the foundation of almost everything else that we perceive about the world. Second, I'll talk a bit about how we perceive motion, or rather how we infer it. Because of the way our brains are built—and frankly because of the way that our universe functions—we can only perceive motion after it's already taken place. We perceive motion as a continuous, real-time experience, but that's an inference. The motions you perceive are, in most cases, already finished before you're able to perceive them. Finally, I'll finish by talking about how we interpret the complex patterns of motion that are delivered to our retina. Motion in the flow of ambient light that's projected onto our retina is caused by a lot of things; the movement of objects out there in the world, for sure, but also by the movements of our own body, the movements of our head, and the movements of our eyes. I'll discuss how our visual system parses this mix of inputs in order to figure out the state of the moving environment around us.

Okay. Let's talk a bit about how important motion information is to our visual system. There's a very famous display called the Ames Room Illusion. Typically with this display, 2 people who are about the same height walk into the Ames room and stand in the back corners of the room, one on the left and one on the right. A third person looks into the room from the front and gets to experience the illusion effect. This viewer will see these 2 people as being greatly different in size, even though they're the same height. For instance, the person on the right might look about 6 feet tall, while the person on the left might look only about 4 feet tall. That illusion is created by the fact that the person who appears to be small is significantly farther away than the person who looks tall. The difference in how far away the people are isn't apparent to the viewer, however, because of how the Ames room is constructed. Indeed, the room is built so that there's a clear perception that the 2 people are not at different distances, but at the same distance from the viewer.

There are certain inferences that your visual system makes when it views the Ames room; or any room, for that matter. For instance, almost every room that you've seen is approximately rectangular in shape. Most windows that we encounter are also rectangular. If there's a tile pattern on the floor—and there is one in the Ames room—that tile pattern is also typically constructed from rectangle shapes. While this rectangular construction principle is used for almost all rooms, it's not present anywhere in the Ames room. The walls, windows, and tiles on the floor of the Ames room are all carefully designed trapezoid shapes; carefully constructed so that, seen from one particular point of view—from the point of view of the viewer of the Ames room— they look rectangular. This Ames room display is something that you can see from time to time in children's museums and science museums around the country and around the world.

The illusion is compelling in photographs, but it works very well in real life. There's something quite amazing about viewing it, unfiltered, with your own eyes. If you do ever see one of these Ames rooms, you'll immediately notice, however, that you aren't allowed to simply walk around and look at the interior of the room from any angle. Indeed, there's usually a single, small viewing hole that's cut into one particular wall of the room. It's always a hole that's big enough to look through with one eye, but no bigger. The entire illusion relies on the fact that you have just that single, small viewing hole to look through. If the hole were any larger, if it was big enough that you could put your whole head in and look around, or even big enough that you could move your eye just a few inches from side to side while still seeing what was going on inside the Ames room, if you could move at all while continuing to look at the room's interior, then the illusion would almost completely vanish.

As soon as you have that relative motion information created by your own movement, that impression that the room is constructed of rectangular shapes goes away; you can see those trapezoids almost instantly. Almost instantly, you would see the 2 people in the back of the room as being the same size, as with the one being seen as farther away than the other.

Studies of illusions such as this have identified many sources of information that influence our perception of size, distance, color, and other aspects of the world. There are many little and not so little inferences that we make when we look at the world around us. Sometimes, these inferences and the sources of information behind them come into conflict with one another; one aspect of an image says one thing while another aspect of it suggests another. And that's what produces most illusions; that's what's going on with this Ames room.

As many different sources of information as there are, however, motion information seems to be the most salient and powerful of them all. If we don't have motion information, our visual system can still do a lot to interpret an image. But if there is motion information that's available, that's what our visual system keys into; that's what it relies upon most. That's why, if you have motion information, all of the other misleading aspects of the Ames room illusion go away. No matter how much the other aspects of the room suggest one thing, if motion suggests something else that trumps it all.

There are good reasons for this reliance on motion. Many people think of them in an evolutionary context. In the ongoing battle for survival among predators and prey, it seems clear that motion has been a major weapon. It's one of the only things that can trump really good camouflage. Imagine that you're walking through the woods and there's a pile of leaves that contains some dangerous animal within it. There are really good systems of camouflage that animals can use to hide themselves in that sort of situation. If you look at these squiggly lines here, I would bet that you can't see that there's a snake hidden within them. However, if we just add just a little bit of motion to the image—if that snake just wiggles a little bit to the side—suddenly it's not only possible to see the snake, it's very, very easy to see it. As soon as the snake stops moving, however, it vanishes again; even though you know it's there, you can't see it. That is, the motion information doesn't just call your attention to the snake; it's the pattern of motion itself that enables you to see it, to recognize it. If the snake moves, you can see the snake; if the snake is still, no more snake.

There are a lot of sources of information that are present in the squiggly line image that you might use to see the snake, but the motion information is enough to find it, see its shape, see its size and location, and ultimately to enable you to avoid it. Now, you might not live in a place where snakes are a frequent hazard, but there's good evidence that snakes have been a source of danger in our evolutionary past and that our ability to use motion information has been important throughout our history.

Motion information doesn't just give us the ability to notice sources of danger. Motion also provides us with a great deal of information about shapes, distances, and depth. Consider something called the Kinetic Depth Effect. Imagine that you had a bent up paperclip, bent into a very irregular, squiggly shape. If you held it up behind a piece of paper, you wouldn't be able to see it anymore. If you turned on a light behind the paperclip, however, you could see a shadow of that paperclip cast through that piece of paper. Now, the lines on that piece of paper—the shadow—are fully 2-dimensional. You could draw a jaggy, squiggly line with a pen that would look just like the shadow. It would be fully 2-dimensional in that situation. In fact, as you hold the paperclip still behind the paper and look at the shadow, as long as that paperclip stays very still, the 3-dimensional shape will seem to go away. If you began to rotate the paper clip, however, the 3-dimensional shape would be immediately apparent again.

At any moment in time, the shadow that you're actually seeing is 2-dimensional; what you're presenting your eyes with is a sequence of fully 2-dimensional images. Your visual system does something pretty incredible with this set of 2D images: It figures out what single, 3-dimensional shape could produce all of these 2D images. As it does, it also tells you how that rigid, 3D shape is rotating in space. This very difficult projective geometry problem is accomplished without any particular effort on your part. You just look at an undulating 2-dimensional image and that 3-dimensional perception pops out at you; and you're pretty accurate at it, actually. It would take some time, but if I showed you a set of shadows—just the shadows—

from a paper clip that I had bent up, you could bend another paperclip so that it would match it; it would match it pretty closely. And it's just the motion information that makes this possible; there are really no other sources of information here telling you about the shape of the bent-up paperclip.

Even in situations in which we have other information available to tell us about the 3-dimensional layout of the surroundings that are nearby us, motion information tends to drive our perceptions. We just considered an example of that, actually, with that Ames room illusion. For the Ames room, without motion—with just a small, round hole to look through—we were totally confused about the size of the 2 people in there. With the motion, the illusion disappears.

So motion perception is important and our visual system is really good at using motion information for finding things and perceiving details about their identity, size, and shape. How does this motion perception work? One of the most interesting things about motion perception is that it's inferred after it's already finished happening. Consider a still image in which a single square is present. Just a square sitting on a screen; no motion here. Consider another image with another square, one that looks just like the first one, located in a different position on the screen. Again, no motion here; just another stationary display.

If I were to rapidly alternate between these 2 pictures, suddenly you wouldn't perceive them as 2 stationary squares but as a single square moving back and forth. This phenomenon is known as "apparent motion" because motion is perceived but there's nothing actually moving; in other words, just 2 stationary pictures. Your sensory system is making another one of those inferences that I keep describing. There's a square in one place, then it vanishes; then at about the same time, another very similar square appears in a different location. It could be 2 different, stationary squares, but your brain concludes that it's more likely that the 2 squares are the same object in 2 different positions. It fills in the motion between them and voilà, apparent motion.

Every time you watch a movie, you're seeing apparent motion. Movies are just many still images presented in rapid sequence. The motion that takes place in movies is fully inferred in between those stationary images. You may have also had a flip book, maybe when you were a kid, where you flip fast through some pages. A figure that's present in there seems to move fast or slow depending upon how quickly or slowly you flip those pages. If you flip too slowly, the illusion's lost; you just see the stationary images. You see them as just that: still pictures. But if you go fast, then you see that apparent motion.

To try to emphasize the notion that this is an inference, this process—that the motion is inferential—let me show you another slightly more complex example. It again consists of 2 stationary images. In one, there's a black square up and to the left, and another one down and to the right of the center of the image. The second image looks just like the first, except now the square on the left is down rather than up, and the square on the right is up rather than down.

If I were to rapidly alternate between these 2 images, there are at least 4 things you might see. First, you might perceive it as 2 images in which there are 2 squares in different positions without any motion at all. That's unlikely, but it's certainly possible; and it is, as I keep pointing out, what's actually present in the images. Second, you might see 2 squares alternately moving up and down. Third, you might see 2 squares alternately moving from side to side. If you were to watch the display long enough, your perception would just naturally change back and forth between these 2 alternatives about every 30 seconds or so, just periodically shifting between them.

If you want, you could force yourself to see the sideways motion by holding up a hand and blocking your view of the 2 bottom square positions. This would force you to see the lateral apparent motion between the 2 top squares, such that if you then pulled your hand away, the bottom square would seem to go side-to-side as well. To force yourself to see the vertical motion, you could hold up a hand and block your view of the left 2 square positions. You would see that vertical motion of the 2 right squares. If you then pulled your hand away, the left square would seem to go vertically as well.

There's even another possibility that I didn't realize when I created this display. A student pointed it out to me after I showed them all of these different interpretations. He raised his hand and said, "There are more." As the displays alternate between these 2 square positions, if you point your index finger at the top left position, then the top right, then the bottom right, then the bottom left and then back around again; if you do this a few times, you'll see this display as rotating in that direction. If you move your finger in the other direction, it can rotate the other way as well.

It's important to note that this is all with exactly the same display. My point in belaboring this one display so much is that there are many different, equally plausible perceptions of it. No one is inherently the right one. Even given that uncertainty, we don't perceive an ambiguous display at any time. Your visual system makes its best guess—an inference—about what event would produce the sensory inputs that you're receiving; and it's that inference that you perceive: not the sensory inputs per se, but the result of that inference. Here, the inference is essentially always motion. My other reason for talking so much about these apparent motion displays is to be clear about the steps involved in a motion inference.

Let's think just a bit more about the simplest apparent motion display: the one in which a single square seems to move from one position to another. I want you to ponder with me the timing of the stimulus presentation and how it relates to the timing of your perception of the event. If I alternate between these 2 square images, we perceive 3 things: First, we perceive the square at its initial starting location one; second, we see the square moving from this location on its way to location 2; finally, we see the square arriving at location 2.

It's really critical here to note that this perception doesn't match the order in which the events actually occur. First, we do see the square in location one; that's the first thing that's presented to your eyes for an apparent motion event. The second thing, however, is the presentation of the square at location 2. It's only at that moment that your brain can begin to fill in the motion event. Even though the inference of the motion doesn't even begin—can't begin—until the motion is finished, we don't experience it that way. Your brain, as we will see with many aspects of perception, seems to construct the world that you experience. It fills things in spatially—as with the blind spot that we discussed back in Lecture 1—and with motion, it also seems to fill things in temporally, and even to shift the order of events when it makes sense to do that.

Okay. So we've talked about how important motion is for our everyday perceptions and discussed the truly inferential nature of motion perception. I want to spend a little time talking in more detail about how your visual system parses and interprets complex motion information. Let's start by considering 3 different situations that produce 3 different inputs on the retina; that is, onto the back of the eye. Let's start simple. First, consider a stationary viewer, looking at a stationary environment, in which one object is moving; for instance a person walking across your field of view. Our perception is obvious for this situation: The world is stationary; the man is moving.

Consider a second situation, however, in which the entire background seems to move leftward across the retina. There are at least 2 possibilities for a sensory input like this; 2 things that could produce it: It could be that everything—the whole room—is moving to the left; but if you watched a movie of this, that wouldn't be your perception. You would perceive it as a stationary world with a rightward moving point of view. You produce this type of display yourself whenever you move your head to the right. In most situations, our visual input and the movement of images that are projected onto our retina are a combination of these 2 types of inputs: motion of things in the environment and motions of our retina through the environment.

Consider one more sensory input; one in which a man is walking, but he remains stationary in the middle of the retina. As he remains in the middle of the retina, however, the entire background drifts leftward across that retina. You produce visual inputs like this yourself whenever you follow a moving target with your eyes.

The point to make here is that just because something is moving across your retina doesn't mean that it's actually moving. Conversely, just because something is stationary on your retina doesn't mean that it's actually stationary. How do we figure out what's moving and what's not? At least part of the answer to this question has to do with a close linkage between the motor systems that move our eyes and the sensory systems that process visual information. When your brain sends a command to your eyes, telling them to move from one place to another, it also sends a copy of that command to your visual cortex. This copy of that motor command is referred to as a corollary discharge. By subtracting out the visual motion caused by your eye movements, your visual cortex is then able to figure out what's moving and what's not.

There are at least 2 really good sources of evidence for this explanation; this idea of corollary discharge. You can do one of the experiments right now on your own visual system. I want you to close one eye, and with your index finger, reach up with your finger and gently press on your lower eyelid. As you do, you will cause your eye to jiggle a little bit as you press on it. Now, this isn't how you usually control your eye movements (with your finger), so there's no corollary discharge—no copy of the message—that's sent from your arm onto the visual cortex. Since there's no corollary discharge signal to tell the visual system to subtract out the motion caused by this eye movement, you'll notice a very particular perception as you press on your eye: The whole world will seem to move up and down! As you move your eyeball down a little, the projection of the world shifts up. If that happens without your eye moving, it would mean that the world has moved up, and that's what you perceive.

There's another very famous experiment—one conducted in a medical laboratory—that really nails this corollary discharge phenomenon. In the 1950s, American psychology was dominated by B. F. Skinner and the behaviorist school of thought. One of the tenets of their theoretical approach was that no thought, perception, or learning can take place without involving the body itself. To test this, a volunteer participated in a somewhat frightening procedure. He agreed to be put on a ventilator while he was injected with drugs that paralyzed his motor system. He needed to be on the ventilator because the muscles that control breathing were paralyzed as well. If the body was needed to control thought and memory, then his thought and memory should have ceased as well until the drugs wore off. Other experimenters showed this paralyzed man during the paralysis procedure images, words, and math problems; and then later, their plan was to test if he'd be able to recall them (and the answers to the math problems) after the paralysis wore off and he was able to talk to them again.

For what it's worth, he was able to think and remember in this state. We now know very clearly that thought can take place without the muscles being involved. Something unexpected happened, however, with this procedure that the man reported as being one of the more salient things that happened when he was paralyzed. As soon as he became paralyzed, he noticed that the world seemed to jump around wildly, up and down and side to side. Eventually, he figured out that this happened whenever he tried to move his eyes. Remember that his muscles were paralyzed, including the muscles that control his eyes, but the corollary discharge system within the central nervous system was still active. When he tried to move his eyes, a signal was sent to his visual cortex telling it to expect a particular eye movement. When it didn't take place, the visual cortex inferred that the objects in the world— indeed the whole environment—had moved in exactly the same direction as the eyes.

Think this through with me for a moment. If you moved your eyes 10 degrees to the right, and if the world around you rotated 10 degrees to the right as well at that same moment in time, what would you see? You would see the same thing before and after the eye movement, right? Twelve degrees up with the eyes and 12 degrees of world movement; same visual input before and after the eye movement. This paralyzed man had this exact experience. No matter where he moved his eyes, the visual input didn't change. The only inference that the visual cortex could make was that the world must be moving in exact synchrony with the man's eyes. That's what the visual system inferred, and so that's what the man perceived.

Your visual system uses a lot of other information to make inferences about motions as well. One simple assumption that it makes is that any motion will follow the shortest path possible between 2 points. This is called the shortest path constraint; a good name for it. In our simple apparent motion example, for instance, any number of different motions could have been inferred between where the square started and where it finished, but you almost certainly perceived it as a straight line motion between the start and end points.

But this rule isn't followed blindly. Your visual cortex can actually be very smart about what it is that's doing the movements that it's observing.

Consider 2 still images of a person with a bent, raised knee. In one, the person's hand is held behind the knee so that you can't see the hand. In the second image, that hand is moved in front of the knee. If this sequence is presented in alternation with a 200 millisecond gap in between those images, most people see the arm as moving around the knee rather than moving along the shortest path, which would be straight through the knee. Many viewers mention seeing a lateral or side-to-side motion of the hand when it's moving around it in front of the leg. That lateral motion isn't in the stimulus; it's constructed by the viewer's visual cortex as it considers the physical, biological constraints of a human body in motion. We know that hands need to go around legs, they can't go through them.

Your brain needs a few hundred milliseconds to fill this in, however. If I were to show the same pair of images without that small hundred millisecond delay in between them, you would notice that your perception of them would change. If there's no 200 millisecond delay between the images, the arm does seem to follow that shortest path constraint, and in so doing move right through the knee. If it's given enough time—and by that I mean a few hundred milliseconds—your visual system even considers lighting and shadows when it infers motion. Consider an event in which a ball rolls across a stage, progressing from the front left to the back right of a platform. If we add shadows and shading that are consistent with that motion, the perception remains about the same. It's possible, however, to add a different shadow; one that moves from left to right across that surface platform as the ball moves. The ball moves just as before. Even without changing the movement of the ball, the perceived path of the ball shifts dramatically. Now the ball seems to float up into the air without changing its position in depth. A bouncing shadow can even make the ball seem to bounce up and down as it moves across the stage.

In all of these situations, the motions of the actual ball remain constant. Only the shadows are changing. But as those shadows do, the perceived motion of the ball shifts dramatically. The human visual system considers the pattern of input and makes its best guess as to what real-world motion would be most likely to produce that pattern. The shadows shift these probabilities and voilà: the perception changes. In general, it's those inferences that you perceive, not the sensory inputs themselves.

Some of those inferences are even based on the internal state of your brain. In Lecture 4, I talked about how your brain contains a large set of retinotopic maps; that is, a set of neurons with spatial organization that matches the organization of the retina. Many of these maps represent information about motion. One map encodes the presence of upward motion; that is, there's activity in every place on the map where there is upward motion present in the retinal input. Another set encodes the presence of downward motion. Another pair encodes leftward motion and rightward motion. For a wide range of directions, there are neurons that encode what areas of the retina contain image elements that are moving in a particular direction. These layers function somewhat independently, but they're also connected together in some interesting ways. For opposite directions of motion, they are connected in an inhibitory fashion. That is, whenever the upward sensitive neurons are active—whenever it's active for a particular place on the retina—they send signals that inhibit the activity of the corresponding downward sensitive neurons, and vice versa. When the downward sensitive neurons are active, they inhibit the upward sensitive neurons for the corresponding position on the retina. It's as if there's this ongoing tug-of-war between these neurons. Whenever one wins the tug-of-war, you perceive motion in that direction.

Imagine watching a waterfall for a few minutes, keeping your eye fixed in the middle of the downward-moving water. For the demonstration to work, you need to keep your eyes fixated on the water for a sold couple of minutes. It's okay if, as you do this, you notice your eyes drifting downward from time to time. As soon as you do notice this, however, just move them back up to the middle and try to keep them held in position there in the middle of the water. I'm going to keep talking, but keep staring at the waterfall. While viewing a waterfall, the downward sensitive neurons are winning that "opponent process" tug-of-war. Opponent process is the name given to this cross-inhibitory connection pattern that I'm describing here. In later lectures, I'll discuss the fact that this system of organization is present for many aspects of sensory processing; not just motion, but color, orientation, and even for more complex combinations of stimuli.

As you continue to gaze at the waterfall, the downward sensitive neurons are receiving a lot of their favorite input: downward movement. They're winning that opponent tug-of-war big time. As they continue to be active, however, they're growing fatigued; and the upward sensitive neurons are getting very, very rested. If, after you fatigue those neurons, you look away from the waterfall at something that's stationary, you'll then give those downward and upward sensitive neurons the same amount of input. When you do this, such that the 2 sets of neurons are receiving that same amount of input, the tired downward sensitive neurons are going to start losing that tug of war, and the upward sensitive neurons will start winning. Your visual system will see this tug-of-war victory and make an inference that there's upward motion. If, after about this amount of time, you look at a stationary stimulus (you can go ahead and do that now), say the middle of a brick wall, you'll see that upward motion. When I do this demo with a big group of students, I usually hear people say, "Ooh!" Hopefully you just did. Even though the stationary stimulus isn't moving, the motion after-effect creates a clear sense that it's drifting upward.

In this lecture, we've explored how you perceive motion. Hopefully I've made clear just how important motion information is, as well as some of the really complex, inferential processes that guide our processing of motion information. In our next lecture, we'll talk about another critical aspect of visual processing and visual inference: We'll discuss depth perception; how your eyes help you to know just where things are located out in the world. As with motion, you'll see just how perceptually intelligent your brain can be. I look forward to talking with you then.

# Seeing Distance and Depth
## Lecture 6

D epth perception is one of the classic mysteries of sensory processing. Our retinas are 2-dimensional, so how can we perceive a world in 3 dimensions? Euclid and his contemporaries in ancient Greece were among the first to ponder the impossibility of depth and size perception.

- If you tip a 2-dimensional rectangle away from the viewer, the Euclidians noted, it appears to be a trapezoid. Tilt the small end of a trapezoid toward you, and it looks like a square.

- For every given shape, there are an infinite number of different projections one can produce. Conversely—here is the "impossibility of perception" part—given any projected shape, there are an infinite number of different 3-dimensional shapes that could produce it.

- A similar story can be told about size and distance. A square has a particular size, but the size of its projection onto a retina (or a video screen) changes as the square moves closer or farther away. For any given projection size, there are an infinite number of different physical sizes that could produce it.

- Yet the early Greek philosophers were incorrect about one thing; perception of size and distance are clearly possible. You know this from experience.

- You also probably realize that your depth perception is not always accurate. Humans are much better at judging nearer distances than farther distances.

- There are many sources of information, called cues, which support our depth and size perception, and depth and size perception interact with one another. What we actually perceive are objects in depth.

- Once again, to fully understand this perception system, we have to understand how the brain integrates many different sources of information to produce a single, maximally accurate perception of the surfaces and objects around us.

- Let's consider an image of Mount McKinley viewed from near Lake Wonder in Alaska. All viewers would likely agree, for instance, that a moose on the near bank is closer to the camera than the low hill or the snow-covered mountain on the far side of the lake.

- There is a salient distance illusion that present in such photographs, however. The mountain on the other side of the lake looks steeper than it actually is because our brain tends to compress greater distances but not greater heights. The farther the distance, the greater our underestimate of it.

- An unfortunately common cause of drowning is visible in this example. In a warm climate, people often look across a lake and decide that the far bank does not seem too far away, not realizing until they swim too far and exhaust themselves that it is several miles away.

- Depth perception is influenced by a great many sources of information, called depth cues. There are so many cues that sometimes depth perception research seems like a series of list-making exercises, and new cues are still being discovered.

- There are 4 broad categories of depth cues: oculomotor, binocular, motion, and pictorial.

- Convergence angle is an oculomotor cue. Your eyes are in slightly different locations. If you look at something in the far distance, you aim your eyes almost parallel to one another out into the distance; if you look at something nearby, however, your eyes turn slightly toward each other.

- Your brain knows both the distance between your eyes and how far the eyes have turned inward and can triangulate the distance to what your eyes have fixated on. This relation between eye rotation and distance is called convergence.

- In an early experiment on convergence, a man named Hans Wallach developed the telestereoscope, basically a pair of periscopes turned on their sides. Looking through the telestereoscope greatly increases the convergence angles between your eyes, as if your eyes were several feet apart.

- When viewers look through a telestereoscope, their perceptions of size change dramatically, making the world and everything in it seem much, much smaller.

- Another oculomotor cue has to do with lens thickening. Recall from Lecture 2 how the eye focuses images onto your retina: For objects in the distance, the lenses in your eyes relax and remain relatively thin. As objects get closer, the muscles in your eye squeeze the lens, causing it to get shorter and thicker.

- As the muscles contract, they send information to the visual cortex about how hard they are pressing on the lens. The more

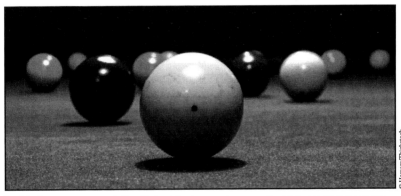

In this image, you can tell which objects are closer and which are farther away by cues such as overlapping and relative size, even with 1 eye closed.

accommodation is needed to create a clear image of something, the closer that object must be, which is another cue to the visual cortex.

- Stereopsis is a binocular cue used with increasing frequency in making 3-D movies. For any frame of the movie, there are 2 images projected onto the screen. The special glasses ensure that your left eye sees one of those images while the right eye sees the other.

- This creates a compelling sense of depth because under normal circumstances, your eyes are almost always receiving 2 slightly different views of the world, which your visual system uses to make inferences about relative distance.

- Two different types of disparity are important here: crossed and uncrossed. To demonstrate these, extend your right arm out to arm's length and keep your eyes fixated on it, then take your left thumb and put it between your eyes and the right thumb.

- As you do so, you will notice that your left thumb appears to split into 2 ghostly images, because there is disparity between where your left thumb is projecting onto your left eye and your right eye.

- Next, keep looking at your right thumb, but focus your attention on the ghostly left thumb. If you alternately close your left and right eyes, the left thumb will seem to jump back and forth. That is crossed disparity.

- As you move the left thumb closer to the right thumb, the amount of disparity between those 2 left thumbs gets smaller and smaller and smaller. If you move it back farther from the point of fixation, the amount of disparity gets bigger. Your visual system is making use of the amount of crossed disparity to figure out how much closer the left thumb is than the right thumb.

- Next, look at your left thumb while moving your right thumb out into the distance beyond it. Now there are 2 images of your right thumb. If you alternately close your right and left eyes, the right thumb seems to jump back and forth. That is uncrossed disparity.

- Based on the amount of crossed and uncrossed disparity present for objects and surfaces in the visual input, your visual system can very precisely determine the spatial layout of nearby surfaces.

- Stereopsis is perhaps the single most studied depth cue in the history of sensory science. You can create a stimulus in which there is literally no depth—just some geometric figures on a piece of paper, for instance—and with stereopsis, suddenly those pictures are jumping off the page.

- It is not true, however, that you need 2 eyes to see depth. There are hundreds of sources of depth information available to us.

- Motion parallax is a very different depth cue, yet it is derived from the same type of relation that drives stereopsis. With stereopsis, you can determine distances because your eyes are at slightly different locations. With motion parallax, you can determine distance as your whole body moves to different locations over time.

- If you have ever looked out the window of a moving car or train, you may have noticed that objects nearby whiz by quickly while more distant objects move by more slowly. There is a direct relation between that velocity and an object's distance.

- Even if other depth information suggests something else, motion parallax tends to dominate our perceptions of distance. In experiments with people who had lost an eye, people's depth perception was slightly impaired just after the injury. But in the following weeks, they developed a tendency to move their heads more to compensate and returned their depth perception to normal.

- Pigeons bob their heads to create more motion parallax to see their environment better.

- The category of monocular cues is by far the biggest. It contains any source of information that can be translated into a picture—that is, one you could look at monocularly and still see depth, like in a photo of Mount McKinley.

- Occlusion, when one object partially blocks another, is in many ways the most robust of depth cues. The object doing the blocking must be closer.

- To understand height in field, imagine that we are standing on a flat surface, looking out at an array of objects as they extend into the distance. If I point at some object that is close up, I point downward. If I point to an object farther away, I raise my arm higher. Thus, if I know how high some object is in my visual field, I can infer how far away it is.

- Height in field can also work as a cue for objects that are overhead. If there are 2 clouds in the sky above me, the closer cloud will be higher in my visual field than the more distant cloud, the reverse of objects on the ground.

- You may have learned linear perspective in an art class. For regularly shaped objects like rectilinear buildings, train tracks, or roads, you can create the impression of depth by marking some point on your drawing paper as infinity and then drawing lines that converge on that point.

- Atmospheric perspective is especially salient on foggy days or in smoggy cities. The light from distant objects has to travel through air before it reaches your eyes. Most air is almost transparent but not completely so. By looking at how hazy an object appears to be, it is possible to estimate its distance.

- Texture density, relative size, and familiar size all work the way these other depth cues do as well. For more distant objects and surfaces, something changes about its projection.

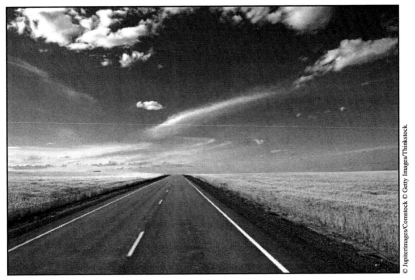

**Linear perspective, often used by artists to create the impression of great depth, is the tendency of straight lines to seem to converge at a point on the horizon.**

- Any object in the environment projects an image of a certain size onto the retina. The object itself also has a particular physical size, and the object is located at a particular location in depth.

- If you know any 2 of the 3—retinal size, physical size, and physical distance—the third can be calculated. Your brain considers the relationship between these 3 things all the time.

- By creating an illusion of closer distance, it is possible to create an illusion of smaller size. The reverse can be done as well. If I make you think that some object is farther away than it actually is without changing the size of its retinal projection, then I can create the illusion that the object is much larger.

- Researchers are discovering new depth cues all the time; here is one subtle example that nonetheless conveys just how perceptually intelligent and flexible humans are. That cue is related to gravity and falling.

- If, on the surface of the planet Earth, you drop a ball, it will fall at a rate of about 4.9 meters per second, and our visual system can easily use falling rate information to determine the distances to things.

- If I put someone in a virtual environment in which things fall a little bit slower than normal, the environment will look bigger. Conversely, if I virtually increase gravitational acceleration for falling objects, the simulated world looks smaller.

- This is really clever work; the research is impressive and elegant, but the researchers who published it pointed out that they were not actually the first people to discover this. A certain group of filmmakers had been capitalizing on it for decades: the makers of monster movies of the 1960s and 1970s.

- In those movies, a 5.5-foot-tall actor in a rubber suit would march out of the ocean and attack some scale model of a city, complete with toy tanks and airplanes. Filmmakers would show these scenes in slow motion, knowing that this made the "monster" seem more compelling because it brought the image more into line with this gravitational constraint.

- Perception researchers have realized that not all depth cues are created equal. Occlusion, for instance, only tells you something is closer, not how close either object is. Other cues work well close up but not at a distance, or vice versa.

- Your visual system seems to have all of this information incorporated into how it combines different sources of information. If you are working with tools to build something, then stereopsis and convergence take over. If you are driving your car, cues like height in field dominate.

## Suggested Reading

Cutting and Vishton, "Perceiving Layout and Knowing Distances."

Pinker, *How the Mind Works.*

## Questions to Consider

1. This lecture made it clear that we consistently misperceive distances, especially beyond a few hundred meters. In the far distance, space is compressed. In the near distance, compression is much less. If that is so, why does the space in front of you not seem to expand as you walk down the street?

2. "When I close one of my eyes, I have no depth perception anymore. The world looks flat." Many people have made this statement, but it is clearly incorrect. Several studies have shown that we can use motion and pictorial depth cues to accurately perceive distances, even with only one eye. Nonetheless, many people share this belief. How is this possible?

# Seeing Distance and Depth
## Lecture 6—Transcript

In this lecture, we'll consider one of the classic mysteries of sensory processing: depth perception. Since the time of the early Greeks—in particular the time of a guy named Euclid—philosophers have pondered how depth perception works. The surfaces of our retina—the surfaces onto which light is projected on the insides of our eyes—are 2-dimensional. Nonetheless, we don't perceive a 2-dimensional world. Even if we close one eye so that we only have a single 2D image to work with, we perceive a precisely structured 3-dimensional environment that surrounds us.

In some of their writings, Euclid and his contemporaries pondered the impossibility of depth and size perception. Consider a rectangular stimulus. If I were to take a rectangle and tip it backwards, it would project not a rectangle, but actually a trapezoid onto your eyes or onto your video monitor. If you were to trace that shape on the video monitor with a marker—please don't, but if you did—it would be a trapezoid projection. If, alternatively, I have a trapezoid shape and I were to tilt the small end toward you at just the right angle, it would look like a square. That is, for every given shape, there are an infinite number of different projections that I can produce. Conversely—and here's the impossibility of perception part—given any projected shape, there are an infinite number of different 3D shapes that could produce it.

A similar story can be told about size and distance. Any square has a particular size, but the size of its projection onto a retina or a video screen changes as the square moves closer and farther away. If I have a small rectangle and move it close enough to you, it would project an image that's the same size as a larger rectangle that's farther away. For any given projection size, there are an infinite number of different physical sizes that could produce it. How do we go from a 2D projection to a 3D perception?

Let me assure you that the early Greek philosophers were incorrect about the impossibility part; perception of size and distance are clearly possible. Actually, you don't have to trust me on that account; you perceive depth accurately all the time. In this lecture, I'll discuss how to untangle this paradox and how your visual system does it every day.

First, I want to point out some ways in which your depth perception is not accurate. In general, our visual system provides us with fairly accurate information about distance, but we're particularly bad at judging very far distances. Second, we'll discuss the "cue approach" to studying depth perception. There are many sources of information, typically called cues, which support our depth and size perception. I'll describe the big categories of these cues and provide examples of some. Third, we'll talk about how depth and size perception interact with one another. If I'm being careful with my terms, I should point out that we don't actually perceive depth, per se. What we actually perceive are objects in depth. If we look out into a big space, no matter how big it is, we won't see anything at all. It's only when there's something, some object, within that space that we can see something. When we see those things—whatever they are—we typically perceive them as having a particular position as well as a particular size. Perceiving that size is integral to our process of depth perception. We'll finish this lecture with a consideration of how we put all these many different sources of information together, combining a large number of separate sources of information to produce a single, maximally accurate perception of the surfaces and objects around us.

Let's consider an image of Mount McKinley viewed from the far side of Lake Wonder in Alaska. There's even a moose in the foreground there to spice up this image. We would all be accurate in judging the relative distances to features in this picture. I think it's safe to assume that we would all agree that the moose is closer than the far side of the lake; also that the green hill on the far side is farther than the moose and also closer than the distant, snow-covered mountain. We could even extend this sort of relative judgment to particular features on the mountain; there'd be a great agreement across many of us if we viewed them. For instance, the base is clearly closer than the peak.

As accurate as this relative depth perception might be, there's a salient distance illusion that's present in this figure. Put your arm out in front of you and tilt it until it matches your perception of how steep the mountain is. That is, if you were to put your elbow at the bottom of the mountain and aim your fingertips directly at the peak, what would the angle be? I think it's actually informative to do that yourself, so please do that. If you're like most people, except maybe if you're a cartographer, your arm is probably angled somewhere around 60 degrees above horizontal. The mountain is very steep, but it's not nearly as steep as it looks. Here's a plot of the actual elevations of Mount McKinley from our viewing location on that far side of the lake all the way up to the peak. The mountain is steep, but you'll notice that the angle is quite a bit less than 60 degrees; it's actually closer to 45. Why is our perception so far off here? Why does the mountain that's this steep actually look much steeper?

The cause of the illusion is our tendency to "compress" far distances. We're very accurate for things out to about 10 meters; less accurate out to 100 meters; and as we get to several miles away, we tend to greatly underestimate distances. Basically, the farther the distance, the greater our underestimate of it. These underestimates serve to compress the layout of those far surfaces and objects. The perceived distances are compressed, but not the perceived heights of things. This serves to reduce the width of the slope, making it seem much steeper than it actually is.

An unfortunately common cause of drowning is visible in this image. This water is very cold—very cold, even in the summer—so you probably wouldn't be tempted to try to swim across. In a warmer climate, however, people often look across a lake and decide that the far bank doesn't seem too far away. They wade in and start swimming, thinking that they have maybe a few hundred meters to traverse in order to get to the other side. The far side of this lake, however, is actually several miles away. Even a very strong swimmer might be too far out before he or she realizes that the far bank doesn't seem to be getting any closer. Hopefully the swimmer will have enough energy to return to the starting point before he or she gets into serious trouble. Your depth perception is accurate under many circumstances, but for far distances, you should consider consulting a map if it's an important decision.

So how does this depth perception process work? Depth perception is influenced by a great many sources of information: depth cues. There are so many of these cues, that sometimes depth perception research seems to be a series of list-making exercises. There are dozens and dozens of relations between depth and the image on the eyes that your brain uses to interpret that depth; and as people continue to study the topic, even thousands of years after the time that those Greek philosophers started thinking about depth perception, even after all that time, there are still new depth cues being discovered. These many different sources of depth information can be considered within 4 broad categories that I'll talk about now: oculomotor, stereopsis, motion, and pictorial. Let's consider each of those categories in turn.

When you look at things, you point your eyes at them. Your 2 eyes are in slightly different locations. If you look at something in the far distance, you aim your eyes almost parallel to one another out into the distance. If you're looking at something that is close, however, your eyes turn inward to fixate it. If you know the distance between your eyes—and your brain does know that—and if you know how far the eyes have turned inward to fixate something, then it's straightforward to triangulate the distance out to that point of fixation.

This relation between eye rotation and distance is called "convergence." It's a very powerful and salient source of depth information. In an early experiment on convergence, a man named Hans Wallach developed something he called the telestereoscope. You probably know what a periscope is; this is a device with some mirrors and some lenses that enable you to look into a tube down near the bottom and see up and around corners through the top. Imagine if I took a periscope and rotated it to the side. I would see the world as if one of my eyes was located at the other end of that periscope, off to the side of my head. If I had 2 of these periscopes off to the sides, I could set them up so that one extended to the left and one to the right. As I looked into those 2 periscopes, I would see what the world would look like if my left and right eyes were located very far apart; as if my head was really, really large. This, in essence, is what a telestereoscope is. By moving the eyes further apart—or alternatively by setting it up so it moves the eyes closer together—Wallach changed the convergence angles produced when people viewed things. As he did, viewers' perceptions of size changed dramatically.

If, for instance, my eyes were a full meter apart from one another, how do you think the world would look; bigger or smaller? Think that through for a second. If things stayed the way they are now while you increased in size, how should they look? If you said "smaller," you're right. Conversely, if the telestereoscope put the eyes very, very close together, then the world would suddenly seem much larger. All that change would be due to the depth cue of convergence.

There's one other oculomotor cue of note here for depth perception: accommodation. Recall from Lecture 2 how the eye focuses images onto your retina. For objects in the distance, the lens in your eyes relaxes and remains relatively thin. As things get closer and closer, however, the muscles in your eye squeeze the lens from the sides, causing it to get shorter and thicker. (Unlike lenses in your glasses or camera, the lenses in your eyes are flexible and rubbery.) As the muscles squeeze down, they send copies of those signals to the visual cortex about how hard they're pressing on the lens. The visual cortex uses that information. The more accommodation is needed to create a clear image of something, the closer that object must be. This has been studied using various lens systems that change the relationship between accommodation amount and distance, but if you've ever put on a pair of new glasses—or maybe someone else's glasses by accident—you probably noticed that the world seemed to change shape. The distances that you viewed things through those glasses appeared different. The thing that causes those perceived changes in distance and shape is the change to the relationship between accommodation and distance.

So those are the 2 oculomotor depth cues: convergence of the 2 eyes and accommodation (the amount of muscle pressure exerted on your lens to focus those eyes). Let's move on to stereopsis. This is the cue that's been used with increasing frequency in 3D movies. When you arrive at the movies, they give you a pair of 3D glasses to wear. For any frame of the movie, there are 2 images projected onto the movie screen. The 3D glasses make it so that your left eye sees one of those—and only one of those—2 images while the right eye sees the other. There are many different techniques used to achieve this, but it always comes back to this one image per eye set-up. The reason that this can create a compelling sense of depth is that under normal circumstances—in the 3D world, as opposed to the 3D movie—your 2 eyes are almost always receiving 2 slightly different views of the world. Your visual system is remarkably adept at using these slight disparities between these 2 inputs to make inferences about the relative distance to elements in the surrounding world. There are 2 different types of disparity that are important here: crossed disparity and uncrossed disparity.

To demonstrate these, you can use your 2 thumbs. I want you to extend your right arm out to a full arms-length and keep your eyes fixated on that distant thumb. While you do that, I want you to take your left thumb and put it in between your eyes and the right thumb. As you do that, especially if you move that left thumb closer to you, you'll notice that it splits into 2 ghosty images. The reason that's happening is because there is disparity between the place that your left thumb is projecting onto your left eye and your right eye. If while you're doing this—so keep looking at your right thumb, but focus your attention on that ghosty left thumb—if you alternately close your left and right eyes, you'll notice your thumb jumping back and forth. When you look at the thumb with your right eye, it's on the left; when you look at the thumb with your left eye, it's on the right; that is, there's cross disparity. If you keep doing this, you'll notice that as you move the left thumb closer to the fixated right thumb that the amount of disparity between those 2 left thumbs gets smaller and smaller and smaller. If you move it back farther from the point of fixation, the amount of disparity gets bigger. What your visual system does is it makes use of the amount of that cross disparity to figure out how much closer the left thumb is than the right thumb, or how much closer objects are in general.

Now for uncrossed disparity, I want you to look at your left thumb; fixate your left thumb while moving your right thumb out in the distance beyond it. The thing you'll notice there is now there are 2 images of your right thumb. If you alternately close your right and left eyes, you'll notice that the right thumb jumps back and forth. When you look with your right eye, the thumb is on the right side; when you look with your left eye, it's on the left side; that is, now there's uncrossed disparity. Based on the amount of crossed and uncrossed disparity present for objects and surfaces in the visual input, your visual system can very precisely determine the spatial layout of nearby surfaces.

Stereopsis is perhaps the single most studied depth cue in the history of sensory science. I think that's at least in part because it's just really fun to play with. You can create a stimulus in which there is literally no depth—just some geometric figures on a piece of paper, for instance—and with stereopsis, suddenly those pictures are jumping off the page. There's been so much work done on this cue that sometimes people say you need 2 eyes in order to see depth. Students of mine will sometimes off-handedly comment that if they close one eye, they lose their depth perception; that the world becomes flat. This is a little bit of a pet peeve of mine. There are, as I've pointed out, hundreds of sources of depth information available to us. Stereopsis is certainly one, and it's a very salient cue at that, but it's certainly not the only one. People with one eye are able to see and judge distances. Even if you covered an eye, you would be able to throw a ball and hit a target. In short, you would be able to perceive depth just fine.

Motion parallax is a very different depth cue, but it's actually derived from the same type of relation that drives stereopsis. With stereopsis, you can determine distances because your eyes are at slightly different locations. With motion parallax, you can determine distance as your whole body moves to different locations over time. If you've ever looked out the side window of a moving car or train, you may have noticed that objects nearby whiz through your visual field very fast. Objects in the distance move across your visual field more slowly. There's essentially a direct relation between the velocity and the distance in the way that objects move across your field of view: the faster the movement, the closer the object. I mentioned in Lecture 5 just how important motion information can be; it's absolutely the case here. Even if other depth information suggests something else, motion parallax tends to dominate our perceptions of distance.

A few moments ago, I mentioned my little pet peeve about people equating stereopsis with all of depth perception. There was an experiment performed by a researcher working with people who had through accident or injury lost an eye; not just covered the eye for the experiment, but actually lost the eye permanently. If he studied these patients shortly after the injury, their depth perception—their ability to judge distances in this case—was slightly impaired. So when you close one eye I guess it is the case the world looks a little flatter. The interesting part came when he studied them later. In both the initial study session and the follow up session several weeks later, this researcher placed a motion tracking device on the participants' heads as they performed their distance judgment task. The patients weren't aware of it, but in those weeks during which they were recovering from their injury, they developed a tendency to move their heads back and forth more. As they did, they generated more motion parallax, and in so doing returned their depth perception abilities to normal.

My other favorite application of motion parallax is that of the common pigeon. If you ever watch a pigeon walk, it seems very inefficient. Pigeons seem to (for lack of a better term) strut as they move, bobbing their heads up and down and back and forth. Studies of pigeons have revealed that they don't do this for show or because they have to do this when they walk, pigeons do this to generate more motion and more motion parallax so that they can see their environment that much better.

Okay. So we've talked about oculomotor cues, stereopsis, and motion parallax. The last of those 4 broad categories to mention is pictorial or monocular cues to depth. This category is by far the biggest. It contains any source of information that can be translated into a picture; that is, one you could look at monocularly as well and still see the depth. When an artist produces a painting, for instance, it's essentially always a 2-dimensional form; there's no depth at all. When we view a great painting or a great photo, however, there's often a compelling sense of a 3-dimensional space. Artists create this sense of space, translating a wide range of depth cues to the canvas. Let's just run through a few of them; I'll talk about occlusion, height in field, linear perspective, and atmospheric perspective in detail, and I'll mention some others.

Occlusion is not thought of as an especially important source of depth information—by most people, anyway—but it's in many ways the most robust of depth cues that are out there. If one object partially blocks or occludes your view of another, then the object doing the blocking is closer; you can guarantee it. If I have 2 really thin pieces of paper and place one in front of the other, you know which one is closer, even though it's only closer by a few thousandths of an inch. Even if I were pretty far away from you—say a hundred yards away—as long as you can still pick out which sheet of paper is the one in front, as long as you can still make out the shapes of those papers, occlusion will tell you which paper is closer. Being able to distinguish a few thousandths of an inch of depth across a range of several hundred yards is remarkably accurate. In terms of relative depth perception, occlusion is certainly the champ of the depth cues.

To understand height in field as a source of depth information, imagine that you're standing on a flat surface, looking out at an array of objects as they extend into the distance. If I point at some object that's close up, I'll point downward. If I move to an object—or to point to an object—that's farther, I'm going to need to need to raise my arm higher. As long as the ground is relatively uniform, the more distant the object, the higher the angle of the point. Even if I don't point with my finger, the more distant the object, the higher that object will be in the projection in my visual field. This depth cue functions by reversing that relation. If I know how high some object is in my visual field, I can infer how far away it is.

At the risk of being confusing, I should point out that height in field can also work as a cue for objects that are overhead rather than on the ground. If there are 2 clouds up in the sky above me, the closer cloud will be higher in my visual field than the more distant cloud. Notice that the relation is reversed relative to what I said for objects on the ground. For objects on the ground, higher in the visual field means farther distance; for objects in the sky, higher in the visual field means closer. In both cases, we're capitalizing on some relation between height in field and distance that exists in the world around us, and we can translate that into a pictorial image.

Linear perspective is another depth cue. I remember being taught this one in fifth grade art class. For regularly shaped objects, like rectilinear buildings, train tracks, or roads, you can create the impression of 3D depth by marking some point on your drawing paper as "infinity" and then drawing lines that converge on that point. Consider the edges of a road in a picture, for instance. As they progress, they get closer and closer together until they would "touch" at some point in the image.

Atmospheric perspective is especially salient on foggy days or in smoggy cities. Before you can see something, the light from that thing that you're trying to see has to travel through the air until it reaches your eyes. Most air is almost transparent, but it's not completely transparent. Even on the clearest of days, light scatters a little as it passes through the atmosphere. The greater the distance, the greater the scatter. By looking at how hazy an object appears to be, it's possible to make an approximate estimate of its distance from you. As with the other pictorial cues, it can be translated to an image. By drawing or painting some objects with hazy edges and colors, you can create a sense of extended depth, even where there's only a flat piece of paper.

Texture density, relative size, and familiar size all work the way these other depth cues do as well. For more distant objects and surfaces, something changes about its projection. For instance, with a repeating texture like bricks, the projected elements get smaller and smaller as they progress into the distance. By showing those smaller and smaller text elements like bricks on a picture, you can reverse this relation and create a perception of depth.

I want to say a quick word about the inherent connection between size and distance perception. Any object that's in the environment projects an image of a certain size onto the retina. The object itself also has a particular physical size, and the object is located at a particular location in depth. Three things there: retinal size, physical size, and physical distance. If you know any 2 of these 3 things, the third can be calculated. For any 2 of these 3 things, once they're specified, the third is also specified. Your brain considers this relationship between these 3 things all the time.

Imagine viewing a photo of a man in the distance. The man will have a particular size; let's say about 6 feet tall. He will be located at some actual distance; let's say about 50 meters from the camera. Given this, he'll project a certain size image onto the camera, or onto your retina. Imagine now that some element of the image is changed; something about its composition. Perhaps a hand is placed in the foreground such that it appears to be holding the man in the palm. The presence of this hand could make the man appear much closer; say about a meter away instead of 50 meters. Now the man will look closer, but the size of the retinal image projection will remain the same. What would your perception be? If something is very close and projects a very small retinal image then it must be physically small as well. By creating an illusion of closer distance, it's possible to create an illusion of smaller size. The reverse can be done as well. If I make you think that some object is farther away than it actually is, without changing the size of its retinal projection, then I'll create the illusion that the object is much larger.

Here we have 2 identical cans. The farther object projects a smaller image— the farther image of the can—but that's because it's farther away. These 2 cans are identical in terms of physical size. They're at different distances, and that's why their retinal image sizes are different. If I use Photoshop to move that piece of the image closer—the distant can up close—I can create the following image. The image of the tiny can is exactly the same as the image of the far can. It appears much, much smaller because, given our perception of depth, it's made to look so much closer. Our perception of size, distance, and object size are intimately connected, essentially all of the time.

Before we leave our discussion of a cue-based approach to depth perception, I want to talk about one more. I mentioned that researchers are discovering new depth cues all the time, and here's one example. It's very subtle, but there's clear evidence that this cue does influence our everyday perceptions. I think it conveys well just how perceptually intelligent and flexible we are as we make sense of the surrounding world. That cue is that of gravity and falling. If, on the surface of the planet Earth (so here, anywhere) you drop a ball, or almost anything, over the course of one second, that object will fall about 4.9 meters. Remember that if I know the retinal image size and physical size of something, I can calculate with some basic trigonometry how far away it is. If I watch something fall for a period of time, I know how big that distance is. I know how big the retinal image size is from the back of my eye; I can calculate the distance.

This has been studied under laboratory conditions, and it's clear that this works. Our visual system can easily use falling rate information to determine the distances to things. If I put someone in a virtual environment in which things fall a little bit slower than normal, the environment is made to look bigger. Conversely, if I virtually increase gravitational acceleration for falling objects, the simulated world looks smaller. This is really clever work; the research is impressive and elegant. But the researchers who published it pointed out that they were not actually the first people to discover this.

A certain group of filmmakers had been capitalizing on it for decades: the makers of monster movies of the 1960s and '70s. In those movies, there's always a scene in which the monster marches ashore and attacks some city. Now in these pre–computer graphics era movies, the monster was not actually some giant creature but a man in a rubber suit, often about 5½ feet tall. He walks out of some water and stomps on a miniature scaled city, often battling miniature toy tanks and airplanes. When this is presented in the theater, the filmmakers present these scenes in slow motion. The slow motion is key here: It makes the monster—actually, the guy in the monster costume—appear to be much larger and more compelling. That's because it brings the image more into line with this gravitational constraint.

So the visual system has a great number of cues at its disposal. There are dozens of different depth cues available, and maybe even more than the many that we've already identified. The human visual system capitalizes on this wealth of information in a very intelligent fashion to determine the layout of the surfaces around us. Given all of the many sources of information, how does the visual system put them together? How do we combine these different sources?

Perception researchers have realized that not all of these cues are created equal. For instance, we discussed occlusion, which works with tremendous accuracy to tell you which of 2 objects is closer—the object that does the occluding is closer, and the object that is occluded is farther—but occlusion doesn't tell you anything else about how close either of the objects is. That is, occlusion is the same for 2 objects on the table in front of you and when the moon occludes the sun during an eclipse. All it tells you is which object is closer.

Other cues work very well close up, but not very well for greater distances. Convergence, accommodation, and stereopsis are in this category. If some object is, say, 10 centimeters away, your eyes have to point very far inward to fixate it. If the object moves just 5 centimeters further away, that convergence angle will change. For an object that's 30 meters away, however, your eyes don't have to point very far inward; they're almost parallel in the direction of view at that point. And if the object moves 30 meters plus 5 more centimeters away, that angle won't change very much at all. For any cue that relies on the differences between the positions of the eyes, the functional range in terms of our sensory accuracy is really only about 10 meters.

Other cues, like atmospheric perspective, do the opposite: They don't work well at all close up like stereopsis and convergence. It's only when the light passes through some great volume of air across a great distance that the cue is even noticeable, let alone usable. Your visual system seems to have all of this information incorporated into how it combines these different sources of information. If you're working with tools to build something, maybe fixing a watch or tying a knot, then stereopsis and convergence take over, dominating your depth perception. If you're driving your car, looking at distant traffic lights and other cars, now stereopsis takes a back seat as cues like height in field begin to take over. In essence, our visual system seems to consider not just what information is available for perception but what we're doing with that information. We'll discuss this impressively flexible system in more detail in the lecture on perception and action control.

In this lecture, I discussed a wide range of methods that our visual system uses to infer the distance between ourselves and objects in the environment. In the final lecture in this unit on visual perception, I'll discuss another type of perceptual inference, this time for color. We perceive a rich world of millions of colors. We use those colors to infer what's beautiful and what's edible, among other things. We perceive millions of colors, but we do so with a system that's really only directly sensitive to 3 specific colors. By knowing the relation between those 3 colors and the infinite range of wavelengths of light in the world, our brains are able put us in touch with this very beautiful aspect of our visual world. I hope that you'll join me for that discussion.

# Seeing Color and Light
## Lecture 7

Colors enhance our enjoyment of other things and can be enjoyable in and of themselves. Many people have strong emotional associations with particular colors. Researchers have argued that color perception is closely linked to our evolutionary past, useful for such tasks as finding reddish fruits among green foliage.

- Most children will tell you that mixing blue and yellow makes green. That is true of paints, but when you mix blue and yellow light, you actually create white light.

- This trichromatic theory of color perception explains very well how color is processed at the level of the retina. The opponent process theory is a better explanation, however, of how color is interpreted at the level of the visual cortex.

- Humans can also achieve color constancy—that is, we are able to perceive colors accurately under a variety of different lighting conditions, a remarkable feat that is so automatic, most of us take it for granted.

- In a purely physical sense, nothing is blue out in the environment; light energy oscillates at a particular wavelength that has an impact on particular chemicals that are present within the light-sensitive cells of your retina.

- If light projects onto the retina with a wavelength between about 390 and 475 nanometers, we see it as blue light. If a wavelength longer than 750 nanometers projects onto the retina, we will not see it at all.

- There's an old philosopher's puzzle that ponders whether I can know if my experience of red is the same as yours. Ultimately, this argument ends up going in circles. We cannot really know.

- It is extremely rare outside of a specialized color perception laboratory for our eyes to be exposed to any single wavelength of light. Most of our color experiences involve ranges of varying wavelengths.

- Light is emitted from some source, such as the Sun or a light bulb. The light comes in contact with some surface, which absorbs some of the energy and reflects the rest.

- The physical and chemical properties of the object determine this reflectance function—that is, which wavelengths are reflected and which are absorbed.

- This is what makes color perception so useful. By looking at the colors that are reflected from something, we can often infer things about the material it is made of. Is it ripe? Is it rotten? Does it contain a lot of water? And so forth.

- As you probably know from high school physics, white light is not the absence of color but rather a mix of all colors, all wavelengths. Early color researchers spent a lot of time on light-mixing experiments.

- They discovered that with only 3 lights—a bluish 420-nanometer light; a yellowish 560-nanometer light, and a reddish 640-nanometer light—all fitted with dimmers, they could create any color they wanted. This is how color televisions work.

- For about 10% of the population, 2 lights are sufficient for complete color matching. These people are often referred to as being colorblind. They lack the full range of human color sensitivity, usually the ability to distinguish red from green.

- These people are usually referred to as dichromats, whereas most humans are trichromats. All dogs and cats are dichromats, as are many other nonhuman mammals. Many birds are quadcromats.

- There are 3 types of chemicals affected to varying extents by different wavelength ranges of light, concentrated in the parvocellular response cells of the retina. They are small, cone-shaped, and within the center of the human field of vision.

- If you hold your thumb out at arm's length and look straight at it, it fills about 1 degree of your visual angle. The fovea, the eye's very small disk of very high-resolution light sensors—takes up about 2 degrees of visual angle. This area provides almost all of the finely detailed visual information that we get from our sense of vision.

- In our peripheral vision, both detail and sensitivity to color are greatly reduced. The vast majority of receptors in the periphery—outside the fovea—respond equally, regardless of the color of the light. They encode brightness differences but are basically colorblind.

- Your peripheral vision is a low-resolution, black-and-white scan, but you do not experience it that way, because as with the other senses, your brain infers a lot of detail and fills it in.

- There are 3 different types of color-sensitive cells in the fovea: Short-wavelength cones that respond best (that is, produce the most action potentials) to wavelengths around 420 nanometers, medium-wavelength cones that respond best around 520 nanometers, and long-wavelength cones that respond best around 580 nanometers.

- All 3 are very similar in appearanceand function. The only thing that differs is the type of light-sensitive chemical they produce. All 3 of these receptors also respond to other light wavelengths but to a lesser degree.

- So, for example, for light at 580 nanometers, the long-wavelength cones might respond at about 80 spikes per second, the medium-wavelength cones at maybe 50 spikes per second, and the short-wavelength cones at about 10 spikes per second.

- This combination of responses—the ratio of different rates of receptor firing—allows the visual cortex to infer that the light is about 580 nanometers in wavelength. That is, there is no particular receptor for this shade of yellow; it is inferred from the pattern of responses.

- In a setup with 2 lights—one at 530 nanometers (greenish) and another at 620 nanometers (reddish)—the medium- and long-wavelength cones would respond strongly, since both of these lights fall relatively close to their preferred wavelengths, while the short-wavelength cones would respond weakly.

- Believe it or not, these combined red and green lights would be perceived as identical to the single yellow light by your visual cortex.

- The short-, medium-, and long-wavelength cones are, for the sake of simplicity, often referred to as blue, green, and red cones.

- Mixing lights is additive color mixing, whereas mixing paints is subtractive color mixing. Blue plus yellow light equals white light, because blue light causes great activation in the blue cones and yellow is produced by activating both red and green cones. All of the cones will respond equally.

- When that happens, our visual system presumes that there's an equal amount of all 3 of these kinds of frequencies—perhaps an equal amount of all of the frequencies. When that is true, things are perceived as white.

- This trichromatic theory of color perception is a good one. For one thing, it is simple. For another, it has been proven accurate in experiment after experiment, combining physiological and behavioral evidence.

- After trichromatic theory was developed, all was well in the world of color perception. All of the big questions seemed to have been resolved except one: afterimages.

- If you stare at an unusually colored image long enough (such as a green, black, and yellow American flag), then look quickly at a white piece of paper, you will see an opposite-colored afterimage for a time (in this case, the flag in red, white, and blue).

- This phenomenon is a result of fatiguing the color-sensitive cells in your visual system. This should remind you of the motion aftereffect demonstration from a few lectures ago and the opponent process concept. There must be opponent process relations with these color-sensitive cells as well.

- Whenever you see green, the activity of particular cells in your visual cortex inhibits red-responsive cells. Red-responsive cells do the same thing to green-responsive ones.

- A similar opponent process relation exists for blue and yellow colors, although it is one step more complex. Yellow light is encoded as equal responses of the red and green cones, so the tug-of-war is between blue on one side and green and red on the other.

- Overall, the opponent process theory of color complements the trichromatic theory of color. The trichromatic theory explains the retinal receptor level, whereas the opponent process theory explains processing in the lateral geniculate nucleus and the visual cortex.

- Color constancy is our tendency to see colors as the same regardless of the conditions of illumination. The light reflected by any surface is some portion of the light that strikes it in the first place. If that light is white, then the reflected light will look very close to the reflectance function of the object.

- If, however, greenish light strikes the object, then mostly greenish light will be reflected at the viewer. It should be the case, then, that if I shine a greenish light on a white sweater, you should see that sweater as green. Amazingly, most viewers still see the sweater as white.

- Fluorescent and tungsten-filament light bulbs are greenish lights. Yet if you are indoors right now, the objects around you probably do not appear greenish.

- How does this work? One theory is related to how shadows can influence your perception of how an object moves—how the visual system carefully encodes light sources and shadows when it is processing moving inputs and uses those to make guesses.

- Your visual system is typically bathed in the same color light that is bouncing off the surfaces you are viewing. The visual system may

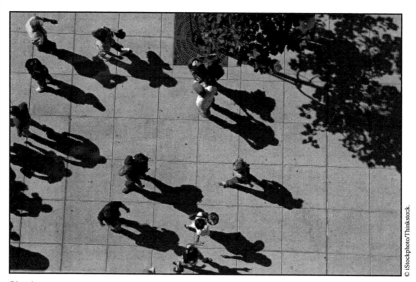

Shadows are not perceived as differences in color because they have fuzzy edges, called penumbra. Block the edges, and that perception changes.

simply compensate for the greenish light to determine what things would look like in broad-spectrum sunlight.

- There is some evidence for this theory: If you shine a red light on both a person and a viewing surface, the color of the viewed surface remains constant. If the red light is only shining on the viewing surface and not on the viewer, then a significantly greater change in color is perceived.

- Shadow perception also fits well within this theory. We very accurately see shadows as things that sit on top of perceived color, not as markings in their surfaces. To do that, we have to consider where the light is coming from and how it interacts with the opaque surfaces in our surroundings.

- At least part of this seems to rely on the fact that shadows have hazy edges—penumbra. If you block out the penumbra, what appeared to be a shadow suddenly seems to be a surface marking, and our perception of the target's coloration changes.

## Suggested Reading

Birren, *Color Perception in Art.*

Gegenfurtner and Sharpe, eds. *Color Vision.*

## Questions to Consider

1. If you were to put on literal rose-colored glasses, the world would look reddish. After a while, however, it would look less and less red. If you kept them on for several days or weeks, the world would look just as it did before you put on the glasses. How does this happen? If you were born with a visual system that responded too highly to red wavelengths, would you ever know it? Are all colors constructed by your brain based on this process?

**2.** Imagine a typical room with a normal variation of colored surfaces, including one particular object that is dark black. If I could somehow shine a bright spotlight onto this black surface without letting you (or your visual system) know that I were doing so, you would perceive the black surface as white. Why?

# Seeing Color and Light
## Lecture 7—Transcript

For many people, color perception is one of the most pleasurable things that our eyes give us; a brilliant rainbow, a fiery sunset, even the wondrous colors in a nice plate of pasta primavera. Colors enhance our enjoyment of other things and can be enjoyable, even all by themselves. I personally get a particularly good feeling just seeing that bright, deep blue of a clear, summer sky. The deep, dark blues of a thick stained-glass window create a feeling that is different, but can be just as strong; almost reverent. And the sparkly blue eyes of my daughter; those are the best of all.

I'm not the only person to have these strong associations to particular colors. Colors are an inherent and important part of how we perceive the world around us, and those connections run deep. Many have argued that our color perception is closely linked to our evolutionary past; for instance, to our ability to find reddish fruits among green foliage. Our visual system seems to have almost been custom built to be especially good at detecting that red-green color discrimination in particular. If you look at a black and white photo of some bushes with fruits on them, it's hard to make out the fruit at all. If you look at a color photo of exactly the same bushes, however, the fruit may not only visible, but in many cases just seems to glow; just seems to jump off the page at you. In some contexts, primate color perception serves almost like a fruit detector.

In this lecture, we'll explore color perception from a variety of different perspectives. I'll discuss some quick physics of light and color here at the beginning, and then discuss the trichromatic theory of color perception in detail. Most children will tell you that mixing blue and yellow makes green. That's true with mixing paints, but when you mix blue and yellow light, you actually create white. Once you understand the trichromatic theory of color perception, you'll understand why. With this older, trichromatic theory of human color perception in hand, we'll then move to the more modern, state of the art theory of opponent process in color perception.

While the trichromatic theory explains very well how color is processed at the level of the retina, the opponent process theory will enable us to understand how color is interpreted at the level of the visual cortex. At this level, the brain encodes and processes colors in opposing pairs; green versus red and blue versus yellow. You've probably experienced colors that are blueish-green or reddish-orange. You've never seen the color greenish-red, however; nor have you ever seen blueish-yellow. There's a reason for that, and it will become clear once you understand this opponent process theory.

I'll finish the lecture by considering how we achieve something called color constancy. We view our environment under a wide range of different lighting conditions. Even when the lights are yellowish or greenish, however, we still see colors as the same. In fact, we're so good at this that most people don't even realize that lighting conditions vary as much as they do. We just perceive the colors as they are; as properties of the objects that we're looking at.

Color, like many things that we perceive, is one of those properties of the world that's constructed by your visual system. In a purely physical sense, there's nothing blue out here in the environment. What there is out here is light energy; energy that oscillates with particular wavelengths. Radiant energy flows through the environment with many different wavelengths. Some of those wavelengths interact with our bodies, and some pass right through. Television and radio signals are propagating through the environment and through you almost all the time. They have very large wavelengths, and mostly pass right through you. Slightly smaller wavelength energies are used for radar systems. Still smaller wavelengths produce heat in what's referred to as the infrared range. When you get a suntan or sunburn, it's even smaller wavelengths of ultraviolet light that are interacting with your skin cells.

All of these wavelengths of radiation are very small. They're usually described in nanometers; that's a unit of measure equal to one-billionth of a meter. For a very narrow range of these different wavelengths—between about 400 and 700 nanometers—this radiation energy has an impact on particular chemicals that are present within the light sensitive cells of your retina. It's the relative responses of these cells that cause us to perceive colors. If light projects onto our eyes with a wavelength of between about 390 and 475 nanometers, we see it as blue light. As the wavelength increases, our color perception changes as well; up through green, yellow, and red. If a longer wavelength projects onto our eyes—longer than about 750 nanometers—then we won't see it at all. The energy is still there—it's not all that different from the energy below 750 nanometers—but it will no longer have an impact upon those light-sensitive chemicals in our eyes, and so we won't see it at all.

There's an old philosopher's puzzle that ponders whether I can know if my experience of red is the same as yours. That is, maybe your visual system is built so that what I see as red looks green to you, and vice versa. Ultimately, this argument ends up going in circles. We can't really know what others are experiencing in terms of perception. (You should recall this from the second lecture in this series, when we discussed how the perception of umami flavor is inherently private as well.) What I can know is that when particular wavelengths of radiation strike either your eyes or my eyes, particular chemicals in our eyes are both impacted, as are the neurons in which those chemicals are produced and stored.

The reason that the question can't really be answered is that the color experience we have is constructed from these wavelengths: The experience of color is all in your head. It's rare—extremely rare outside of a very specialized color perception laboratory—for our eyes to be exposed to any single wavelength of light. Most of our color experiences involve ranges of varying wavelengths. These mixtures of wavelengths are produced and delivered to our eyes in 3 particular stages. First, light is emitted from some source, such as the sun or a light bulb. This light emanates in every direction from wherever it was emitted through the air until it comes in contact with some surface. At that point, the surface absorbs some of the energy and reflects the rest. The physical and chemical properties of the object determine this reflectance function; that is, what portion of the energy is reflected and what portion is absorbed at different wavelengths.

Actually, this is what makes color perception so useful. By looking at the colors that are reflected from something, we can often infer things about the material that it's made of. Is it edible? Is it rotten? Does it contain a lot of water? The pattern of reflectance lets us perform a quick and often accurate chemical analysis of the objects around us just by looking at them. Ripe tomatoes, for instance, absorb most radiation in the 400–550 nanometer range, and reflect most radiation from 625 nanometers on up. It's for that reason, because that range of different frequencies and wavelengths of light are reflected, that we perceive tomatoes as being reddish. A blue shirt absorbs most of the long wavelength energy but reflects short wavelengths; that's why we see it as blue. If you see something as white or gray, it means that whatever that object is, its material is reflecting light equally well across the whole visible spectrum, regardless of its wavelength.

As you probably know from high school physics, white light is not the absence of color, but rather a mix of all the colors; all the wavelengths put together. Early color researchers spent a lot of time working with light mixing experiments. For instance, imagine that you had 3 lights: a bluish one that emitted mostly light around 420 nanometers; a yellowish one that emitted mostly 560 nanometer wavelengths; and a reddish light, mostly around 640 nanometers. If you shine those 3 lights onto a single white surface, the 3 colors of light mix together. That is, the light that's reflected onto the eyes will be a sum of all 3 of those lights. Imagine next that these 3 lights all have dimmer switches on them; that is, you can vary the amount of each of these 3 lights mixed into this color combination. The breakthrough discovery of these early color researchers was that if you have these 3 lights—just these 3—you can make any color you want, just by varying the brightness of these 3 lights; 2 lights doesn't work, that's not enough; 4 lights is more than you need; 3 lights, they found, is the key.

If you look closely at most color television sets, you'll notice that there are many sets across the screen of 3 color-emitting lights: 1 red, 1 blue, and 1 green. As the color picture is projected onto that TV screen, the color of any given place on the image is created just by varying the brightness of these 3 colors. Color TV hardware is directly based on these 3-light color mixing experiments.

Actually, for some people, about 10% of the population, 2 lights is sufficient for color matching. That is, they will, after adjusting just 2 of the dimmer lights, feel perfectly comfortable that they have perfectly matched the color of some test patch. These people are often referred to as being colorblind. They aren't actually colorblind in the sense that they can't see any colors at all; they can see colors. They're simply lacking 1/3 of the color sensitivity—

usually the ability to distinguish red and green—that most humans have. These people are usually referred to as dichromats, whereas most humans are trichromats.

There's a simple test for this disorder, this dichromatism, in which a number is presented in green dots amidst a background of red dots. If the ability to distinguish red and green is missing, then no number can be seen; it just looks like a mix of dots. If you can see the number, then your red-green color perception must be functioning.

All dogs and cats are dichromats, as are many other non-human mammals. Many birds are quadromatic; they would require 4 lights to match colors if they could do those color-matching experiments. There are many colors that look the same to us humans that would look very different from each other for birds. The behavioral evidence of needing 3 lights to match colors maps very well onto physiological studies of those light-sensitive chemicals in the human retina. There turn out to be exactly 3 types of chemicals that are impacted, to varying extents, by different ranges of light wavelengths.

In Lecture 4, I talked about magnocellular and parvocellular response cells in the retina. The parvocellular cells are the color-sensitive ones that I'm talking about today. The receptors are smaller, cone-shaped, and concentrated within the center of the human field of vision. If you just hold your thumb out at arm's length and look straight at that thumb, your thumbnail fills about 1 degree of visual angle. That is, in the 360° world around you, if you had 360 thumbs and you lined them all up next to each other at this arms-length distance, you could make a full circle all the way around your head. If you hold both thumbs together at arm's length out there, your thumbnails now fill 2° of visual angle. This is about the range of view that's called your fovea. There's this very small disk of very high resolution light sensors—one on each eye's retina—that provides almost all of the finely detailed visual information that we get from our sense of vision. Whenever you look at something, when you fixate it, what you're doing is aiming your fovea right at that point in space.

When you read a book, you point your eyes at the letters that you're reading; as you read you move your eyes rapidly from left to right, then go down to the next line and repeat. If you ever try to read without shifting your eyes to the right, you'll notice that you can't. You can read the first few letters, the things that you're fixated on; but if you try to read things that are in your peripheral vision—things that are away from that fovea—you can't. Away from that fovea, you can only gather a much lower resolution scan of the visual world around you. It's also the case that for our peripheral vision, sensitivity to color is greatly reduced. The vast majority of the receptors in the periphery—outside this fovea I'm talking about—respond equally, regardless of the color of the light. They encode brightness differences; but in essence, these peripheral vision cells are truly colorblind.

In this course, I've continually talked about how our perception of the world is, to a large degree, inferred from your sensory input. Many of the things that you see aren't actually your sensory input, they're filled in; educated guesses, really, based on partial information. That's really salient here with this fovea and peripheral vision. I think in the context of this, if you're thinking about it, there's this tiny disc right in the middle of your visual field. There, based on that small region that's presented at a very high resolution with fully detailed color, you can see the world. But that's not how we experience it. For the rest of your visual field, what you actually sense is a low resolution scan that's largely black and white. None of us experience it that way. We see a clear, well-colored, detailed environment all around us. That clear and detailed perception isn't in our visual input at any given moment; it's not in our eyes; it's only in our heads.

Let's be more specific about this trichromatic theory of color perception. Within the fovea, there are these densely packed sets of visual receptors. There are 3 different types of color sensitive cells in that fovea: There are those short wavelength cones; they respond best to wavelengths around 420 nanometers. There are medium wavelength cones; they respond best to light around 520 nanometers. And there are long wavelength cones; they respond best around 580 nanometers. All 3 of these receptors are very similar in their appearance and their function. The only thing that differs is the type of light-sensitive chemical that they produce. All of these cells respond best at these 3 particular wavelengths I keep mentioning: 420, 520, and 580 nanometers. This is the wavelength of light that produces the most action potentials for these receptor neurons. All 3 of these receptors also respond, though, to other light wavelengths; it doesn't have to be exactly those 3 wavelengths. The greater the difference between the light wavelength that's striking the cell and their preferred wavelength values, the less will be the response.

Let's consider for a moment how the cells would respond to light at 580 nanometers. The long wavelength cone would love this, perhaps responding to it at about 80 spikes per second because it's so close to its preferred wavelength. For the medium wavelength cones, this isn't the perfect stimulus, but it's not so far off. They would perhaps respond with maybe 50 spikes per second. For the short wavelength cones, this 580 nanometer light is a long way from its preferred 420 nanometer light, but it's still light; and so you would expect it to respond with about 10 action potentials per second. This combination of responses—the ratio of different rates of receptor firing—allows us to infer that the light that's being perceived, the light that's being projected onto the eyes, must be about 580 nanometers. This is how this particular yellow color is perceived. That is, there's no particular color receptor just for this shade of yellow, it's inferred from the pattern of responses of the 3 types of cells.

That's how it responds to a particular frequency of light; let's try to imagine this trichromatic setup responding to a mixture of light. Let's mix 2 lights: 1 at 530 nanometers and another at 620 nanometers. Seen separately, these would be a greenish light and a reddish light, respectively. What would they look like if they were mixed together in about equal quantities? For the 530 nanometer greenish light, the long wavelength cones would respond quite a bit: about 30 spikes per second. The medium wavelength cones, the ones that like greenish light, for those the response would still be quite high: about 30 spikes per second. For the short wavelength receptors, the ones that prefer blue light, there would be a little response, but not very much since 530 nanometers is not very blueish. We would expect to see about 6 spikes per second there.

How about that 620 nanometer light? This reddish light would stimulate the long wavelength cones a lot since it's very close to their preferred wavelength: about 50 spikes per second. The medium wavelength cones, the ones that like greenish light, for them the response would be substantial as well: about 20 spikes per second. For the short wavelength receptors, the ones that prefer blue light, there would be very little response: about 4 spikes per second.

Consider for a moment what would happen if we presented both of these lights—the 530 and the 620 nanometer lights—at the same time, in the same places, and in about equal quantities. The 2 responses from the different types of cones would be added together. For the long wavelength cones, 30 spikes per second for the 530 nanometer light plus 50 spikes per second for the 620 nanometer light gives us 80 spikes per second. For the medium wavelength cones, 30 plus 20 gives us 50 spikes per second. For the short wavelength cones, 6 plus 4 gives us 10 spikes per second. Overall then, we would see 80 spikes per second for the long wavelength cones, 50 for the medium wavelength cones, and 10 for the short wavelength cones.

If this response to a summation of 530 and 620 nanometers light looks familiar, it should; it's the same pattern of response I described for a single 580 nanometer wavelength. If you were to look at 2 patches of light, 1 with the 580 nanometer light and another with this mix of 530 and 620 nanometers, they would look identical to you. They don't contain identical amounts of light, but in terms of how our visual system responds to them, it would be identical. For light mixing purposes, red plus green equals yellow. Again, it's this combination of responses—the ratio of the amounts of short, medium, and long wavelength cone responses—that determines the color we perceive. The short, medium, and long wavelength cones are, for the sake of simplicity, often referred to as blue, green, and red cones. I'll start doing that now myself, actually, to make the description of this a little bit simpler.

I mentioned in my introduction to this lecture that blue plus yellow equals white; that's true if you add together colored light. It's also true that blue plus yellow equals green; that's true when you mix paints or other colored pigments. The key difference here is that mixing lights is additive color mixing, whereas mixing paints is subtractive color mixing. Blue plus yellow equals white; let's think that through. It applies in this additive color mixing domain. Here the blue light causes great activation in the blue cones; it's at their preferred wavelength of this particular receptor class. Recall from our previous mixing example that yellow is produced by activating both red and green cones. If the right combination of blue and yellow is added together, then, all of the cones will respond equally. When that happens, our visual system presumes that there's an equal amount of all 3 of these kinds of frequencies; perhaps an equal amount of all of the frequencies. When that's true, things are perceived as white.

Let's do subtractive color mixing: blue plus yellow equals green. It applies when we mix paints together, or any kind of a colored pigment. Remember that most pigments absorb some light and reflect the rest; that's how we end up seeing the colors of things. Most blue paints actually reflect mostly blue and also some green. They absorb all the other frequencies of light; in particular, they absorb yellow light. Most yellow paints reflect mostly yellow and some green. They absorb all the other frequencies of light; in particular, they absorb blue light. When you mix these 2 paints together, you get a new compound that absorbs all of that yellow and blue light, subtracting them both out. The only thing that both of these pigments don't absorb is green light. When you mix them together, voilà; it appears green. This subtractive color situation applies for most paint mixing wherein blue plus red is purple, red plus yellow is orange; things like that. For additive color mixing, in which lights are added together, we need to consult those 3 response curves for the short, medium, and long wavelength cones in order to really figure out what will be perceived.

This trichromatic theory of color perception is a really good one. For one thing it's simple: I've just described the whole thing from start to finish in just a few minutes. Also, it's accurate: It enables us to really precisely predict just what colors people will perceive given that we know the physical properties of the stimulus. It also combines physiological and behavioral sets of evidence really well; there's a nice dovetailing of those 2 approaches to understanding color perception here.

After this theory was developed, all was well in the world of color perception. All of the big questions seemed to have been resolved. There was just one sticky problem: afterimages. Imagine staring at an American flag picture with unusual coloring. The red and white stripes of the flag are replaced with green and black stripes. The white stars on the flag are colored black, and the usually blue field in the upper corner that contains those stars is colored yellow instead. If you stare at this figure long enough, you'll fatigue the color-sensitive cells in your visual system. It's important for one of these color afterimage experiments that you keep your eyes very still. For that reason, the demonstration flag usually has a white dot, as this one does, right in the middle where you should fix your gaze and hold it there while I continue talking. If you're doing this demonstration, you should keep fixating on that target for a good 2 minutes or so. As I said, I'll keep talking, but you should keep staring while you're listening.

This demo should remind you of the motion aftereffect demonstration that we completed just a few lectures ago; the one in which you stared at a downward moving waterfall for 2 minutes and then saw an upward drifting motion aftereffect. As in that case, there are particular cells involved that are growing fatigued. You're probably also thinking about opponent process relations; we talked about those with the motion aftereffect demo. There must be opponent process relations with these color-sensitive cells, but that was a mystery at the time that the trichromatic theory of color perception was first coming about. We'll talk about what this means for opponent process relations in just a minute. For the moment, just keep staring at that flag.

Okay, that should be about long enough to fatigue your color sensitive systems. The systems you're fatiguing, by the way, are in the lateral geniculate nucleus and in the visual cortex. What you would do now for this demonstration is to look at something with a neutral color background; ideal would be a white wall. As you look at the white wall, you should blink a few times. For some reason, this tends to bring up the color afterimages and make them more salient. If this has all worked properly, you should see an afterimage of a properly colored American flag now. Where you've been staring at yellow, now there's a blue afterimage; where you've been staring at green, now there's a red afterimage; where you've been resting your visual response cells by staring at relatively dark gray or black, there should be a white color. Not only are these the colors of the American flag, they're the opponent process relations that seem to be present in the human visual system. Whenever you see green, there are particular cells in your visual cortex that are active, and those cells use that activity to inhibit red responsive cells. Red responsive cells do the same thing to green. In just the way that upward and downward motions are encoded as the result of a stimulus-based tug-of-war, so are red and green colors as well.

Actually, you might notice that you've never seen a reddish green or a greenish red color, for that matter. That's because you can't. This opponent organization for color perception means that redness is, in essence, a lack of green and vice versa. A similar opponent relation exists for blue and yellow colors, although it's one step more complex. Remember that yellow light is encoded as equal responses of the red and green cones; so for blue and yellow, the tug-of-war is between blue on one side, and green and red on the other.

Overall, the opponent process theory of color hasn't disproven or replaced the trichromatic theory of color. In many ways, they're complementary theories. The trichromatic theory explains one aspect of color perception—at the retinal receptor level—whereas the opponent process theory explains later levels of processing in the lateral geniculate and the visual cortex. There's something very satisfactory about that. It's good perceptual science.

The last topic that I want to consider in detail is here is called color constancy. This is our tendency to see colors as the same regardless of the conditions of illumination. Recall the 3 steps that I described that lead to a color perception event. First, light is emitted and scatters from its source of emission until it strikes some surface. Then the surface absorbs some portion of the energy and reflects the rest. Finally, this light reaches our eyes and we perceive the color of it. What's reflected by the surface is always going to be some portion of the light that's emitted in the first place; it can't reflect things that aren't shone onto its surface to begin with. If that light that's emitted is bright—if it's, say, bright white sunlight—then the light that's reflected back will look very close to the overall reflectance function of the object. If, however, there's a lot of greenish light, then mostly greenish light will be reflected. If there's only a very little bit of blue-range light projected onto the surface to begin with, then there's very little of it that can be reflected back to the eyes.

It should be the case, then, that if I shine a greenish light on a white sweater, you should see that sweater as green. The amazing thing is that except in very carefully controlled and unusual circumstances, you don't see it as green; the sweater still looks white. If you're outside in the sunshine right now then (a) good for you, and (b) you're being bathed in a light that's almost truly white;

that is, it's a broad, balanced mix of all of the visible frequencies of light. If you're inside, probably under the illumination of fluorescent or tungsten filament light bulbs, then you're bathed in greenish light right now. Most commercially produced bulbs just don't produce much of the bluish range of light that we see when we're out in the sunlight.

This color constancy applies not only to a white sweater, but to everything as you look around you. Probably, things don't look green. In fact, if you were to move everything around you—clothes, furniture, carpet, the cat, whatever's in the space around you—if you were to move all of that out into the bright, sunny environment, the colors would look pretty much the same as they do now.

How does this work? One theory about this is related to something we discussed in the lecture on motion perception, when I talked about how shadows can influence your perception of how an object moves. In that example, I described how a ball moved the same way every time, but a changing shadow created the impression that its path of motion was changing: from moving in depth, to floating up in the air, and even bouncing as it moved across the stage. The idea there is that our visual system carefully encodes light sources and shadows when it's processing moving inputs, and it uses those to determine its best guess about the state of the external world.

The same idea applies for color perception. Your visual system is typically bathed in the same color light that's bouncing around the surfaces that you're viewing. In the greenish light situation, maybe the visual system simply compensates for the greenish light to determine what things would look like in broad spectrum sunlight. Once it's figured that out—figured out its best guess about those surface colors—that best guess becomes your perception of the colors of the surrounding surfaces. There's some evidence for this account: If you shine a red light on both a person and a viewing surface, the color of the viewed surface is pretty consistent; it remains constant. If the red light is only shone on the viewing surface and not on the viewer, then there's significantly greater change in the color that's perceived.

Shadow perception also fits well within this theory. We very accurately see shadows as something that sit on top of perceived color. We essentially never see shadows on objects as markings in their surfaces. In order to do that, we have to consider where the light's coming from and how it interacts with the opaque surfaces in our surroundings. At least part of this seems to rely on the fact that shadows have hazy edges; they're referred to as penumbra. If you block out that penumbra, what appeared to be a shadow does suddenly seem to be a surface marking; a change in the perception of the target's coloration.

This is the last of the lectures in this unit on what are thought of as the mainstays of vision research. We've considered motion, depth, and color perception. In the next unit of lectures, we'll start focusing on the non-visual modalities of the senses: taste, smell, touch, and hearing. I think you'll notice that many of the lessons learned as we considered how visual perception functions will apply for these other senses as well.

I started this lecture by describing some of the strong associations that exist between emotional responses and color perception. I also talked about how there seem to be deep, evolutionary foundations for how we perceive these aspects of the world around us. In our next lecture, I'll discuss another aspect of sensory processing that's very much related to our emotions and to our survival: taste and olfaction. I hope you'll be there, and come hungry.

# Your World of Taste and Olfaction
## Lecture 8

For the next 6 lectures, we will focus on nonvisual sensory modalities, starting with taste and olfaction. The senses are often described and thought of as independent and separate from one another. But in fact, the senses almost always work together.

- It is a rare thing for us to eat a meal without also looking at it. Our experience of food is inherently multimodal. Similarly, for many real-world tasks, touch and vision go together.

- Just as our visual system combines the output of different visual modules to arrive at an overall inference, the brain regions involved in different sense modalities tend to be combined as well.

- Flavor perception is one of the most multimodal sensory experiences that we have. Taste and smell are senses with which most people associate great pleasure.

- From an evolutionary perspective, this makes perfect sense, because energy is necessary for survival. We are all the descendants of creatures who liked to eat.

- From a behaviorist, operant-conditioning point of view, our love for eating also makes sense. If any action is followed by a physiologically meaningful reward, the frequency of that action will tend to increase in the future.

- Humans are born with some basic flavor preferences. A newborn infant will make a happy, cooing face if a drop of sugar solution is placed on his or her tongue and will crinkle up his or her face when given lemon juice.

- Much more of our idea of what tastes and smells good is learned, however, and flavor preferences change drastically over a person's lifespan.

- A researcher named Paul Rozin has suggested that flavor preferences emerge as our bodies learn what is nourishing in our own particular habitat. Every time you eat, your body is affected by that food—for good, ill, or not at all. Which foods have which impacts may change over the course of your lifespan as well.

- The body of a child and the body of an adult are similar in many ways, but there are obvious differences in their nutritional needs and the tolerance of their bodies for certain types of chemicals.

- Our brains seem to keep track of all this and generate flavor preferences based on it. On the flip side, our bodies also learn to avoid foods that seem to cause bad side effects.

- Rozin has expanded on this idea to consider how different regional cuisines may have developed—evolved, really—as people within different cultures, living in different physical environments, learned not just what tasted good but how to make things their bodies craved.

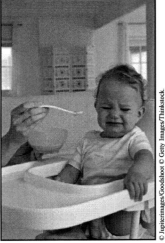

- The loss of smell is often called anosmia; however, your sense of smell is in many ways also your sense of taste. People with anosmia tend to experience a much greater incidence of depression than the general population.

**Babies seem to have innate flavor preferences.**

- They also have, on average, a significantly reduced lifespan after losing their sense of smell from food-borne illness, toxic exposure, smoke inhalation, and so forth.

- The ability of humans to detect faint odors of chemicals in the air is impressive, typically characterized in units of parts per billion. For the chemical *t*-butyl mercaptan, which chemical companies add to otherwise odorless methane so we can detect a leak in our homes, we can detect a mere 0.3 parts per billion.

- As impressive as our sense of smell is, humans are actually quite a bit less sensitive than many animals. Dogs can be an amazing 10,000 times as sensitive to odors as humans.

- The number of olfactory sensors available to the dog is the key to this sensitivity. While humans have an impressive 10 million receptors in their olfactory epithelium, dogs have as many as 1 billion.

- There is some evidence that humans and other animals can be influenced by smells that we are unaware we can detect. If several women live together, it is commonly observed that their ovulation schedules will synchronize. Other studies suggest that our perception of how attractive someone is interacts with subthreshold olfaction.

- More important than the absolute threshold of human smell—how much of a given stimulus is detectable—is how much an odor has to change before we can tell it is stronger or weaker than before.

- If I smell cookies and I want to know where they are, I might walk in one direction. If the aroma grows stronger, I will continue that way; if it fades, I change directions. Humans need about a 10% change in aroma magnitude to notice a difference.

- Note that this is a percentage of the relative strength; it is not an absolute amount like parts per billion.

- This proportional factor comes up for all of the senses. For a very bright light, you need a correspondingly large change in brightness for it to be apparent, and so forth.

- Let's delve more deeply into the transduction process associated with olfaction. Transduction converts energy from the environment into action potentials. In this case, it is energy in the chemicals we are able to smell.

- Humans have about 350 different olfactory receptor types, and they are slightly different for every person depending on your olfactory experiences.

- Androstenone has been widely studied. This steroid compound is excreted by many mammals, but only about 10% of humans can smell it. Most of these people have been exposed to farms that raise pigs or other livestock.

- The mechanisms behind this phenomenon are not completely understood, but at least in part, repeated exposure seems to cause the body to produce receptors that match the androstenone molecule.

- It is believed this works with many other chemicals as well. It seems that, quite literally, your nose can learn new things.

- Your scent receptors sit at the surface of the olfactory epithelium, embedded in a layer of mucous inside your nose. Each receptor has a particular shape, and a chemical must fit into that shape perfectly to cause the receptor to fire off a train of action potentials, like a key fits a lock.

- This lock-and-key system is unique to the senses of taste and smell. It is worth highlighting that olfaction only works when some piece of the thing you smell makes contact with the inside of the nose.

- The axons connected to these receptors project to a subcortical structure in the brain called the olfactory bulb and then on to the olfactory cortex for additional processing.

- Unlike the other senses, the sense of smell also projects directly to a subcortical structure called the amygdala, the center of human emotional processing. The amygdala also plays some role in decision making.

- This direct connection between olfaction and emotion fits with what many people report: Certain aromas have the capacity to inspire strong feelings.

- As with the other senses, smells seem to be encoded based on a pattern of responses rather than in terms of single neurons. If you smell pineapple, you have not activated some pineapple neuron but a set of neurons that encode the different chemical substances present in pineapple.

- Remember Müller's doctrine of specific nerve energies: What you perceive is a direct function of where your brain is active. Here, it seems that what you smell is caused by where in your olfactory cortex the neurons are activated.

- Taste works very much like olfaction, except with many, many fewer types of receptors—just bitter, sour, salty, sweet, and umami.

- Like smell, our perception of tastes seems to be based on the pattern of responses across these receptor types—the combination of salty, sweet, sour, and so forth—not an individual tomato soup neuron, for example.

- The taste receptors connect to the brain near many of the same brain areas, as do those associated with olfaction. The receptors make one subcortical pause in the thalamus before projecting into the cortex.

- It is common knowledge that taste and smell are closely related. You may have done an experiment in school where you tasted different foods holding your nose and then again with your nasal passages open.

- There is often a dramatic change in complexity between the plugged and unplugged experiences, but you do not experience the change as smell. When you release your nose, it somehow feels as if your tongue is working better.

- When we inhale through our nose, we experience orthonasal olfaction. Chemicals from out in the environment are pulled into the nose and onto the olfactory epithelium.

- We also smell things through the other opening in our olfactory tract: the throat. When you chew things, small bits of the chemicals in the food diffuse up through the back of the throat and retronasal olfaction proceeds, accounting for most of our experience of taste.

- Olfaction is not the only thing that gets lumped into the taste experience. If you eat very hot, spicy peppers, much of the burning sensation is actually conveyed by a stinging that occurs in your eyes.

- There is even evidence that the eyes and the center of the brain that encodes your level of hunger get in on the act of taste. If food looks good, it literally tastes better; conversely, if you are hungry, the areas of your brain that encode flavor ramp up their responses.

## Suggested Reading

Gilbert, *What the Nose Knows*.

Zald and Pardo, "Emotion, Olfaction, and the Human Amygdala."

1. A theory states that our flavor preferences emerge over the course of our lives as we eat things and experience the physiological consequences that follow. If something has a distinctive taste, and after eating it you feel good, then your brain will make the connection and cause you to crave that flavor in the future. Can you tell a similar story about the emergence of particular kinds of cooking in different cultures around the world? Why might some cultures favor spicy foods, while others seem to prefer more bland flavors?

2. Olfaction seems to be strongly linked to memory in humans, and even more so to emotional memories. What types of memories are the makers of scented candles trying to inspire in their customers?

# Your World of Taste and Olfaction
## Lecture 8—Transcript

Hello. We've spent most of the course so far talking about visual perception. For the next 6 lectures, we're going to focus on those other non-visual sensory modalities. First, we'll talk about taste and olfaction in this lecture, then hearing. We'll spend another lecture talking in particular about how hearing functions in the important context of language. I'll then talk about the sense of touch and how we use it to actively gather information from our environment. We'll then spend a lecture on kinesthetic perception, the sense that enables us to know the positions and postures of our body parts, even without looking at them. We'll finish this unit with a discussion of how we sense pain, and some of the ways in which our sense of pain can go wrong.

The senses are often described and thought of as independent and separate from one another. That's certainly how most books on perception are organized and also how I've organized this course, with specific lectures about these sensory modalities. It's worth noting at this point, however, that the senses almost always work together. For instance, today I'll be talking about taste and olfaction, but it's a rare thing for us to eat a meal without also looking at it at the same time. Chefs go to great lengths to make sure that the food looks good as well as tastes good, and with good reason: Our experience of food is inherently multimodal. Similarly, for any real-world tasks, touch and vision always go together. Just as our visual system combines the outputs of different visual modules together to arrive at an overall inference about what's out there, so the different brain regions involved in other modalities in those separate senses tend to be combined as well.

With that concept in mind, however, let's focus for the moment on taste and olfaction. In this lecture, I want to talk about how important taste and olfaction are, and consider where our flavor preferences come from. Why do some people like strange foods while others detest those exact same foods? I'll then turn to olfaction in particular, and talk about transduction for our sense of smell in more detail. I'll consider how smells are processed in the brain. I'll also discuss why aromas have the capacity to inspire the recall of powerfully emotional memories. I'll then consider taste perception and how it interacts with our sense of smell and vision. Flavor perception is one of the most multimodal sensory experiences that we have.

Why are taste and smell so important? Taste and smell are senses with which most people associate great pleasure; most people greatly enjoy eating. From an evolutionary perspective, this makes perfect sense. If there once were creatures that didn't like to eat, they probably didn't survive and thrive to produce a great many offspring. We're all the descendants of creatures who liked to eat. From another perspective—from a behaviorist, operant conditioning point of view—our love for eating also makes sense. After eating, our body receives nourishment in the form of calories and nutrients. If any action is followed by a physiologically meaningful reward such as this, the frequency of that action will tend to increase in the future.

Humans are born with some basic flavor preferences right from the beginning. For instance, a very newborn infant, just in the first minutes after being born, will make a happy, cooing face if a drop of sugar solution is placed on his or her tongue. Newborns will also make crinkled up facial expressions that we associate with eating something very sour if they receive a drop of lemon juice on their tongue. There's no doubt that they recoil and are made unhappy by bitter flavors; you can recognize that facial expression right away.

While some basics of our flavor preferences seem to be inborn, much more of our idea of what tastes and smells good are learned. In the world of art, it's common for people to say that, "There's no accounting for taste." That's often said when some painting that looks very bad to some people is sold for a great amount of money to someone else who presumably likes that same painting a lot. One might say the same thing about our tastes for different foods. Some people love spicy food; the hotter and more burning the better. Others detest spicy food, preferring—even relishing—foods that have more subtle, bland flavors. Some love to eat something called lutefisk, a dish from Norway in which white fish are soaked in lye until it has a tremendously strong and pungent odor. As much as some people love this, most people detest even the smell, let alone the thought of eating it. Haggis is a Scottish dish in which organ meats are simmered for many hours in the stomach of a sheep. The famous comedian Mike Meyers once commented that a lot of

Scottish cuisine seems to have been developed based on people daring others to eat things. And flavor preferences change drastically over the lifespan. During some phases of our lives, things like sauerkraut might seem almost inedible. Later in life, we may come to absolutely crave that very same food.

How could this amazing range of preferences exist for human eaters? One idea, associated with a researcher named Paul Rozin, is that flavor preferences emerge as our bodies learn what's nourishing in our own particular habitat. Every time you eat, your body is affected by that food. After eating some food, you may experience a boost of energy. After eating other food, you may feel ill. Some food will have good impacts on your body, others little or none. Which foods have what impacts may change over the course of your lifespan. The body of a child and the body of an adult are similar in many ways, but there are obviously big differences in their nutritional needs and the tolerance of their bodies for certain types of chemicals. Your brain seems to keep track of all of this every time you eat, and generates flavor preferences based upon it. Peanut butter may not always smell especially good to you, but if you're very hungry—in particular, if your body has a current pressing need for protein, vitamin E, and magnesium—3 things that are very rich in peanut butter—that peanut butter aroma may suddenly smell fantastic.

On the flip side, our bodies also learn to avoid foods that seem to cause bad side effects. If you ever experience some novel food flavor, you try something new you've never had before, and then become nauseous afterwards—even if you know for a fact that that nausea wasn't produced by the food, it was produced by a rollercoaster ride that you went on right after you ate—even if it's unrelated to the food, you'll probably never like that novel food again. Rozin has expanded on this basic idea about where flavor preferences come from to consider how different regional cuisines may have developed—evolved, really—as people within different cultures and who live in different places have learned not just what tastes good for them, but how to make those things that their body craves.

In general, our perception of the positive or negative valence of some smell or taste seems to perform a very specific, functional role in maintaining our health and maintaining the well-being of our bodies. This is especially apparent for people who have, unfortunately through accidents or injury, lost their senses of taste and smell. The loss of smell is often called anosmia; this is the more common of the things that would happen. As we'll discuss in a moment, however, your sense of smell is in many regards also your sense of taste. These patients don't just lose their ability to make fine discriminations between 5-star and 2-star restaurants; they tend to experience a much greater incidence of depression than the general population. They actually have, on average, a significantly reduced lifespan after losing that sense of smell.

Most people take for granted that their senses of taste and smell can tell them, for instance, when food has spoiled. You could just read the sell-by date on the milk; there's no real need for smell there, right? That's not quite true. At a few times in your life—maybe a few dozen—you will somehow be presented with food that has decayed and often been invaded by bad bacteria. These bacteria sometimes produce toxins that can be extremely harmful to your health. If you've ever gotten a mild case of food poisoning, let alone a bad case, you'll understand this. The sense of taste is important not only for our enjoyment, but in a very real sense for our survival.

The ability of humans to detect faint odors of chemicals in the air is impressive. Our absolute sensitivity is typically characterized in units of parts per billion. This is a very small unit of measure: One drop of ink placed into a large tanker truck full of water would be about one part per billion. For the chemical methanol, the primary component of rubbing alcohol, we need about 141,000 parts per billion; that's still a pretty small concentration. We need that much in order to be able to detect that that odor is there. For the chemical acetone, just 15,000 parts per billion is enough. For the minty smell of menthol, we need only 40 parts per billion.

Many appliances, like gas stoves, run on a flammable gas called methane. If it leaks into the outside air, it can lead to fires and even explosions (this is dangerous stuff) Pipelines are carefully constructed, of course, but leaks are an inevitability in a network of pipes this large. Unfortunately, methane is odorless; we have no receptors in our olfactory system that respond to it. In order to make the detection of leaks possible, utility companies add a chemical called T-butyl mercaptan to methane. It's used for at least 2 reasons; one, it doesn't create much of an odor after it's burned along with the methane. But it is amazingly detectable in its unburned form for the human sense of smell. Humans can detect this chemical at a concentration of only 0.3 parts per billion. That's 3 parts per trillion. Imagine if I had 1000 tanker trucks of liquid now and put 3 drops of some material into them. Humans would still be able to smell that natural gas odor, even at that very tiny concentration. For the right substances, human olfaction is very sensitive.

As impressive as our sense of smell is, humans are actually quite a bit less sensitive than many animals. Rats are 8 to 50 times as sensitive as people. Dogs can be an amazing 10,000 times as sensitive to odors as humans. When a dog is tracking a fugitive, in many cases they're smelling the tiny amounts of odorants that come off the skin and through the bottoms of the shoes into the grass. That's a small amount of stuff. The number of olfactory sensors available to the dog is the key to this sensitivity. While humans have an impressive 10 million receptors in their olfactory epithelium, dogs have as many as 1 billion.

In humans and other animals, there's some evidence that we can be influenced even by some smells that we're unable to detect. If several women live together, it's commonly observed that their ovulation schedules will synchronize. This is caused by the release of certain pheromones that can't be consciously detected. Something in the female olfactory systems is clearly able to detect it, however. There've even been studies suggesting that our perception of how attractive someone is interacts with sub-threshold olfaction. In an experiment that some people think of as a little gross, a group of male participants was recruited and asked to wear a t-shirt for 24 hours and then to not wash it. These t-shirts were handed in to the researchers and stored for later smell tests. Photos of the men were also taken and they were rated by one group of participants. The participants viewed those photos and scored them on a scale of 1 to 10, from very unattractive to very attractive. Other participants smelled the shirts and rated the shirts on that same sort of scale, from unattractive to attractive smells. Studies like this consistently find a positive correlation between these ratings. People who look good seem also to smell good.

So far, the olfactory sensitivity that I've been describing here is about the absolute threshold of human smell. That is, in the stimulus that's being delivered to you, how much do you need to be able to detect that there's something there at all? A more important measure of sensitivity is actually how much an odor has to change before we can tell that it's stronger or weaker than before. If I'm smelling some cookies and I want to know where they are, I might walk in one direction. If the aroma grows stronger, I'll keep going that way; if it's growing weaker, then it's time to change directions and go back the other way. For humans, we need about a 10% change in the magnitude of some aroma in order to tell the difference.

You'll notice that the measure I'm giving there for a relative perception threshold is no longer in parts per billion or any other measure of concentration. The amount of change you need in order to sense a difference is a proportion of the strength of the stimulus that's there in the first place. If you're smelling some weak odor of something—around 1000 parts per billion; something really weak now—then changing it to only 1100 parts per billion (an extra 10%) will be enough to sense the change. If the odor is strong, however—something at a concentration of 100,000 parts per billion—then I'll need a much larger change, an increase of about 10,000 parts, shifting it up to 110,000 parts per billion in order to sense that change.

This proportional factor is actually not specific to olfaction; it's one of those general properties that comes up for all of the senses. In the visual domain, if you're looking a very dim light, then even a very small change in brightness will be apparent. For a very bright light, you need a correspondingly large change in brightness in order for it to be apparent. This is even true in the domain of haptic and kinesthetic senses that we'll learn more about when we discuss the sense of touch. If you're given 2 paperclips, with one weighing about 1 gram and the other just a tiny, tiny bit more, you can pick out the heavier one even if that difference is amazingly small. If you give the same person 2 bowling balls, where one weighs about 12 pounds and the other is a tiny bit more, that tiny bit more is actually going to have to be pretty substantial before they're able to tell which one of those 2 very heavy bowling balls is heavier.

I've been discussing some general characteristics of olfaction performance. I want to delve a little more deeply now into the transduction process associated with olfaction. Transduction, you know by now, is the process of converting energy from the environment—in this case for olfaction, it's energy in the chemicals that we're able to smell—into patterns of action potentials (these are the signals that your brain uses to process information). For vision, we've talked about 4 different receptor types: There were those 3 different color receptive cells, plus a non-color sensitive peripheral vision receptor. For touch, we've talked about 6 different types of receptors for things like pressure and vibration. For hearing, there's really only one type of receptor; it's connected to the cochlea in your inner ear in those different locations, but it's really just one type of receptor. For olfaction, there aren't 5, 10, or even 20 receptors; there are about 350 different receptor types, and they're a little different for every person depending on your olfactory experiences.

One example of this that's been studied a lot is the case of androstenone. This is a steroid compound that's excreted by many mammals; pigs, it turns out, excrete a whole lot of androstenone. Only about 10% of humans are able to smell androstenone. If I made a strong androstenone solution and handed it to you, you would most likely, if you smelled it, say it didn't smell like anything; maybe it just smelled like plain water. If I handed this around the room to a large number of people, almost everyone would agree with you; they would smell it, and it would just smell like water. Every once in a while—about 1 in 10 people—I would find someone who would take a whiff and not only would they smell something, they would recoil at the strength of the smell. If I interviewed these people who could smell the androstenone, I'd find that a substantial percentage of them had spent time on or near farms that raise pigs or other livestock. If you're exposed to androstenone on a regular basis, your olfactory system seems to learn to smell it. The mechanisms behind this perceptual learning phenomenon are not completely understood, but at least part of it seems to be because as you're repeatedly exposed to this androstenone, your body begins to produce receptors with a shape that will receive that androstenone molecule. There's a belief that this works with many chemicals other than androstenone. It seems that, quite literally, your nose can learn new things.

All of these receptors sit at the surface of what's called the olfactory epithelium. It's embedded in a thick layer of mucous in your nose. The receptors all have a very particular shape to them, and a chemical has to fit into that shape almost perfectly in order to cause the cell to fire off a train of those action potentials. Most theories think of this as a lock-and-key type system. Any given molecule has a particular 3-dimensional shape. That 3D shape has to match the 3D receptacle of the receptor like a key fits a lock. Only one side of the molecule has to fit in, so the actual chemistry of predicting what a particular chemical will smell like is still pretty complex. This lock-and-key type system is really unique to the senses of taste and smell.

I think it's worth highlighting here that olfaction only works when some piece of the thing you're smelling makes contact with the inside of the nose where these receptors are located. Some trace parts of the substance you're smelling has to waft through the air from whatever the object is and into your nose. If you can smell those delicious cookies, then you're actually ingesting at least a few molecules of those cookies into your body. For pleasant odors, this doesn't concern me too much. But when I smell something that I find very unpleasant, I always find this fact kind of disturbing.

Regardless, the axons connected to these receptors project to a part of the brain referred to as a subcortical structure called the olfactory bulb and then on to the olfactory cortex for additional processing. Unlike the other senses, the sense of smell also projects directly to a subcortical structure called the amygdala. The amygdala is the center of human emotional processing. It also plays some role in decision making, but most studies suggest that if you feel happy, sad, angry, proud, or any of the tremendous range of human emotions—if you're feeling a strong emotion—it's likely connected with patterns of activation located in this amygdala brain region. This direct connection between olfaction and emotion fits with what many people report. Certain aromas have the capacity to inspire strong feelings.

Like most parents, when my son was very young, just a few weeks old, we washed him with baby shampoo; Johnson and Johnson baby wash was our brand, I think. During a lot of nights, my wife and I got very little sleep as we carried this baby around the house, singing lullabies, telling stories; basically doing anything that we could do to get him back to sleep. Now that he's older, of course, we haven't had to do this in a long time. We were cleaning out an old cabinet recently, though, and happened upon some of his old baby blankets. The aroma of that baby shampoo—it was just a weak little aroma, but detectable—came wafting into my nose. For a moment, when that happened, that smell took me back in time. I remembered those nights so clearly in that moment. The nostalgia was overpowering. I've talked to many people who report similar kinds of experiences. Smells are very distinctive; more lock-and-key-like than any other sensory experience we have. It makes sense that memories, emotions, and emotional memories would be encoded in this direct way through human olfaction.

As with the other senses, smells seem to be encoded based on a pattern of responses rather than in terms of single neurons. If you smell pineapple, it's not that there's some pineapple neuron that's activated, but rather a set of neurons that encode the different chemical substances present in pineapple. It's worth reminding you of the Mueller doctrine of specific nerve energies here again, something we talked about back in the second lecture. Recall that this concept is that what you perceive is a direct function of where your brain is active. Here, it seems that even what you smell is caused by just where in your olfactory cortex the neurons are activated. It's still all just action potentials, but they're encoding particular properties of the chemicals that are wafting into your nose.

Taste works very much like olfaction, except with many, many fewer types of receptors. Remember that there are 5 receptor types here: bitter, sour, salty, sweet, and the relatively newly discovered umami. We've also talked about the fact that all of these receptor types are present throughout the tongue; they aren't localized to only particular places on the tongue as had been erroneously believed. Also like smell, our perception of tastes seems to be based on the pattern of responses across these receptor types. The combination of salty, sweet, sour, etc. is what tells us what we're tasting; not an individual tomato soup neuron, for example.

The taste receptors connect near many of the same brain areas as do those associated with olfaction. The receptors make one subcortical synapse in the thalamus before projecting into the cortex itself. It's pretty common knowledge that taste and smell are closely related to one another, but I think it's worth reviewing that in this context. There's an old demo that I remember hearing about and trying for the first time when I was about 10 years old. You blindfold someone and plug their nose with a clothespin. Then you tell the person that you're going to give them a bite of an apple. Instead, according to the instructions, you feed them a bite of an onion. Most people don't realize how juicy and sweet onions are, actually, because the smell of onions is so pungent. If you plug your nose, however, and take a bite, you get all of the flavors very clearly. A good, firm onion even has a texture that's not so far off from apples. Whether you've tried this apple-onion trick or not, I don't recommend that you do it. I especially don't suggest that you do it to someone else. When you do eventually unplug your nose—and eventually you will—the odor and stinging sensations are really pretty awful. This is clearly as much a kid practical joke as it is a taste experiment.

If you would like to explore how taste and smell interact, I recommend using jelly beans, the kind that come in that rainbow of different flavors from berries to pineapple to hot-buttered popcorn. If you hold your nose and put one of these jelly beans in your mouth, you'll certainly taste something. You'll get the sweet, maybe a little sour, and the grainy texture of the sugars. After you bite down a few times, release your nose and breathe normally. The dramatic change in the complexity of what you're eating will be utterly striking. The other thing to note as you do this is that you won't experience that striking change as a change in smell, often not at all. When you release your nose, it somehow feels as if your tongue is working better. When we inhale through our nose, we experience what's called orthonasal olfaction. Chemicals from out there in the environment are pulled into the nose and onto the olfactory epithelium and the process of smell progresses. We also smell things through the other opening in our olfactory tract, however: Not the nostrils, but in the throat. When you chew things, small bits of the chemicals in the food diffuse up through the back of the throat and to that olfactory epithelium, and olfaction proceeds. This is called retronasal olfaction.

Most of our experience of taste takes place through this orthonasal olfaction. With the jelly bean task, almost everyone reports that when your nose is plugged, almost all of the many jelly bean flavors in that combo pack pretty much taste the same. It's only when you release your nose, allowing that orthonasal air to flow, that the jelly beans taste different at all. It's no wonder that many people don't feel like eating when they have a stuffy nose, perhaps along with a cold. Without the air flowing through your nose—without that orthonasal olfaction—food can be pretty bland and boring.

Olfaction isn't the only thing that gets lumped into the taste experience. If you eat very hot, spicy peppers with your meal, you may feel as if you're tasting them with your tongue; and you are to some extent. But much of the burning, hot sensation that seems to be conveyed on your tongue is actually conveyed through a stinging sensation that occurs in your eyes. When I've said "taste" in this lecture, I've essentially always been referring to the tongue and what it does. In general, however, the concept of flavor perception seems clearly to be a very multimodal experience. There's even evidence that the eyes and even the center of the brain that encodes your level of hunger get in on the act. If food looks good, it literally tastes better. Similarly, if you're hungry, then the areas of your brain that encode flavor ramp up their responses as well.

In this lecture, we've considered taste and olfaction, both in terms of how they function and in terms of how we use them. I've discussed how taste works in concert with olfaction, blending with it so seamlessly that we can't actually tell where smell ends and taste begins. These sensory modalities are very fundamental. They make very direct connections between particular chemicals—the chemical needs of our bodies—and memories that we associate with particular chemical contexts. As much as any other modalities, taste and smell are directly linked with your happiness, enjoyment, health, and survival.

In our next lecture, I'll discuss another important non-visual modality: the sense of hearing. Hearing provides us with information that's similar to that of vision in many cases—things like the identity of objects that are out there or the locations of those objects—but hearing also provides us with other very specialized information as well; information that's unique to that hearing modality. Hearing is also the primary conduit of language, something that distinguishes us from other animal species as much as any other facet of our existence. It's been said that vision connects us with the world around us, but hearing connects us with other people. I look forward to making those connections with you in the next lecture.

# Hearing the World around You
## Lecture 9

Your ears sample high frequency vibrations from the air around you, from which your brain infers a variety of important things. It infers what objects, people, and events are around you, as well as where those things are located. A sound-rich environment can even contribute to your depth perception.

- It can be an interesting exercise to sit in a restaurant and close your eyes for a minute, take in the sounds, and explore the space by moving your head and directing your auditory attention.

- You will notice you do not just perceive sounds; you perceive a sort of soundscape, an environment with a certain shape that happens to have sounds within it.

- Hearing is in some ways like an extension of the sense of touch. As the inner ear samples sound, it performs a Fourier transform on it before passing it on to the brain for more processing.

- You probably know already that sound results from waves of pressure in the air. Imagine I were standing in front of you holding a large piece of wood; if I pushed that wood forward and then pulled it back, it would create a wave of pressure in the air.

- If I moved the board back and forth repeatedly, a series of these pressure waves would be created.

- If I could move the board 10 times per second, you would start to feel a vibration on your skin. If I could move the board about 16 times per second, you would start to hear a low humming noise.

- If I placed a device between us that could measure air pressure at any given moment in time, it would show a sine wave with a baseline at 15 pounds per square inch.

- Sine waves show up in a variety of scientific and mathematical applications. Their shape is determined not so much by sound in particular but by the nature of our universe.

- Certain properties of sound perception are determined by the shape of this sine function. If the peaks and troughs are very high and low, the sound will be very loud, whereas if they are small, it will be quiet.

- Sound volume, or amplitude, is typically quantified in decibel units. The sound of rustling leaves is about 20 decibels. Conversation is about 60 decibels. A space shuttle launch registers around 140 decibels from a few miles away.

- The rate, or frequency, at which the pressure waves are produced is encoded as pitch. If I were to move my board back and forth 20 times per second, you would hear a low hum; at 4000 times per second, you would hear something like the tone of human speech.

- The number of back-and-forth motions per second is usually referred to as cycles per second, and the unit is hertz (Hz).

- There is an interaction between amplitude and frequency. Human auditory systems are constructed to encode certain sound frequencies much better than others.

- We can hear very quiet sounds in the range of frequencies that human speech occupies, even sounds that are less than a single decibel. For very low pitches, like 20 Hz, or very high pitches, around 15,000–20,000 Hz, a sound has to be 80 decibels or more before our ears will register it.

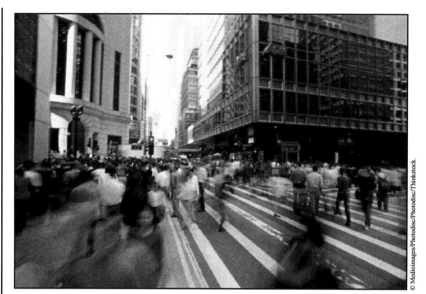

**Under real-world conditions, we rarely hear a single, isolated sound frequency at any time. We are constantly surrounded by complex auditory input.**

- Sounds consisting of a single frequency of oscillation are called sine tones because they produce single pressure functions. These are relatively rare in the real world.

- Adding several sine tones to make a complex sound is straightforward. What results is a repeating function that has a much more complex shape.

- We usually represent those functions as bar graphs. The height of each bar indicates the amplitude of the sound at each frequency.

- When the same singe note is played on different musical instruments, it has a different distribution of energies among the sound frequencies, which is referred to as the timbre of the instrument.

- Your auditory system has to take these frequencies apart to make sense of them. This process is called a Fourier transform, named after the mathematician Joseph Fourier who made important contributions in this area in the 16th and 17th centuries.

- This analysis is conducted right at the level of the auditory receptors in the cochlea in the inner ear. Sound waves enter through the auditory canal and reach the eardrum, which conveys vibration through a set of tiny bones called the ossicles.

- The vibration is amplified as it is transferred from the relatively large eardrum to the substantially smaller oval window located at the end of the cochlea.

- To understand Fourier analysis, you first need to understand sympathetic vibration: If 2 strings of a guitar are tuned to the same note, when I pluck one, both will vibrate. Think of the cochlear membrane as consisting of thousands of different guitar strings tuned to thousands of different notes.

- At the narrow end of the cochlea, the strings are sympathetic to high notes; at the wide end, they are sympathetic to low notes. Between those 2 extremes are strings that correspond to the full range of human hearing.

- Next to each of these strings is a tiny, motion-sensitive neuronal cell that fires its action potentials when the string vibrates.

- If I were to play a sound for your cochlea with tones at 440, 880, and 1320 Hz, since there is more energy in the low frequencies— that is, more amplitude—the amount of movement would be correspondingly larger for the low tone, and so would the train of resulting action potentials.

- Your cochlea sends these signals on through several subcortical synapses until they reach the auditory cortex near the middle of your brain. Müller's doctrine of specific nerve energies particularly applies here, as it does with the other senses.

- With vision, I talked a lot about retinotopic maps. For hearing, the representation is a tonotopic map. The individual frequencies and their loudness are maintained from the cochlea into the auditory cortex.

- The tonotopic map is dynamic over the course of a person's lifespan. It can be especially influenced by experience. Expert musicians typically have larger, more precise tonotopic maps than nonmusicians, for example.

- An old philosophy puzzle is relevant here: "If a tree falls in the woods and no one is there to hear it, does it make a sound?" Hopefully you understand the actual meaning of this question already based on our discussion of vision.

- There is no color in the world, only energy our brains interpret as color. The same is true of sound. If a tree falls in the woods, it will cause air to vibrate, but if there is no one there to transduce the vibration, there is no sound.

- We do not hear sounds in a vacuum but as coming from particular places. The auditory system has its own what-versus-where system in the temporal lobe, located on the side of the head and in the frontal lobe just above the forehead. This system also makes many connections with the visual what-versus-where system.

- As with vision, your auditory system determines identities and locations of objects, and it seems to do so with 2 different areas of the brain.

- Sound localization, the "where" system, capitalizes on the fact that we have 2 ears in 2 slightly different locations that sounds project to slightly differently, just as light projects slightly differently to the 2 eyes.

- At least 2 aspects of sounds are different between your ears as a function of the sound source's position: First, it will be slightly louder in one ear than the other. Second and more importantly, it will arrive at one ear slightly earlier than it arrives at the other.

- You may have noticed that it is harder to figure out the source of some sounds than others. In terms of using differences between the ears, the head must create a bit of a sound shadow—that is, it must interfere with the sound as it passes between one ear and the other.

- The auditory shadow is much more defined for high-frequency sounds than for low-frequency sounds.

- If you think of sound as waves in the water passing by the support for a pier, the reason for this may become apparent. Big, wide waves in the water move around obstacles much more easily than do little, thin waves.

- Interaural timing and interaural amplitude differences are not quite enough information to help us locate sound sources. If I close my eyes and listen, I have no trouble knowing when a sound source is directly in front of me, behind me, or overhead, yet such sounds reach both ears at the same time.

- Holophonic recordings are made using microphone systems of a similar shape and density as a human head, with microphones placed at the base of 2 auditory canals and 2 pinnae shaped like those of the human outer ear.

- Pinnae are the key to this effect. They create a compelling soundscape via a head-related transfer function. The pinnae selectively attenuate different frequencies to particular extents in predictable ways based on the sounds' location.

## Suggested Reading

Repp and Knoblich, "Action Can Affect Auditory Perception."

Schnupp, Nelke, and King, *Auditory Neuroscience*.

1. When you listen to music at a concert hall, it always seems to sound better than listening to a recording of it at home. Given your knowledge of hearing, why do you suppose that is so? Would holophonic recordings of an orchestra reduce the magnitude of this difference?

2. Your brain seems to encode the presence of particular frequencies with the activations of particular locations of the auditory cortex— the tonotopic map. Can you think of another way that it could be represented? Could the location indicate volume and the magnitude of response represent frequency? Would this be better or worse?

# Hearing the World around You
## Lecture 9—Transcript

Hello. In this lecture, I'll be talking about our sense of hearing. Your ears sample high frequency vibrations from the air around you; or, if you're swimming, from the water around you. As your hearing does this, it infers a variety of important things from that pattern of vibration. It infers what's out there—what objects, what people, what kind of events—and it also tells you where those things are located. In a sound-rich environment, your hearing can actually give you a very good sense of depth perception; of the layout of the surfaces around you.

It can be very interesting to sit in a restaurant and close your eyes for a minute or 2. As you take in the sounds, actively explore them by moving your head a little bit and directing your attention to different things in the environment around you. As you do, you'll notice that you don't just perceive sounds, you perceive sort of a soundscape; an environment with a certain shape that happens to have sounds within it.

In the last lecture of this course, I'll talk a bit about some technological devices that have been developed to enable blind people to see. Some of those devices transform the light-based information that we normally get from vision into sound patterns and then deliver those to a blind person through headphones. It's worth noting that in a lot of cases, blind people aren't interested in using these devices. The headphones do provide that visual information, but they also interfere with normal hearing. As technologically marvelous as some of the devices are, and as important as vision information can be, there's a lot of important stuff that comes in through our ears already. Most blind people aren't interested in giving that up, trading a visual deficit for an auditory one.

In this lecture and the next one, I'll be talking about this important sense of hearing in some detail. In this first lecture on the topic, I'll start with some quick physics about the nature of sound and discuss how the auditory system transduces that sound into patterns of neural activity. I'll argue that hearing is, in at least some ways, like an extension of our sense of touch. As the inner ear samples that sound, it performs something called a Fourier transform on it before passing it on to the brain for more processing. I'll explain what that Fourier transform is and what it can tell us about what we can and can't hear.

I'll then talk about sound localization; about how our auditory system infers the location of different sound sources. We accomplish this by comparing how the sound arrives at the 2 ears, sort of like stereopsis did with the 2 eyes. To figure out the location of some sound source, we also make use of these rubbery pinna that are attached to the sides of our heads. For any given pinna, there's something called a head-related transfer function. I'll talk about how our auditory cortex uses that transfer function and what happens if it's abruptly altered by changing the shape of the outer ear.

Let's start with a quick description of what sound is. You probably know a lot of this already; I'll be quick about it, and the structure of my description will be such that it will fit well with how I'll describe the function of the auditory system. Sound perceptions result from waves of pressure in the air. Imagine I were standing in front of you holding a large piece of wood. If I pushed that wood forward and then pulled it back, it would create a wave of pressure in the air. If I were standing waist-deep in some water with that large board and pushed it back and forth, you'd be able to see that pressure wave on the surface of the water. The water would bulge upward in the places where the pressure was high, and the bulge would move across the water to your location.

Even if I'm not in the water, there's still a pressure wave. You can't see it, but it's there. As I push that board out, it pushes the wave forward; it moves rapidly through the air until it bumps right into you. If the board were big enough, and if I moved it back and forth fast enough, you might actually feel it as a quick puff of wind going by. If I moved the board back and forth repeatedly, a series of these pressure waves would be created. If I went fast enough—say I could somehow move that board back and forth about 10 times per second—you'd start to feel a vibration on your skin. If I could go even faster—about 16 times per second—you'd start to hear a low humming noise. This is exactly how electronic speakers work, actually. They don't have big pieces of wood, of course; they have pressure plates that move back and forth; they're usually pushed back and forth very quickly with a magnetic force.

Okay, imagine I have my board again and it's moving back and forth. If I placed some device between us that could measure the amount of air pressure at any given moment in time, I'd see a very particular shape to that resulting pressure function. As any individual pressure wave passed by the device, the pressure would start at some baseline level of air pressure, about 15 pounds per square inch. The pressure would then increase gradually and then decrease just after it passed back down to that baseline level, and then below the baseline, then back up to baseline again. It would produce what's called a sine wave function. This shape shows up in a variety of scientific and mathematical applications. It's determined not so much by sound in particular, but by the nature of our universe. Certain properties of the sound perception that you have are determined by the specific shape of this sine function. If the peaks and the troughs of the sine function are very high and very low, then the sound will be experienced as very loud. If the peaks aren't very high and the troughs aren't very low, then it will be relatively quiet.

Sound levels are typically quantified in decibel units. A very quiet sound, say the sound of rustling leaves, will produce sound at about 20 decibels. The ambient noise level in a typical residential neighborhood is usually around 40 decibels. Most people speak in conversations at about 60 decibels. If you stand a few miles from the space shuttle when it launches, you'll hear noise at around 140 decibels. It's worth noting that this decibel scale isn't a linear progression of loudness increase but an exponential one, so that ambient neighborhood noise at 40 decibels is actually about 100 times as loud as those rustling leaves. The space shuttle, at 140 decibels, is about 10 million times as loud.

The height of the pressure function—of that sine wave—is encoded by our brain as loudness. The rate at which the pressure waves are produced is encoded as pitch. If I were to move my big board back and forth at 20 times per second, you'd hear a low hum; very, very low. If I were to move the board faster, around 100 times per second, you could hear the pitch of the sound rise tremendously. To make the sound sound kind of like what you hear in most human speech, I'd have to make that board oscillate about 4000 times per second. The number of back and forth motions per second it usually referred to as cycles per second. The unit that's used here is called Hertz. I would say that most human speech sounds are around 4000 Hertz.

Amplitude of pressure change corresponds to loudness, and frequency of vibration corresponds to pitch. In terms of human hearing, however, there is an interaction between these 2. Our auditory systems are constructed to encode certain sound frequencies much better than others. For instance, in the range of sound frequencies that human speech occupies—somewhere between 3000 and 5000 Hertz—we can hear very quiet sounds, even sounds that are less than a single decibel. For other sounds—very low pitches, like 20 Hertz; like when I was moving the board back and forth at 20 times per second—that sound has to be really loud; it has to be about 80 decibels or even more before our ears will even be able to register that there is a sound. Similarly, for very high pitches—up around 15 or 20,000 Hertz—we can still hear them, but they need to be very, very loud in order for our ears to pick up on them.

Our ears are good at encoding all sorts of sounds, but they're particularly attuned to speech sounds. Alternatively, one might say that the human vocal tract is particularly constructed to produce the type of sounds that we hear best. However you prefer to think of it and say it, there's this close correspondence between speech and hearing.

The sounds I've been describing so far consist of a single frequency of oscillation. If you hear one of these, it's called a sine tone, because of the shape of that pressure function. The closest a human can get to producing one of these is with a high-pitched whistle. If you were plot the sound pressure function of that sound, it would look very much like the ones we've been discussing.

These types of sounds are relatively rare in the real world, however; the single frequency sounds. Usually, what we hear are combinations of many different frequencies all mixed together. It's a straightforward thing to add together several different sine tones. You can see what it would look like to add a loud 440 Hertz tone, a quieter 880 Hertz tone, and a still quieter 1320 Hertz tone. What results is a repeating function that has a much more complex shape.

For the purposes of describing more complex sounds, we usually represent those functions as bar graphs. The height of the bars on the graph indicate the amplitude of the sound—the amount of energy, the amount of change in pressure level—that's present at each of these 3 frequencies. We can make these bar graphs for complex, real-world sounds. The composition of the sounds of a single note being played on 3 different instruments: a guitar, a bassoon, and an alto saxophone. Let me emphasize: It's exactly the same note being played on all 3 of these instruments. It looks very different, however, in terms of how the energy is distributed among those sound frequencies. The distribution of energies at those frequencies is referred to as the timbre of the instrument. The mix of these frequencies is the thing that makes the same note sound different when it's played on different instruments.

Okay, so we've seen how we can put different sound frequencies together, adding them up to create a more complex sound form. Your auditory system has to do the opposite somehow: It has to take them apart again. Your ears don't get that bar graph as an input; they get the complex wave form itself, and somehow have to decompose it and make sense of it. Your ears do indeed parse these wave forms. The process is called a Fourier transform; it's named after the mathematician Joseph Fourier who made important contributions in this area in the $16^{th}$ and $17^{th}$ centuries. This analysis is conducted not in the auditory cortex or up in the central nervous system at all, but right at the level of the auditory receptors, in a snail-shaped structure called the cochlea; it's located in your inner ear. After they're emitted, sound waves reach your head, they pass down through the auditory canal, and ultimately reach the eardrum. This is a relatively large structure, about the same size as the auditory canal. It conveys this vibration through a set of tiny bones, the smallest bones in the human body, called the ossicles. The vibration is amplified as it's transferred from the relatively large eardrum to the substantially smaller oval window located at the end of the cochlea. This cochlea is where the Fourier analysis is performed.

If you were to unroll the cochlea, you would have a cone-shaped organ with a thin membrane stretched down the middle. At one end of this membrane, it's very narrow. As you move down to the other end of the cochlea, that thin membrane progressively gets wider and wider. To understand the Fourier analysis that's performed in this cochlea, you first need to understand something called sympathetic vibration. Before we talk about it in the ear, let's discuss sympathetic vibration in something simpler: the guitar.

If I were to take a guitar and use just 2 of the strings on that guitar—no real music today; we're just going to focus on these 2 strings—I can tune them so that they will play the same note or 2 different notes. If I play 2 different notes on the strings on the guitar, there are 2 notes. If I play just one of the notes, you'll notice nothing really surprising happening. One of the strings is playing a note and the other string is silent; there's no reason that plucking one string should influence the one next to it. If, however, I tune these 2 strings so that they're tuned to exactly the same note, now if I pluck one of the strings, you'll notice something unusual happens: Even though I've only plucked one of the strings, both of the strings are vibrating. I can even pluck one of the strings and then stop it, and the second string will continue vibrating. If 2 guitar strings are tuned to the same note, not only do they make the same note when they're plucked, they're actually set up just right to receive that note. This is something called "sympathetic vibration."

You can think of the cochlear membrane as consisting of thousands of different guitar strings tuned to thousands of different notes. At the narrow end of the cochlea, you have strings that will sympathetically vibrate when there are high pitches present. At the other end, you have low note strings; these will vibrate sympathetically with low frequency pitches. In between those 2 extremes are all the strings that correspond to the full range of sound frequencies that humans can hear.

Next to each of these strings within the cochlea is a tiny, motion-sensitive neuronal cell. If the string associated with that cell begins to vibrate, then that cell will move and it will fire off a train of action potentials that are then delivered to the brain. If I were to play that complex tone for your cochlea—the one that we talked about before that was the summation of the 3 tones at 440, 880, and 1320 Hertz—you would get those sympathetic strings vibrating at just those 3 pitches; those 3 locations within the cochlea. Since there's more energy in the low frequencies—that is, more amplitude— the amount of movement would be correspondingly larger for the low tone, and so would the train of resulting action potentials. Voilà, your Fourier transform is complete.

Your cochlea sends these signals on through several subcortical synapses until they reach the auditory cortex, which is tucked into one of the primary folds in your cortical surface, near the middle portion of your brain and head. Mueller's doctrine of specific nerve energies particularly applies here, as it does with the other senses. If a particular sound pitch is produced, a particular part of the auditory cortex is activated. If I were to reach in and somehow stimulate just that same part of the brain, that particular sound would be heard.

With vision, I talked a lot about retinotopic maps. These were brain representations that maintained the spatial representations of the projection found at the level of the retina. For hearing, the representation is a tonotopic map. The individual frequencies, and the amount of loudness at each one of them, are the aspects of the stimulus that are maintained from the cochlea on up into the auditory cortex.

It's worth noting also that this tonotopic map is dynamic over the course of the lifespan. It can be especially influenced by experience. Expert musicians, for instance, typically have larger, more precise tonotopic maps than non-musicians. You might remember the part of Lecture 2 in which we discussed the somatosensory cortex; this is the area that processes information for the sense of touch. In that lecture, I noted that more somatosensory cortex space is devoted to a single fingertip than to the whole back, enabling very precise encoding of touch sensations on that fingertip. The larger tonotopic map for expert musicians is directly analogous to this. By devoting more brain space to encoding sounds, more precise information processing can take place. Musicians need, and use, that more precise information about sounds in order to be good at what they do.

I keep talking about old philosophy puzzles in this course, and there's another bigee here: "If a tree falls in the woods, and there's no one there to hear it, does it make a sound?" I remember hearing this as a student and thinking that this was just about the nuttiest thing I'd ever heard. Of course it makes noise when a tree falls! Do you think that things stop making noise when people aren't there? Do trees look around to see if there are people nearby and then decide, "Oh, I see some people over there having a picnic; I better make some noise when I fall down"?

Hopefully you understand the actual meaning of this question already—certainly better than I did when I first heard it—based on things you've learned in our discussions of vision, color vision in particular. In that case, I mentioned that there's no color out there in the world. There's energy that propagates with certain wavelengths, and some of those wavelengths impact the light-sensitive chemicals in our eyes; some of those wavelengths have differing effects on the different types of chemicals; and based on that we construct the notion of color. I think I used the phrase, "Color is all in your head."

A similar story can be told about sound here. If a tree falls in the woods, it will cause air to vibrate; of that I'm very, very confident. If there's no human there to transduce the vibrations into sound, however, then no matter how much vibration that tree creates when it falls, if there's no one in the woods to hear it, it doesn't make any sound.

The last topic I want to address in today's lecture is sound localization. We don't just hear sounds in a vacuum, just as we don't see light without a context around it. We hear sounds as coming from particular places. I mentioned that many of the things discovered about visual perception apply to the other senses as well. That's really true here, certainly in terms of the what-versus-where system that we discussed in Lecture 4. The auditory system seems to have its own what-versus-where system, located in the temporal lobe (on the side of the head) and the frontal lobe (just above your forehead). This auditory what-versus-where system also makes many connections with the visual what-versus-where system; it makes sense that our vision and our hearing would work together in this regard. As with vision, your auditory system determines both the identities and locations of objects that are out there, and it seems to do that with different segments of brain tissue.

When you look at the world, you seem to look at it with 2 separate visual systems; energy travels to 2 different areas of your brains up there, encoding and processing different things first, before they collaborate to coordinate those sets of information. With auditory information, the same thing seems to happen. It's as if there are 2 auditory systems up here in the brain listening to sound in 2 very different ways before working together to produce our full perception of the world around us.

With sound localization, I want to focus on this where system for the moment. How can it figure out know where a sound source is located? Many studies have characterized how our auditory system capitalizes on the fact that we have 2 ears, in 2 slightly different locations. Sounds project to these 2 locations slightly differently. It's analogous to the fact that light projects slightly differently to the 2 eyes because they occupy 2 slightly different locations.

With the ears, there are at least 2 aspects of the sound that are different between the 2 ears as a function of the sound source's position. First, if the source is off to one side—even a little off to one side—it will be slightly louder in one ear than the other. As sound propagates away from its source, the farther it goes, the quieter it becomes. There may not be a great deal of loudness change between the arrival of one ear and the other, but it's big enough that the ears can reliably use this information to figure out first, if the sound is located to the left or to the right; and second, by the amount of the difference, how far to the left or the right that sound source is. Second—and this is actually the more important source of information when comparing the sounds in the 2 ears—if the sound source is off to one side, it will arrive at one ear slightly earlier than it arrives at the other. Sound travels very fast, about a mile per second, but it's not infinitely fast. If sound is coming from the right side, then it will arrive at the right ear a few milliseconds before it reaches the left.

For both of these interaural sources of information—that's referring to the comparison between the 2 ears—the ear is encoding first, if the sound is located to the left or the right; and then also how far to the left or right. It can calculate both of those things based on these differences.

You may have noticed that it's harder to figure out the source of some sounds than others. There was a buzzing in my office at William and Mary every so often about a year ago that used to drive me a little crazy. It would start, sound for about a minute, and then go away. It was a low-frequency hum; a vibration really. I ultimately did find it, almost by accident, and not while it was actually making noise. It was behind a filing cabinet on the floor. It was an old alarm clock with a vibrate function that would go off every day at the same time.

Given what we know about how sound localization functions, it actually isn't surprising that this hard-to-find sound was low-frequency. In terms of using these differences between the ears, we need the head to create a bit of a sound shadow, if you will. That is, the head has to somehow interfere with the sound as it passes between one ear and the other.

It turns out that the auditory shadow is much more defined for high frequency sounds than for low frequency sounds. If you think of sound as waves in the water passing by a vertical log, maybe the support log for a pier or something, the reason for this may become apparent. Big, wide waves in the water, things that are very long, move around obstacles much more easily than do little, thin waves. The same is true with sound moving around your head. The high frequency sounds are far easier to locate for this exact reason.

So far I've talked about interaural timing and interaural amplitude differences—that is, differences in when the sound arrives and how loud it is when it gets to the 2 ears—and we can use this information to figure out how far to the left or right some sound source is. If you think this through, however, it's just not enough information. We perceive more about the source of a sound than its approximate direction. Consider for a moment the idea that maybe something is right in front of me; maybe the sound source is directly ahead. If that's the case, then there will be no timing difference; the sound will reach both ears simultaneously. Also, there will be no loudness difference; the sound is traveling exactly the same distance to get to my 2 ears. These timing and loudness differences—or lack of differences—are present if the sound source is right in front of me; it should be able to tell me if the sound is right in front of me. On the other hand, they're exactly the same if the sound is directly overhead or even behind me. If I close my eyes and listen, however, I don't have any trouble knowing when something is in front of me, when it's behind me, or when it's overhead. There must be something else that our auditory system is doing to figure out where sound sources are.

One of my favorite demonstrations of how good human auditory localization can be comes from something called holophonic recording. To make one of these recordings, you need a very special microphone system. The microphone system looks a lot like a human head. It's the same size and shape as a head, and it's constructed from material that approximately matches the density of a human head. On each side of the head, an auditory canal is drilled into the model head. The depth and width of the hole that forms those auditory canals is made to match how big they should be in a regular head. Two small, high-performance microphones are placed at the bottom of each of these auditory canals.

If I stop here, with the head built as I've described it, sound can be recorded that has those interaural differences in timing and loudness, and there's a sense of space that's produced if you listen to recordings in the microphone. But there's a last step of this holophonic microphone construction that is absolutely key: To finish it, you need to attach 2 rubbery pinna, one on each side of the head. A pinna—the one that you attach to the microphone—needs to be shaped approximately like that of a human outer ear, like the one we have. With this feature added, the sound recordings take on an eerily accurate spatial quality. I'm going to pause here for a moment and let you hear one of these recordings. If you listen with your regular television or computer speakers, you'll just hear the sounds themselves; they won't sound especially magical. What you need to do is listen to them with headphones. If you put the headphones on, now you'll be listening to them such that the sound that's recorded from the right ear of the holophonic microphone is going to your right ear, and just your right ear, and the sound from the left is going to your left.

When you put on those headphones, you'll hear this eerily compelling spatial world. You'll hear exactly where the sounds are coming from; you'll hear how they're moving around the world. You'll even hear when they get very close to your skin; when they get very close to your virtual head. When they do, it's not uncommon for people to feel goose bumps stand up in that place. Why does this pinna matter so much; why does this little rubbery thing influence our sound perception so much? How does it create this compelling soundscape?

The answers are related to something called a head related transfer function. I mentioned having trouble finding that alarm clock in my office a few minutes ago. I had trouble finding it because its frequency was so low. Because of the low frequency, my head didn't cast a good enough auditory shadow. This relation between sound frequency and the amount of interference created as it passes through and around solid surfaces is the information that we're talking about with the pinna. If a sound source is directly in front of us, then the pinna will selectively attenuate different frequencies to particular extents. As the sound source moves up or down, this amount of attenuation changes in specific, predictable ways and your brain seems to know what they are. By looking at the relative proportion of different frequency information in the sound input, your auditory cortex can figure out just how high or low—or left or right, for that matter—some sound source is.

Some interesting studies have been performed on this topic, in which experimenters filled the pinna of their study participants with putty. They then cut out a hole for the auditory canal so the participants could hear. When they did this initially, the ability of the participants to figure out where sound sources were all but vanished. Interestingly, if the participants kept these in after the initial experiment—if they walked around with them for about 3 weeks—the brain seemed to figure out this new head-related transfer function. As the brain figured this out, sounds could be localized again. As with the tonotopic maps, it seems that this head-related transfer function processing is dynamic and flexible as our bodies and the environment change over time.

In this lecture, I've described auditory transduction in detail and discussed how it capitalizes on the physics of sound and sympathetic vibration to encode auditory input. I've also described how we figure out how sounds are localized. In the next lecture, I'll talk about a particular, important way in which we apply our auditory perception: in the domain of speech perception. I hope you'll join me and perceive at least a little more of my speech.

# Speech and Language Perception
## Lecture 10

In terms of what your senses can perceive, language is the most amazing. I have some idea in my head, I make some noises and wave my hands around, and viola—suddenly you have the idea in your head, too. Speech distinguishes humans from all other species on Earth.

- Animals communicate with sounds and gestures. Some researchers have devoted decades to teaching chimpanzees and other nonhuman primates picture and sign languages, with limited success.

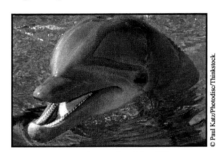

- Humans not only use words, we use them spontaneously. You do not have to teach children language explicitly. They just pick it up when exposed to it.

The most complex animal "talk" cannot touch human language.

- Unlike nonhuman animals, we also use language flexibly, inventing new words all the time.

- By the time we finish high school, most people know about 30,000 different words and regularly use about half of them. The sentences we form with these words are incredibly variable.

- Language seems to be infinitely productive; think of all the unique written works in the world.

- In terms of language perception, therefore, we have to perceive speech in a generalized, on-the-fly fashion. It cannot simply be memorization at work. Yet each language is constrained by many rules.

- Many of these rules are implicit; you may not be conscious of the rules per se, but if someone breaks these rules, it interferes with your speech perception.

- Humans speak quickly and well, using tens of thousands of words that convey countless ideas and interpreting these words through hundreds of rules. Yet the English language contains only about 47 different sound units, called phonemes, the smallest units of meaningful speech sound.

- The power of the language lies in its ability to combine this limited range of sounds, and the power of the auditory system is its ability to distinguish, very rapidly and accurately, between different sound units.

- The human vocal tract is a wonder of high-speed precision, able to produce phonemes at a rate of dozens per second. Often as it is making one sound, it is readying itself to make the next few. This is called coarticulation.

- Your auditory system makes use of coarticulation as well. If I took recordings of the words *soup* and *soon*, both of which contain the phoneme /u/, and spliced the /u/ from *soup* into *soon*, it would sound strange and the word would be harder to perceive, because the /u/ would not be coarticulated properly.

- In general, your vocal tract functions by making sounds and then filtering them. Your vocal cords make a broad mix of frequencies. As you open and close your mouth, move your tongue, constrict your throat, and so forth, you change that mix of frequencies.

- Speech information is visually represented on graphs called spectrograms. The horizontal axis of a spectrogram represents time. The vertical axis represents frequencies and energy at those frequencies.

- Essentially every vertical slice of a spectrogram is a momentary Fourier transform. The slices change over time as the word is formed and pronounced.

- The spectrogram for even a simple sentence starts to look very complicated. Linguists usually refer to those swoops as formants and the shifts between them as transitions.

- These aspects of speech are the building blocks of how we perceive what is actually being said. Their shapes matter more than the absolute frequency values.

- When your auditory system recognizes the meaning of some speech, these shapes are the building blocks. Speech-recognition software is programmed by using these graphs, but humans are still much better at speech recognition than any computer.

- Before you can recognize a word, you need to know where it starts and ends, yet in real speech, there are no gaps. Research suggests our brains use transitional probabilities to make these determinations.

- A researcher named Jenny Saffran created strings like the following: *bida, kupa, doti, gola, bubi, daku, gola, bupa, doti.* These strings of seemingly random syllables are set up so that, for example, the likelihood of /ti/ is much greater after the sound /do/ than it is in general.

- Such transitional probabilities are small but significant in natural languages. These statistics seem to be the way we learn to find word boundaries.

- There is even some suggestion that reading may work in this fashion. Researchers who study this type of phenomenon suggest that as you read the first part of a sentence, or even a word, your brain is already developing a set of expectations about how it will end.

- Another facet of speech perception that seems to enable its high level of performance is its categorical nature. Categorical perception actually applies to many of our senses. We see distinct stripes in rainbows, even though they are actually smooth, continuously changing arrays of colored light with no stripes.

- In auditory perception, we use categorical perception with phonemes all the time, sometimes dozens of times per second. Consider /da/ and /ta/. They are both made by pushing your tongue up against the roof of your mouth, releasing it, and exhaling slightly. The difference is that you engage your vocal cords right away for /da/ and wait 30 milliseconds for /ta/. This delay is called the voice onset time.

- If you take recordings of someone saying /da/ and increase the voice onset time, your brain would sort every recording with an onset time shorter than about 30 milliseconds into the /da/ category and anything longer into the /ta/ category, even though they are all different.

- This turns out to be quite important for our speech perception. Not only do we not attend the minor variations, most people cannot attend to them even if they try. The few people who can sense the difference all have one thing in common: They are younger than 6 months of age.

- We seem to be born with a fully flexible language-perception system, able to learn any categorical boundary structure that is important for a particular language. Through those first few months of life and language exposure, a particular categorical boundary gets set into place.

- Our eyes help us to perceive speech. When the audio of me saying /ba/ was dubbed into the video of me saying /ga/, you should have perceived me as saying /da/, even though /da/ was nowhere in the recording. This is called the McGurk effect.

- When you look at someone's face, you not only hear the speech; you see the speech. If you are having trouble hearing someone speak for any reason—say, at a loud party—watching the person's mouth can metaphorically turn up the speaker's volume for you.

- Although the McGurk effect is very visual, it is not perceived visually at all. It gets mixed into the audio input and is fully perceived as something you are hearing. Once again, you are not perceiving the stimulus but your brain's best guess about the stimulus.

- Incidentally, the McGurk effect gives you /da/ from /ba/ and /ga/ because of where you constrict your vocal tract when you make each sound. For /ba/, you constrict your vocal tract at the front of your mouth; for /ga/, you constrict your vocal tract at the at the back of your mouth.

- If you were to average between those positions—somewhere in the middle of your mouth—that is where you normally form /da/.

## Suggested Reading

Doesburg et al., "Asynchrony from Synchrony."

Moore, Tyler, and Marslen-Wilson, *The Perception of Speech.*

## Questions to Consider

1. The McGurk effect demonstrates that we "see" speech as well as hear it. Why do you suppose that the mix of sound and light is perceived as sound? Could it not be the other way around?

2. When we read, we activate some of the same areas of our brain involved in perceiving speech. Does this mean that we are reading aloud in a sense, even if we are expert readers who can read silently?

# Speech and Language Perception
## Lecture 10—Transcript

In this lecture, I want to talk with you about language and speech perception. Throughout this course, I've highlighted aspects of your sensory processing that are amazing: your ability to perceive objects and scenes in less than 100 milliseconds; your ability to perceive millions of colors with only 3 different types of photoreceptors; your ability to detect the faintest of aromas; things like that. In terms of amazing, we're about to discuss a biggie. Speech and language are almost magical when you think about what they do. I have some idea in my head, I make some noises and wave my hands around, and voilà, suddenly you have the idea in your head, too. Written language is, in a sense, even more amazing. I have an idea, I make some squiggly blobs of ink on a piece of paper, and voilà, someone else has the same idea in his or her head. The extra thing that writing has is time travel. I can look at squiggly blobs of ink made by people hundreds of years ago and the ideas they had in their heads when they made those squiggly blobs will travel through time to my own brain.

But let's focus on speech perception for the moment; it's amazing in its own right. Our speech and communication are things that distinguish us from all other species living on the planet Earth. Other animals communicate, of course, with chirps and barks, and even some very complex sounds. Some researchers have devoted decades to teaching chimpanzees and other non-human primates, teaching those animals picture-based languages and sign language. These endeavors have been somewhat successful, but they've also been strikingly limited. Humans not only use words, we use them spontaneously. You don't have to teach a child language explicitly for years and years, they just naturally pick it up when they're exposed to it.

Unlike nonhuman animals, we also use language very flexibly. We invent new words all the time. The word "email" didn't exist even a few decades ago, and now it's both a noun and a verb and gets used all the time. "I'll email you later, I just have to clear all of this spam out of my inbox and Skype my BFF." ("BFF" stands for "Best Friends Forever"; I had to ask my 10-year-old about that). I'm not sure if you caught all the words in that sentence, but your typical 10-year-old will know exactly what I was talking about.

By the time we finish high school, most people know about 30,000 different words and regularly use about half of them—15,000—in conversations. The sentences we form with these words are incredibly variable. Language seems to be infinitely productive. Imagine that you go to the library, go to a random floor, a random shelf, pick a random book, open it to a random page, and read the first sentence there. Except in rare circumstances, you will be unlikely to be able to find that exact same sentence anywhere else in the library. We almost never say the same thing the same way more than once. In terms of language perception, then, we have to be perceiving speech in a generalized, on-the-fly fashion. It can't be just memorization that's at work at all.

While we're extremely productive and variable in our speech and language production, we're also very constrained by the rules of our language. We conform to them almost all the time, and there are a tremendous number of those rules. Some of them you may know explicitly; things about subject-verb agreement, for instance. I can't say "The boy go to school"; I must say "The boy goes to school." There are also a whole lot of rules that you know implicitly; rules that you follow all the time; rules that, if someone else broke them, would interfere with your speech perception. You follow the rules and rely on them, but you don't always know that you know them.

My favorite is the unwritten rule that you can make "going to" into a contraction version of "gonna." If I were talking to you and telling you about my plan for the day, I could say, "I'm going to work for 8 hours." I could also say, "I'm gonna work for 8 hours," and that would sound just fine. Okay, first part's ok; so "going to" is allowed to change to "gonna." But it's not quite that simple: You're only allowed to use this rule—and you know this already; you know this implicitly—you're only allowed to use that contraction when "going to" is followed by a verb. If I was talking to you and said, "I'm going to New York," you would get that. If I said, "I'm gonna New York," something is off, and you would know it right away.

Another similar rule helps to mark when you've finished one sentence and you're starting the next. When you start a sentence, you raise the pitch of your voice. As you speak, the pitch gradually drops over the course of the sentence. When you start the next sentence, the pitch rises up again and then drops down over the course of the sentence. No one ever taught you this rule; you just implicitly learned it as you mastered the English language. There are literally hundreds of similar rules that you follow whenever you speak and whenever you interpret the speech of others.

In this lecture, I'll be describing how we perceive this impressively flexible, productive, and grammatical language. I'll explain some things about how we produce it along the way. I'll describe phonemes, the simplest units of speech, and how we're able to communicate a wealth of ideas with only a relatively small number of basic sounds. I'll talk about spectrograms, representations of speech that consider the presence of different amplitudes, at different frequencies, over the course of time. In essence, how the information in speech is present at the level of the cochlea and the auditory cortex. I'll talk a little about formants—components of speech that you can see in a spectrogram—and transitions in these spectrograms as well. I'll also talk about the roles that these play in speech perception. I'll describe the problem of speech segmentation; of finding where one word ends and the next word begins. By looking at how infants accomplish this task as they learn their first language, we can better understand how adults perform the task as well. Finally, I'll consider one of those intermodal, intersensory interactions. In the lecture on taste and olfaction, we considered how things we experience as taste—on the tongue—can sometimes actually come from things that are happening in your nose. For speech perception, I'll show you how things that you think are being perceived by your ears are actually sensed by your eyes.

Okay, so humans speak very fast and very well. We can communicate 30,000 or more words and an even greater number of ideas. We follow hundreds of rules as we form and interpret speech. How many sounds do you think we make as we do it?

Most people are surprised to know that the English language contains only about 47 different sound units. These are called phonemes, and they're the smallest unit of meaningful speech sound. Every word you've ever said; every word you've ever heard; all of it consisted of strings of these 47 different sounds, put together in different ways. The great power of our language is in the ability to put these different sounds—this small set of sounds—into complex, meaningful combinations. The power of our auditory system is its ability to distinguish, very rapidly and accurately, between those different sound units.

Before we delve into speech perception, I should say a few words about how we produce speech. The human vocal tract is a real wonder of high speed precision. It's able to produce these phoneme sound units at the rate of dozens per second.

Speech always begins with your diaphragm, which produces pressure, pushing air out of your lungs and through your throat. Already, at this first step in speech production, precise control is already exerted. The timing and particular patterns of pressure produced by the diaphragm are critical to producing clear, audible speech. If you've ever tried to talk to someone when you're winded from some physical effort, you'll certainly appreciate this.

As the air is pressed through your throat, the muscles around your vocal cords in the larynx sometimes press the air across those vocal cords. As they do, they cause the vocal cords to vibrate. To make high-pitched tones, the vocal cords are stretched very taut. For low tones, the vocal cords are only slightly stretched. In essence, these muscles tune your voice like a guitar string. An excellent singer will have tremendous control over the vocal cords, being able to produce precise notes with just the right timing and duration. That said, everyday speech, regardless of your vocal training, requires tremendous control over these vocal cords. You communicate excitement, emphasis, even uncertainty with you tone of voice. Even sarcasm comes across in part with the particular notes you hit as you express yourself through speech.

These larynx muscles also regulate how much of the airflow is pushed onto the vocal cords, and how much passes around them. The breathy tones that you make when you talk sometimes are a product of this aspect of the control. As with many things in the motor domain, we typically take all of these things for granted. From a perception perspective, we almost always take them for granted. All we perceive is the meaning behind those sounds, behind the speech that we're listening to, without focusing much at all on the sensory information that leads us to that understanding.

The diaphragm and the larynx are critical to speech production, but the real action begins in the speech articulators—the lips, the tongue, the cheek, the jaw, and our teeth. The vocal cords emit a broadly distributed range of frequencies. As we change the note that we're emitting, this distribution changes, shifting higher or lower, but it's always a broad distribution of low-, medium-, and high-range frequencies. By reshaping our vocal tract, we filter this broad range of frequencies, allowing certain sound pitches to pass right through to the outside world, and largely blocking others. For instance, with the vowel sound /ah/, we open our vocal tract up almost completely, allowing the sounds of the vocal cords to be heard with very little interference. In order to make the vowel sound /ee/, however, we close our mouths a bit, and lift and spread our tongue across the middle of our mouth. This posture of the vocal articulators blocks much of the high frequency sounds produced by the vocal cords. They absorb those vibrations rather than allowing them to be emitted and then picked up by the ears of anyone who happens to be listening.

The auditory system is very sensitive to those frequency distributions that are emitted. By encoding them, the listener is able to tell if you're saying "mall" or "meal." Even if you say the word very quickly—"mall" or "meal"—there's plenty of time for the ears to pick up that information. For some vowels, a single distribution isn't enough. For instance, if I want to say "mile," I'll need to make an /i/ vowel sound. This is accomplished by starting with that /ah/ posture and then shifting to an /ee/ posture. There are dozens of tiny rapid moves that you make with your mouth in order to filter the frequencies emitted by the vocal cords, and thus produce one of the phonemes that make up our language.

The one other big category of vocal articulator move that you make comes with the sound produced by pressing air through your teeth as you speak. If I want to make an /s/ sound, I accomplish this by pushing a short burst of air through my teeth. If I push my lips forward just a bit, however, and the sound is filtered again, turning a /s/ sound into a /sh/ sound. Again, the ears of a speech perceiver—the brains of the perceiver, actually—are attuned to picking up this subtle categorical distinction. "Sealed" and "shield" have very different meanings. Even if I speak those words very rapidly, you can effortlessly tell that difference.

All of these different pieces of the vocal tract perform with remarkable consistency, accuracy, and precision at an individual level. Perhaps even more impressive is that they all work in precisely-timed synchrony, working together with one another to produce the speech that we utter—ultimately the speech that we hear. Even when you speak the simplest of everyday sentences—Good morning. How are you doing?—there are dozens of critical actions taking place in this vocal tract, about which we're never aware.

Often, as the vocal tract is making one sound, it's already getting ready to make the next one or 2. For instance, the sound /u/ is a part of the words "suit," "soup," and "soon." If you take out just the /u/ sound in those 3 words, however, they sound different. As your vocal tract is getting ready to make the /t/, /p/, or /n/ sound that goes with that "suit," "soup," or "soon"—as it's getting ready to make that after the /u/ sound—it has to slightly change itself to sort of get set to make the next one. This is called co-articulation, since you're articulating one sound but also getting ready to articulate the next.

What's even more interesting is that your auditory system makes use of that co-articulation information. If I swap the /u/ sounds in those words between "soup" and "soon," if I were to take those and splice them so that the sound went with the wrong word—I took the "soup" /u/ and put it with "soon"—it would sound strange; it would be harder to perceive; it would take us longer and we would be less accurate in terms of figuring out what the word was. When your auditory system hears the /u/ that precedes the /t/ sound, for instance, it seems to use that information to get ready to process the /t/. If the co-articulation information is wrong or even if it's just missing, speech perception is much more difficult.

In general, your vocal tract functions by making sounds and then filtering them. Your vocal cords, when activated, make a very broad mix of frequencies. Recall from the last lecture—specifically the topic of head related transfer function—that different frequencies are differentially able to move around and through spaces of a certain shape. With the head related transfer function that we talked about, the shape was that of the irregular but constant shape of your pinna, these flaps of cartilage on the sides of your heads; things that actually we refer to as "ears." For speech production, that shape is constantly changing as you open and close your mouth, reshape your mouth, move your tongue up down and back and forth; as you make constrictions at the level of your throat. As we make all these very rapid and accurate movements, we're constantly changing the mix of frequencies that are emanating from your mouth.

I should say that the one other thing we do is force sound through our teeth and lips at times to make sounds like /s/, /sh/, and /t/.

Here's what this speech information looks like at a frequency and time based level. The horizontal axis of a spectrogram represents time. The vertical axis represents frequencies and energy at those frequencies. We discussed the Fourier transform that your cochlea performs during the last lecture. For the spectrogram, essentially every vertical slice of that figure is one, momentary Fourier transform. Those slices change over time, of course, as the word that's being said is formed and pronounced.

The spectrogram for even a simple sentence starts to look very complicated. For instance, if we look at how frequency distributions evolve over the course of the sentence, "Roy read the will," we can see how there's an initial distribution of sound during the /r/ phoneme that swoops up during the /oy/ sound then drops it down again for the /r/ in "read." Linguists usually refer to those swoops as formants and the shifts between them as transitions. These aspects of speech are the building blocks of how we perceive what's actually being said. It's their shapes that matter more than the absolute frequency values.

I could say "Roy read the will" and I could say "Roy read the will" and you would have no problem knowing that I'd said the same thing twice. The frequencies involved would be totally different, but the shapes of the formants and transitions would be constant. When your auditory system recognizes the meaning of some speech, it's these shapes that are the building blocks.

When someone writes a piece of software that's able to understand human speech, the information on this graph is the input that it gets. This is one of those areas where there's been a lot of progress made in recent years, but humans are still much better than any computer that's out there. This is a really tough computational problem. One of the hardest things to deal with is the fact that before you can recognize a word, you need to know where it starts and ends. We discussed this briefly in the first lecture; that there aren't gaps in between words when we speak, yet somehow our auditory system is able to find those word boundaries. If you look at a spectrogram of the sentence, "I owe you a yo-yo" for instance, you can probably tell right away that the sounds never stop; they never pause at all in between those words. "I owe you a yo-yo" is a kind of a weird sentence, but in this regard it's not. "Hi there, whadayadoin" is something that people would say a lot. If I were to say that as "What … are … you … doing" it would actually be harder to understand, not easier. Again, there are no pauses to look for. There's certainly no obvious way to look for the individual letters that might be used to actually spell these words.

I mentioned a moment ago that before you try to recognize a word, you'd want to know where the word starts and ends. There's some fascinating recent research with young children—as young as 5 months of age—that suggests how we might do this based on something called a transitional probability. Imagine that you're a child listening to a complex new language, one that you don't understand. This problem is faced by every young infant, actually. For the experiments, a researcher named Jen Saffran created strings like the following: Bida, Kupa, Doti, Gola, Bubi, Daku, Gola, Bupa, Doti. Did you hear the word boundaries? If I played a string like this for a 7 month old, or even a 5 month old, for as little as 2 minutes, the baby would know where those word boundaries are. These strings of seemingly random syllables are set up so that the likelihood of some particular sound—in this case /ti/—is much greater after the sound /do/ than it is in general. That is, there's a relatively high conditional probability that if you just heard /do/ that the next sound will be /ti/. These transitional probabilities are small in natural languages, but they're there. After any given sound there are many other sounds that could follow, but not all of them. For instance, after the sound /bay/, there's a slightly elevated probability of the next sound being /bee/. The word "baby" is thus easy to pick out, even if you don't know what "baby" actually means.

These statistics seem to be the way that we learn to find those word boundaries. One can even look at these transitional probabilities at the level of those spectrogram formants that we discussed. It certainly seems that our auditory perception systems do.

Just being exposed to the speech seems critical. Teaching very young infants particular words might be fun, but that's not the path to word parsing. It seems mostly driven by the statistical mechanisms within our speech perception system. There's even some suggestion that reading may work in this fashion.

This is a little off topic, but it illustrates this point and I think it's just fascinating. For this short paragraph, the first and last letters of each word are left in place, but the middle letters of the word are scrambled. It's really interesting how little this actually disrupts your ability to read it. Researchers who study this type of phenomenon suggest that as you read the first part of a sentence, or even the first part of a word, your brain is already developing a set of expectations about how it will end. We thus may not need to read every letter to understand things. We need the first part, and then enough information to pick between the alternatives that we already have in mind. With reading, that's the last letter. With speech, it might be just a very rough encoding of the last sound.

Another facet of our speech perception that seems to enable its high level of performance is its categorical nature. Categorical perception is actually a concept that applies not just to speech perception but to many of our senses. If you've ever looked at a rainbow, you've probably seen it as having a red stripe, and an orange stripe, and a yellow stripe, and so on. That is, there appear to be parts of the rainbow—these stripes—where the color is about the same, and then there are transitions between the stripes from one color to another.

That's not physically what's present in a rainbow. Rainbows are produced by the differential refraction of different light wavelengths as they pass through some medium at an unequal density at some angle (that was quite a sentence). For the moment, let's just say that something like a prism bends a ray of white light. It bends long wavelengths of light less than short wavelengths, such that the individual colors present in the white light fan out and produce a rainbow.

The key here is that a smoothly, continuously changing array of colored light is present in a rainbow; there are no stripes. To the extent that you see those stripes, it's because you're grouping similar colors together categorically.

In auditory perception, we do this categorical perception process with phonemes all the time; sometimes dozens of times per second. Let's consider 2 syllables: /da/ and /ta/. (I talked about /ba/ and /pa/ in a previous lecture as an example of 2 sounds that are made using almost identical motions of the vocal tract.) For both /da/ and /ta/, you push your tongue up against the roof of the mouth and build a little pressure behind it; then you release it and exhale slightly. The only difference is when you engage your vocal cords for /da/ and /ta/. For /da/, you make the sound part (the /a/) right away; /da/. For /ta/, you wait just about 30 milliseconds before you engage your vocal cords; /ta/.

You can see this clearly if you look at the spectrogram for these 2 sounds. Both have a pressure release component at the beginning; for /ta/, there's a gap between that pressure release point and the onset of that low frequency /a/ sound. I could actually make a /ta/ sound into a /da/ sound by just deleting the segment of the recording in which that pause takes place. In so doing, I would be reducing the voice onset time to 0.

Okay, imagine now that I created a sequence of these sounds in which the voice onset time varied slowly; say, about 4 milliseconds per presentation. If I presented this sequence of sounds, they would be changing every time. Even though every one of those stimuli would be different, they would all sound the same. All of them, that is, until I reached that threshold around 30 milliseconds of voice onset time. At that point, quite abruptly, one sound would come out as /da/ and the next would come out as /ta/. Let's listen to that sequence. Somewhere right about there, it switched for me. After that point the stimulus keeps changing, but now it sounds consistently like /ta ta ta/.

You perceive this sequence of sounds categorically. Even though they're all different—every stimulus was different from every other in that sequence—you lump one group of them together (the small voice onset time group); the others (the long voice onset time group) are lumped together as well.

This turns out to be quite important for our speech perception. We perceive almost all phonemes in this fashion. It happens very fast and unconsciously, and we throw out the pre-categorical variations after we do it. Not only do we not attend to things like that voice onset time variation, we're actually incapable of doing it, even if we really try.

Interestingly, there are some people who can still perceive these differences. They can tell the difference between, say, a /da/ with a 10 millisecond voice onset time and another one with an onset time of about 20 milliseconds. Remember that these are on the same side of that categorical boundary for you, so we would be unable to do it. The people that can sense this kind of difference all have one particular thing in common: they're younger than 6 months of age. We seem to be born with a fully flexible language perception system, able to learn any categorical boundary structure that's important for a particular language. Through those first few months of exposure, however, a particular categorical boundary gets set into place.

The last topic I want to touch on in today's lecture is how our eyes help us to perceive speech. To demonstrate this, I'm going to show you a video of me saying a particular syllable over and over again, about 10 times. First, for this first presentation of it, I want you to close your eyes and just listen. (Audio customers should refer to their guidebook for figures detailing this demonstration.) Please close your eyes now, just for about 20 seconds; I'll tell you when to open them again.

/ga//ga//ga//ga//ga/

/ga//ga//ga//ga//ga/

You can open your eyes again. I'm now going to replay that same video again. This time, however, I'm going to mute the sound. You'll see me speaking, but you won't hear anything.

/ga//ga//ga//ga//ga/

/ga//ga//ga//ga//ga/

Hopefully, when you closed your eyes and listened that first time, you heard me saying /ba/ (saying /ba/ over and over again; /ba//ba//ba/). When you watched the video, you may or may not have been able to read my lips as saying /ga/. For this next run through, I'm going to show you video of the /ga/ (/ga/ video) dubbed with audio of /ba/.

/ga//ga//ga//ga//ga/

/ga//ga//ga//ga//ga/

If this has worked, you should have perceived the sound /da/. /Da/ is nowhere in the recording; it's something that happens when you add the visual /ga/ with the audio /ba/. Let's play it one more time. This time, close your eyes for the first few /ba/ sounds, then open your eyes for the last few. You should experience a rather abrupt change in the sound when you open your eyes.

/ga//ga//ga//ga//ga/

/ga//ga//ga//ga//ga/

What you're seeing demonstrated here is something called the McGurk effect; named, like many such effects, on its discoverer. It clearly demonstrates that our vision plays an important role in our language perception. When you look at someone's face, you don't just hear him speak, you see him speak.

As I've grown older and my hearing has started to fade a little, I've found that sometimes I have trouble hearing quiet, conversational tones when I'm in a loud, silverware-banging dinner party. When I was first starting to have this problem, I discovered that if you just smile and nod a lot you can get pretty far in most conversations, even if you can't hear what the other person's saying. More recently, however, I've found a better solution to this problem: If I really want to hear what someone's saying, I just make a point of looking down at his or her mouth. You don't want to be too obvious about this; it can make you look creepy to look down, staring at someone's mouth. But if you just make sure that the mouth is within your field of vision, suddenly it's like someone turned up the volume on that person doing the speaking.

Another fascinating part about this McGurk effect, I think, is that it's a very visual effect; it's not perceived visually at all. That is, we clearly are seeing speech here, but it gets mixed into the audio input and fully perceived as something that you're hearing; something with your auditory perception. As with many, many things in the domain of perception, it seems that what we perceive is not actually the stimulus—or in this case, multiple stimuli—what we perceive is our brain's best guess about what's happening in the world around us. It's those inferences that are our perceptions.

The way the McGurk effect works, by the way—what the explanation for why, if you put together /ba/ and /ga/, you should hear /da/—has to do with where you constrict your vocal tract when you're making those 2 sounds. If you're making a /ba/ sound, you're constricting your vocal tract at the front of your mouth; you're building up that pressure behind your lips and making /ba/. If you're making a /ga/ sound, you're building up pressure and releasing it just like with /ba/, but now you're making that constriction all the way in the back of your mouth, at the position of your throat. So you're presenting a visual /ga/ with the constriction at the back of your throat and an auditory /ba/ with the constriction at the front of your mouth. If you were to average between those 2 positions, it would come out somewhere in the middle of your mouth. If you do that—if you build up a pressure behind a constriction at the middle of your mouth—it actually comes out as /da/, so it's sensible then that /ba/ plus /ga/ would equal /da/.

Our senses enable us to make contact with the world around us in a figurative sense. In our next lecture, I'll talk about the sense that literally makes contact with the world around us: touch. I've described all of our senses as embedded within a moving body. We almost never passively receive sensory inputs. We're always moving our eyes, ears, and nose for that matter. With touch, that active, exploratory characteristic is very salient. I hope you'll join me next time for a discussion of "Active Touch."

# Touch—Temperature, Vibration, and Pressure
## Lecture 11

I t is said that seeing is believing, but one might add that touching is being absolutely sure. There is something fundamental and direct about touch perception. Touch, like all senses, is the brain's best guess about the environment, and there are many different types of touch receptors in your skin.

- Distributed throughout your skin's surface are 2 very different types of temperature-sensitive cells. One population, the cold cells, responds strongly to stimuli in the range of 10–30°C, then slow and stop responding as temperatures rise.

- Another class of receptors, warm cells, does not respond to cold much at all; rather, they respond when a warm stimulus is present, between about 30 and 45°C. Colder or much warmer than this, and these receptors slow down and stop responding.

- Two receptor systems: If one is active, you can infer that something out there is cold. If the other is active, you can infer that something out there is warm. But burning makes both types of cells active.

- If you heat neurons so much that they are about to be destroyed, they typically make a last intense burst of action potentials. Cold and warm receptors both do this, so if both are active, your brain makes a particular inference—something is very, very hot out there.

- The so-called thermal grill illusion results from this organization of the inferential temperature-sensing system. To try it, you will need 2 forks, 2 cups, some warm water, and some ice water.

- Soak one fork in the ice water and the other in the warm water for a few minutes. Then intertwine the tines of the forks and press them lightly against the surface of the skin. Your perception will be they are intensely hot.

- In the regions where the warm and the cold tines are very close together, both the cold and the warm receptors are responding at the same time; therefore, your touch-perception system infers that something is burning you.

- When we are babies, touch is the primary sense we use to explore the world. They put things in their mouths as much to feel them as to taste them. Eventually, children switch to using their hands as the primary instrument of haptic exploration.

- Most early developmental theories argued that human infants use their sense of touch to educate their sense of vision. For instance, children would hold and move an object, and only then would notice that its retinal image size grew larger and smaller as they did this.

- The brain actually infers the state of the surrounding world on the basis of a wide range of different specialized receptor systems imbedded in your skin. Some areas provide detailed, high-resolution touch information, such as the surfaces of the fingertips.

- Recall that the transduction process for touch is accomplished by many different types of receptors located at different locations below the surface of the skin. In addition to having different locations in depth, the cells' structure gives them different receptive properties.

- We only experience one conscious perception of touch, but it is derived from many different types of information capture. For instance, Merkel receptors lie near the skin's surface, just beneath the epidermis.

- They are small and in some places quite densely packed. This gives them the ability to encode fine details of a pattern of pressure when something presses against your skin, like the precise textures and shapes in the bark of an oak tree versus a maple tree.

- Compare the Meissner corpuscles at about the same depth in the skin. These cells are substantially larger and do not encode fine details but vibration—or more accurately, changes in pressure.

- If you press on a Meissner corpuscle, it responds for a few milliseconds, after which it turns off. If you release that pressure, it responds again.

- Because the cells respond so quickly, rapid, repeated increases and decreases in pressure (that is, vibration) activate them best. If you were to run your fingers along that tree bark, your emergent perception of texture would be derived from the patterns of vibration sensed by your Meissner corpuscles.

- In most situations, different types of neurons work together. Imagine the seemingly simple task of holding a raw egg. The shell is fragile, but the egg has a substantial weight. You need enough pressure to keep the egg from falling but not so much that you crack the shell.

- Grasping the egg very lightly, only a small response is produced by your Merkel cells. If the pressure grows too light, the egg will slip a little and the Meissner corpuscles will respond. You will then increase your grip pressure, to keep the egg in your grasp.

- This interaction between the muscles that control your actions and the tactile receptors in your fingers is impressive, yet as with so many things that are automatically controlled by our nervous system, most people think of them as quite simple. It is only when we try to duplicate that process with machinery that we realize the depth of information processing occurring in our sensory systems all the time.

- Ruffini cylinders are located a bit deeper within the skin. These encode stretching movements when skin is pulled as a result of our own actions from passive contact with some surface. They seem especially important for kinesthetic perception—our sense of our body's posture.

- Pacinian corpuscles are located even deeper, in the layer of fat underneath the skin. They work much like Meissner corpuscles, sensing vibration rather than pressure, but whereas Meissner corpuscles respond best to vibration in the range of 3–40 cycles per second, Pacinian corpuscles prefer 10–500 cycles per second.

- The relative responses of these types of cells enable us to infer the actual rate of a given vibration. If the 2 types are responding equally, then the vibration is probably in the middle of their preferred ranges; if only Meissner cells are responding, a slower rate of vibration is present. If there is a lot of Pacinian corpuscles response and no Meissner cell response, then a high rate of vibration is present.

- One of the key tests of how well you can sense touch is called the 2-point threshold. If your eyes were closed and I gently touched 2 pins to your fingertip (not breaking the skin), if the pins' tips were close enough, you could not tell whether there was 1 pin or 2.

- In fact, if the pins' tips were closer than 1 millimeter apart, you would be essentially at chance in guessing whether there was 1 pin or 2. Only when we get to about 2 millimeters apart does the presence of 2 separate points become clear.

- Yet we can and do resolve details about objects that are much smaller than 2 millimeters across. How? By using vibration information.

- For parts of the body other than the fingertips, this 2-point threshold is much larger. For the back of your calf, the 2-point threshold is about 5 centimeters apart—a little less than 2 inches.

- We can draw an analogy to our visual experience here. Recall that our peripheral vision is very low resolution both in terms of seeing fine details and in seeing colors. Almost all of our clear visual information comes from the fovea.

- Nonetheless, we have a perception of a clear visual field all around us, not just in the fovea. That fine detail is perceived, but it is not sensed.

- Your vision system takes in information through your senses and uses it to infer the state of the world. One small area of the visual field is good at picking up fine details and a larger area is good at detecting changes, like movement.

- The sense of touch seems to be organized in an analogous fashion. Some small regions of the skin's surface are very good at picking up finely detailed information—our hands, our fingers, and our mouth. The rest of the skin is very sensitive to the presence of even slight touches, but mostly it serves to call our attention to things that are happening in the world, things on which we might want to focus our more detailed touch perceivers (our hands or our fingers).

- So the 2-point threshold varies a lot across the skin surface; it also maps nicely onto the representation of touch sensations in the somatosensory cortex—the area of the brain that stretches horizontally across the middle part of the top of your head, where touch of any kind is processed.

- Particular locations in the brain correspond to particular locations on the skin. Some areas of the body command a large area of the cortex, such as the fingers and the tongue. Other areas of the body, like the calf, are physically larger but occupy small region of somatosensory cortex.

- The size of the area of somatosensory cortex is directly proportional to this 2-point threshold: The bigger the area, the greater the sensitivity.

- The somatosensory map has a dynamic, changing structure. The sensory cortices are hardwired to particular areas of the skin, but they also pass through complex neural networks in the spinal cord and the hindbrain. Recent evidence suggests that this neural network is quite flexible.

- The more you use some particular part of the skin, the more your brain devotes to encoding information about touch in that particular region.

- Experimenters worked with macaque monkeys, whose brains and sensory systems are similar to those of humans. They identified the touch regions of the macaque somatosensory cortex and provided hours and hours of stimulation to a particular fingertip.

- They found that areas of the brain that had previously encoded touch for areas of the skin adjacent to the fingertip had shrunk, while the brain area that mapped this particular finger had grown tremendously, increasing by almost 400%.

- An extreme version of this remapping often takes place when someone loses a limb. Right after the limb is lost, such patients still have a somatosensory cortex that contains neurons devoted to representing the sense of touch for that arm and often report an odd sense that the arm is still there, which doctors call a phantom limb.

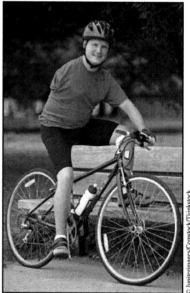

- Over time, adjoining areas of the somatosensory cortex typically expand, taking over this cortical real estate that the lost limb was using. Even after this happens, however, the phantom limb

**When a limb is lost, other body parts can use that limb's brain real estate.**

often does not completely disappear. This persistent phantom limb suggests that our mental representation of our own body must reside somewhere other than this somatosensory cortex.

- In some cases, patients with phantom limbs report that the phantom limb feels pain—or worse, feels itchy. To scratch that itch, patients can scratch the region of the body that adjoins the missing limb on the somatosensory cortex. In the case of a missing arm, scratching the face can sometimes relieve a phantom itch.

- Touch not only connects us to the world but to ourselves. The link between our mind—our sense of who and where we are—and our body is influenced by many senses, but touch is the most important.

- Consider the rubber hand illusion, in which a participant's real hand is hidden from sight and replaced with a rubber hand. The experimenter takes 2 paintbrushes and gently strokes the rubber hand and the hidden hand in synchrony. The participant begins to have a strange sensation that the rubber hand is his or her hand.

- The strength of the illusion is measured by threatening the rubber hand—for instance, with a hammer. Unconscious fear response mechanisms are activated, and the subject will jump and startle the same way she would if a hammer struck one of her real hands.

- The participant typically explains that he she knows that the rubber hand fake and feels no pain, but some part of the brain is not convinced.

- We can even generate a whole-body version of the rubber hand illusion by faking a sort of out-of-body experience using goggles with video screens inside them that show the participant a view of the back of his or her own head. The experimenter then brushes and pokes the chest of the participant while moving another brush in the same way in the bottom part of the video camera that's behind his head.

- The participant sees someone poking just below the field of view and feels the sensation of those poking movements. No spirit has left the body here, but an inference has been made: The participant infers that he or she is outside of the body looking in.

## Suggested Reading

Drewing and Ernst, "Integration of Force and Position Cues."

Tsuchiya et al., "Vib-Touch: Virtual Active Touch Interface for Handheld Devices."

## Questions to Consider

1. When I reach into my pocket, I can find my keys and even the very key that I need to open my front door. What information do I have at my disposal to aid in this precise object recognition? Pressure pattern? Vibration? Sense of inertia when I move the key chain? Knowledge of my keys?

2. Touch is commonly thought of as an active sense in which we obtain information by reaching out and exploring things with our hands. Many argue that we can describe vision in the same way—that we scan the environment to pick up information with our eyes. In what ways is this a good analogy? Can you think of ways in which it is not?

Lecture 11: Touch—Temperature, Vibration, and Pressure

# Touch—Temperature, Vibration, and Pressure
## Lecture 11—Transcript

I've often heard it said that seeing is believing. That might be true to some extent, but I've always thought there should be an add-on to that expression: Seeing is believing, but touching is being absolutely sure. There's something very fundamental, something direct, about touch perception. As primates, our brains are very focused on visual inputs; but touch still provides the most concrete, direct information about the world around us. Our sense of touch, like all of our other senses, gathers information from different sources and then combines those sources to produce our perceptions. Our brain makes its best guess about what's happening in the world around us, and it's that best guess that you perceive. This is very apparent in the domain of touch perception, especially since there are many different types of touch receptors in your skin. I want to start today by talking about 2 of them: cold sensors and warm sensors.

Distributed throughout your skin's surface are 2 very different types of temperature-sensitive cells. One population—I'll call them the cold cells— responds a lot to stimuli that are in the range of 10–30°C. As the temperature rises, however, these cells slow down and stop responding. Another class of receptors doesn't respond to cold much at all, they respond when a warm stimulus is present; I'll call these warm receptors. They respond most between about 30 and 45°C. If the temperature is colder than this, or even a bit warmer, these receptors slow down and stop responding.

Two receptor systems: If one is active, then you can infer that something's cold out there. If the other is active, then you can infer that there's something warm; pretty simple so far. There's one other thing that makes both types of cells become active: burning. If you heat neurons up—if you heat them up so much that they're about to be destroyed—they typically make a last intense burst of action potentials before they do so. Cold receptors and warm receptors both do this; so under ordinary circumstances, if both the warm and the cold sensors were active, then there's a particular conclusion, a particular inference, your perceptual system would make: there's something very, very hot out there. In fact, rather than just being aware of this, you'd probably act, pulling your skin away from whatever was causing that stimulation.

There's a fascinating little illusion—the thermal grill illusion—that results from this organization of your inferential temperature-sensing system. You can try this at home or see a version of it at several museums around the United Sates. For the in-home version of this thermal grill illusion, you'll need 2 forks, 2 cups, some warm water, and some ice water. Soak 1 fork in the ice water and the other in the warm water for just a few minutes. Note that 1 fork will grow cold and the other warm. If you're going to try this out on a friend, make sure that he or she isn't carrying something heavy at the time. Probably they should also be seated. Intertwine the tines of the 2 forks and press them lightly against the surface of the skin. The perception will be that you have just touched that skin with something intensely hot. If the person you try this on isn't watching and doesn't know what you're doing, the reaction can be quite intense.

I should be clear here that there's nothing hot on the skin; nothing that's doing any damage to anything. But in the regions where the warm and the cold tines are very close together, both the cold and the warm receptors are responding at the same time; and they're both responding a lot, because there's something cold and something warm. Except in the context of this thermal grill illusion, except in this particular context, this only happens under 1 circumstance: the presence of something very, very hot. Your touch perception system makes the inference that there must be something scaldingly hot out there; and, voilà, you perceive that inference.

In this lecture, we'll be exploring the processes of inference that lead to our rich, detailed sense of touch. There's something very primary about our sense of touch; something very fundamental; something we trust a lot. When we're babies, it's the primary sense that we use to explore the world. Kids put things in their mouths; in part to taste them, but also to feel them in their mouth. Eventually kids switch to using their hands as the primary instrument of haptic exploration. That's a good thing, of course: The hands can reach farther away, and there are lots of things that we might want to touch but don't especially want to put into our mouths. Most early developmental theories argued that human infants use their sense of touch to educate their sense of vision. For instance, children would hold an object and move it back and forth, and only then notice that its retinal image size grew larger and smaller as they did this. In the future, perhaps they would make use of the visual cue of relative size by itself. But according to the theory, it was the active touch and object exploration that started this process.

In this lecture, I'll discuss how the brain infers the state of the surrounding world on the basis of a wide range of different specialized receptor systems, all of which are imbedded in your skin. I'll focus particular attention on our haptic exploration of the world; information that's derived from touch sensors as we're actively moving the hands to manipulate and touch surfaces around us. The skin has some areas that provide very detailed, high resolution touch information, such as the surfaces of the fingertips. Large regions of the skin are sensitive to some kinds of touch but not very detailed in the information that they provide about what or even where that touch contact was made. I'll draw an analogy between this scheme for organizing touch and the organization of the visual systems around foveal and peripheral vision. We'll spend some time considering how we combine touch information with our actions, both to control our actions and to actively explore the surfaces around us. I'll finish this lecture with a consideration of how the sense of touch grounds the other senses, providing a foundation from which they encode their information. I'll describe how touch can be used to induce an out-of-body experience, and we'll have a little fun inspiring some in the minds and bodies of some volunteers.

In Lecture 2, I discussed transduction in general, the process by which energy in the world is converted into neural impulses. Just to remind you, the transduction process for touch is accomplished by many different types of receptors located at different locations below the surface of the skin. In addition to having different locations in depth, the cells' structure gives them different receptive properties. We only experience one conscious perception of touch, but it's derived from many different types of information capture. For instance, Merkel receptors live very close to the surface of the skin, just beneath the tough outermost layer of skin called the epidermis. They're small, and in some areas of the skin they're very densely packed together. This gives them the ability to encode very fine details of a pattern of pressure when something presses against your skin. If you touch the bark of an oak tree by pressing your fingers against it, you'll be able to feel the precise texture, the precise shapes, of the tiny features that make up that surface. If you touch a maple tree, the bark will feel different. It's the Merkel cells that provide you with that finely detailed information that's derived during that continuous pressure experience.

Meissner's corpuscles are located at about the same depth within the skin. These cells are substantially larger than Merkel cells and thus can't encode fine details very well. What they can encode is vibration. If you press on a Meissner's corpuscle, it would respond but only for a few milliseconds, after which it would turn off. If you release that pressure, it responds again. In essence, what the Meissner's corpuscles are encoding is not pressure per se, but changes in pressure. Because the cells respond so quickly, the best thing to stimulate them is vibration; the rapid, repeated increase and decrease in the amount of pressure. If you were to run your fingers along those oak and maple trees, feeling their bark as you move their hands across their surfaces, you would feel the individual details to some extent, but your primary experience would be that of an overall texture. That emergent perception of texture is derived from the patterns of vibration sensed by these Meissner's corpuscles.

If you're engaged in a manual activity, like using pliers or a screwdriver, it might feel as if you're using pressure information as you do this; but it's the dynamic changes in pressure caused as you move that are most important for controlling your actions. In most situations, these different types of cells work together. Imagine the simple—or seemingly simple—task of just holding a raw egg. The shell of an egg is fragile, but the egg has a substantial weight to it. How hard should you press your fingers together as you hold that egg? What you need is enough pressure to keep the egg from falling downward, but not so much that you crack the shell. In this type of situation, you would grasp the egg very lightly, such that only a small amount of response was produced by your Merkel cells. If the pressure grows too light, the egg will begin to slip just a little. As it does, the Meissner's corpuscles will begin to respond, telling you that the egg is starting to fall, and you will automatically increase your grip pressure, just slightly, to keep the egg in your grasp.

It's actually quite impressive that we can hold an egg lightly between our fingertips and move our hand around. Every time I move my hand up, the inertia of the egg creates a downward force. As it does, I slightly increase the pressure of my grip to keep a hold on the egg. When I stop moving, the same thing happens again. If I grip too tightly, the egg will break; so I need to control that force very, very precisely, and it feels very easy to do so. This preciously controlled interaction between the muscles that control my actions and the tactile receptors in my fingers is downright impressive. (It's not just the muscles and fingers of me, of course, but those of anyone who can do this.)

As with many things that are automatically controlled by our nervous system, most people think of them as quite simple. As with other things we've talked about in this course, however, it's only when we try to duplicate that process—in this case, to build a robot to accomplish the same task— that we realize the depth of the information processing that's occurring in our sensory systems all the time. As simple as this task is—waving an egg around—there are essentially no robots out there that can do it. Human perception and action are amazing.

There are even more classes of receptors in our skin. Ruffini cylinders are located a bit deeper within the skin. These encode stretching movements whenever our skin is pulled, either as a result of our own actions or as a result of a passive contact with some other surface. These cells seem to be especially important for kinesthetic perception; that is, our sense of our body's posture. I'll be talking about this in more detail in Lecture 15.

Pacinian corpuscles are located deeper, in the layer of fat underneath our skin. These receptors work very much like the Meissner's corpuscles, sensing vibration rather than simple pressure. The Meissner's corpuscles respond best to vibration in the range of 3–40 cycles per second; Pacinian corpuscles prefer 10–500 cycles per second. As with color vision, the relative responses of these 2 different types of cells enable us to infer just what the actual rate of vibration that's out there in the world is. If the 2 cells are responding equally, than the vibration is probably in the middle of their 2 preferred ranges; if only the Meissner's cells are responding, then a slower rate of vibration is present; lots of Pacinian corpuscle response and no Meissner's cell response, then probably a high rate of vibration is present. We only feel one rate of vibration, but it's derived from a combination of the rate of action potentials being produced by these multiple-cell systems.

Let's talk about one of the key tests of how well you can sense touch, something called the 2-point threshold. Imagine that I closed your eyes so that you couldn't see, and while I did I took 2 pins and then pressed them lightly onto the skin of your fingertip. (In this experiment I would just press lightly, the pins would never break the skin.) If the pins were small enough, and if I placed those 2 pins directly next to one another, you wouldn't be able to tell if it was 1 pin or 2. Indeed, if the points were right next to each other then it would be just like pressing 1 pin against the skin. Imagine that I moved the pins slightly apart—1/10$^{th}$ of a millimeter—and then pressed them against your fingertip again. If they were closer than 1 millimeter apart, you would be essentially at chance in guessing whether there was 1 pin or 2. Only when we get to about 2 millimeters apart—about 1/3 of an inch—does the presence of 2 separate points become clear.

It's worth noting that this is a pretty big gap for our fingertip. We certainly have the impression that we can resolve details about objects that are much smaller than 2 millimeters across; and we can. I mentioned that we use vibration information as we move our hands across some surface. In order to perceive a texture, we use this vibration information. Given this relatively high 2-point threshold, the importance of that motion information becomes clear. For fine perceptual distinctions between textures, it's the vibration that we're really sensing, not the pressure.

For other parts of the body, this 2-point threshold is much larger. The champion in this regard is the back of your lower legs; the skin over your calf muscles. If you can, I recommend trying this with someone at home sometime. Take 2 pins, and put them 3 centimeters apart; a little over an inch. Tell the person to close their eyes, and then press the pins lightly against the skin, sometimes pressing 1 pin and sometimes pressing 2. As you do this, ask the person to guess which is which, whether it's 1 pin or 2. You'll find that they're terrible; that they really just can't do this. Only when the pins are more than 5 centimeters apart—a little under 2 inches—will there be a clear perception of 2 separate pressure points. This is very surprising to most people; we don't realize just how limited some of our pressure-sensing abilities are.

I can't resist relating this to our visual experience, to at least some extent. Recall that our peripheral vision is very low in resolution, both in terms of seeing fine details and in seeing colors. Almost all of our clear visual information comes from the fovea, that region in the middle of our visual field that spans about 2° of visual angle. If you place your 2 thumbs side by side at arm's length, your thumbnails will all but fill the part of the visual field where you can see clearly and well. Nonetheless, we have a perception of a clear visual field all around us, not just in this little area right in the middle of our visual field. That fine detail is all perceived, but it isn't sensed.

Let me take a moment to spell out what I mean by this: When I speak of your perception of the world around you, I mean your conscious experience of your surroundings; of the surfaces, objects, people, and the events that are going on around you all the time. When I speak of your sensations of the world around you, I mean the activities produced at the level of the receptors for your different sensory modalities. As we've seen throughout this course, your perceptions are based on your sensory inputs, but they're much more. Your vision system takes in information through your senses and uses it to infer the state of the world, the situation that would have been most likely to give rise to those incoming sensations that it has to work with; and it's that set of inferences that you perceive. In the case of vision, you only sense a detailed color image in one part of your visual field, but your visual system infers colors that it's unable to sense directly; and it's those inferences that you perceive: a visual field that's filled with color and precise detail.

What we have, then, is one small area of the visual field that's good at picking up fine details and a large area that's good at detecting changes, like movement. Once we know, or once we sense, where in the visual field there's something interesting to look at, then we direct that high-resolution set of detectors over to it by looking at it.

The sense of touch seems to be organized in an analogous fashion. There are some small regions of our skin surface that are very good at picking up the very finely-detailed information; so things like our hands, our fingers, and our mouth. (For kids, that mouth, remember, is very important for touch; for adults, we tend to rely on the fingers.) The rest of our skin is very sensitive to the presence of even slight touches, but mostly it serves just to call our attention to things that are happening in the world; things to which we might want to focus our more detailed touch perceivers (our hands or our fingers). If you're in complete darkness and something furry brushes up against your leg, you'll very likely reach down and find the cat or dog with your hands. (If you don't have a cat or dog then you might move your leg away from whatever it is very quickly). As with all of the senses, very different types of receptors work together to produce our understanding of the world around us.

This 2-point threshold that I've discussed here varies a lot across the skin surface. It also maps very nicely onto the representation of touch sensations in the somatosensory cortex that we've discussed. You'll remember that's the area of the brain that stretches horizontally across the middle part of the top of your head. If you perceive pressure on your skin or touch of any kind, it's processed in terms of activations in the body map in this area of the cortex. Particular locations in the brain correspond to particular locations on the skin. Remember that the mapping of body to brain is not uniform in scale here. Some areas of the body command a very large area of the cortex; for instance, the fingers and the tongue. Other areas of the body—for instance, the skin on the calf—are physically larger but only connect to a relatively small region of somatosensory cortex. The size of the area of somatosensory cortex is directly proportional to this 2-point threshold: The bigger the area, the better your sensitivity.

It's become apparent to researchers in recent years that this somatosensory map has a dynamic, changing structure. Most people think of the sensory cortices as hardwired in a sense to particular areas of the skin. To some extent that's true, but the connections to the cortex only arrive there after passing through some complex neural networks in the spinal cord and the hindbrain located near the back of your head. Recent evidence suggests that this neural network is quite flexible. The more you use some particular part of the skin, the more your brain devotes to encoding information about touch in that particular region. To test this, experimenters worked with macaques, a type of monkey with a brain and sensory system that are very similar to those of humans.

First, using recording electrodes, the researchers identified a particular region in the somatosensory cortex of the macaques that encoded touch sensations. Second, they provided the monkey with hours and hours of stimulation to the fingertips, the areas that encoded touch for that particular area of the somatosensory cortex, several hours a day for several weeks. Then, the experimenters recalculated which regions of the monkeys' brain responded to touch in that region. They found that the regions that responded before the extra stimulation still responded like they did at the beginning of the study, but much new brain area had been recruited, in a sense, as well. Areas that had previously encoded touch for areas of the skin adjacent to the fingertip had shrunk. The brain area that mapped this particular finger had grown tremendously, increasing in area by almost 400%.

This was an experiment in a laboratory with an unusually intense regimen of finger stimulation, but it only occurred over several weeks. Imagine that you were an avid violin player. You might spend time every day practicing this violin. As you master the ability to play your music, you become very attuned to the feeling of pressing on particular strings in just the right way to make the violin produce just the right sound. You would get better at playing the violin for many reasons, but one of the causes seems clear here: Your sense of touch would improve. After several months of practice, you would quite literally have a different, improved sense of touch. Your 2-point thresholds on your fingertips would drop. Your brain would have reconfigured itself to better support the things that you want to do. I think that's pretty cool.

An extreme version of this remapping often takes place when someone loses a limb due to injury or disease. After the limb is lost—say, an arm—these patients still have a somatosensory cortex that contains neurons devoted to representing the sense of touch for that arm. In many cases, these patients report an odd sense that the arm is still there. Doctors often refer to it as a phantom limb. There's little to no stimulation delivered to this area, of course, since the peripheral nerves that used to be in the missing arm are gone. There's still normal touch stimulation, however, delivered to the areas of the somatosensory cortex nearby. Over time—a few weeks or months after the amputation—these adjoining areas typically expand, taking over this cortical real estate that nothing else is using. In essence, the brain recycles this somatosensory cortex tissue.

It's interesting to researchers in this area that, even after this happens, the phantom limb often doesn't completely disappear. There can be a sense for the patient that the arm is still there, especially when they aren't looking at it; if they don't have a visual sense that there's the arm missing. In Lecture 15, I'll talk a bit about kinesthetic perception; our sense of where our body parts are located and what our body posture is. This persistent phantom limb suggests that our mental representation of our own body must reside somewhere other than this somatosensory cortex.

In some cases, patients with these phantom limbs report that the phantom limb feels pain; or even worse, it turns out, that it feels itchy. This can be especially maddening since the region of the body that has the itch is no longer present. It's literally an itch that you can't scratch. But it turns out that you can. If you look at the map of the somatosensory cortex, you'll notice that the areas that represent the arm are directly next to the areas that represent the face. If the arm is taken away, the face part of the somatosensory cortex expands into the region that used to be stimulated by the arm. This knowledge leads to what must be the simplest, least expensive neurological therapy ever discovered. If your phantom limb itches, there's a way to scratch it: scratch your face. In a great many cases, this gives these phantom limb patients tremendous relief.

We've discussed a lot about how the touch system works to this point in the lecture; how you and your brain gather information about temperature, pressure, and vibration and use that information to infer the state of the world around you. As with the other senses we've discussed in this course, there are inferential processes that lead us to those perceptions. We don't just perceive sensations, but rather the inferences that arise from them. I've mentioned, however, that there's something very fundamental about our sensation of touch. It doesn't just tell us about the world around us, it connects us with it. I'm going to argue here that touch doesn't just connect us to the world but to ourselves. The link between our mind—our sense of who and where we are—and the body in which our mind resides is influenced by many senses, but touch is the most important for this.

Let's consider something called the rubber hand illusion. In this display, a participant sits with her hand resting palm-down on the table in front of her. An experimenter places a screen up on one side that blocks her view of one of her hands. The experimenter places a rubber hand on the table in a location that replaces the real hand that's hidden. To strengthen the illusion, the experimenter typically drapes a cloth over the space between the participant's body and the rubber hand. If you looked at this setup—if you just walked in and looked at it—you'd see a person sitting at a table with one regular hand and one rubber hand resting on the table. The experimenter then takes 2 paintbrushes and gently strokes the rubber hand and the hidden hand in synchrony, moving the brush in the direction at the same time on corresponding parts—corresponding fingers, for instance—of the hidden hand and the rubber hand. As this happens, the participant begins to have a strange sensation that the rubber hand is her hand; that she's feeling that brush from its touch on the rubber hand. If I see something touch a hand that's located adjacent to my body, and if at the same time I feel that touch sensation via my sense of touch, my brain reaches one of those inferences: that the hand I see is me.

How do we know this is happening; how can we measure the strength of this illusion? One way involves threatening the rubber hand. If the rubber hand is threatened—for instance, with a hammer—unconscious fear response mechanisms are activated, and the subject will jump and startle the same way she would if a hammer struck one of her real hands. You can find a demonstration of this on the internet if you just search for "rubber hand illusion."

This phenomenon had been noted for many years, but some recent studies have provided some scientific evidence for the psychological reality of it. The participant's blood pressure and heart rate will rise; adrenaline begins to course through her veins. The participant typically explains that she knows that the rubber hand is just that, a rubber hand; she knows that her real hand is behind the occluding screen; and no matter what happens to the rubber hand, she'll feel no pain. She knows this. Consciously, cognitively, and rationally the participant is completely aware of this setup, but some part of the brain is not convinced. Even as the participant is completely convinced that the rubber hand is not her own, she'll often ask the hammer-wielding experimenter to please stop doing that; it's very uncomfortable.

The rubber hand illusion creates the sense that the false hand is connected to the body, but that's still not our whole sense of who and where we are that I'm suggesting here arises from touch. Could we generate a whole-body version of this rubber hand illusion? It turns out that we can. Many people report of having out of body experiences. They describe floating up and away from their bodies and being able to look back at the body from some position that's separated from it. With the rubber hand illusion as a starting point, we can generate one of these out of body experiences very easily.

In the standard set up for this, a participant wears goggles with small video screens inside of them. These tiny screens are hooked up to a video camera. If, for instance, the experimenter were to take that camera and walk down the hall, the participant would see a view of what it would look like to move down the hall. To get the out of body experience, the experimenter places the video camera not in a hall but behind the participant, looking back at it. With the camera in this position, the participant's able to see the back of his own head.

Nothing dramatic so far, right? What comes next is the key. The experimenter then brushes and pokes the physical chest of the participant while moving another brush in the same way in the bottom part of the video camera that's behind his head. The participant sees someone poking just below the field of view and feels the sensation of those poking movements. As in the rubber hand experiment, the subject actually feels a touch sensation with his own body, which is hidden, and he sees movements that would suggest brushing and poking just off-screen, presumably on the body in the video. Just as the sense of touch with the hand connected it to the body, so this experience seems to transport the viewer out of the body to the position of the video camera. No spirit has left the body here, but an inference has been made: The participant infers that he's now outside of his body looking back in.

The same type of threat measures used in the rubber hand situation confirm this here. Even though the participant might know exactly what's going on, he feels connected to the point of view of that camera. If the experimenter swings a hammer just below the video camera, the participant will brace for impact. Our sense of touch doesn't just tell us about the world; it seems that our sense of touch tells us about ourselves.

In this lectures, I've described the sense of touch and how it provides us with information about the world around us. I've talked about how certain areas of our skin are much more sensitive than others, and about how that sensitivity is achieved in the somatosensory cortex. I've discussed how that cortical representation changes as a function of injury and, more commonly, through experience. In this last section, I've talked about how fundamental touch perception seems to be; not just for perceiving the world, but for perceiving ourselves within it. As I like to say: Seeing is believing, but touching is being absolutely certain.

In the next lecture, we'll consider a particular application of touch perception: pain perception. Most people think of pain as something bad; something to be avoided; something that we wish we didn't have to experience. I'll argue that as long as it's working properly, pain is one of the most important senses that we have. I'll look forwards to joining you for a pain-free discussion next time.

# Pain—How It Works for You
## Lecture 12

In high school and college, I was a pretty serious cross-country and track-and-field runner and I learned a lot of things about pain. My coach would, of course, shout, "No pain! No gain!" as well as more creative slogans like "Pain is inevitable, suffering is optional!" The philosophy behind such clichés, which I think pervades our understanding of pain, is that pain is an enemy, something to be overcome. In fact, our ability to feel pain is extremely valuable and important to our well-being.

- Pain is annoying, yes, but it is also a continuous monitoring system that provides us with information about when something is damaged or malfunctioning in our body. A stomach ache is bad, but it teaches us about what to avoid eating in the future.

- Perhaps the best evidence for the claim that pain is our friend includes examples from the lives of people who cannot sense pain—people with congenital analgesia. They do not learn from stubbing their toes or eating spoiled food and are frequently injured.

- All of that injury typically leads to infections and complications. Most patients with congenital analgesia die before they reach the age of 20. It is clear that pain helps you to modify your behavior to enable you to thrive.

- There are 3 main types of human pain perception, 3 different systems that cause pain signals to be sent to the brain: nociceptive pain, inflammatory pain, and neuropathic pain.

- We have talked about how touch perception activates particular cells in the skin and sends information on to the brain. The same basic principle applies for nociceptive pain. Extreme heat, cold, or pressure will activate those receptors. Some receptors also seem to specifically encode damage to the skin, especially cuts.

- If almost any neuron is damaged or destroyed, the last thing it will do is fire off a very strong train of action potentials. The brain knows to interpret these as an indicator that the body is being damaged. You experience it as pain.

- When you exercise a lot and feel sore afterwards, that soreness is inflammatory pain. If you stub your toe, the immediate pain is nociceptive, but the ache in the days that follow is inflammatory pain.

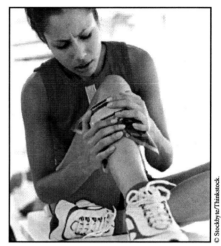

The type of lingering soreness caused by exercise is inflammatory pain.

- As your body works to repair damage to your muscles, skin, and other tissues, it sends a lot of extra blood and fluid to that area in part because blood contains the materials needed to make the repairs. This causes swelling and pressure on surrounding tissues, in turn causing pain.

- It is important that this swelling causes pain. It reminds your brain to avoid using that body part while it is under repair. Congenital analgesia patients do not have these reminders; their injuries, even small ones, do not heal properly, leading to other complications.

- Neuropathic pain results from damage to the nervous system itself, which can swell and require repair. The most common example in Western society is carpal tunnel syndrome, which results from typing and other tool use.

- Many of the muscles that move your fingers are not in your hands but in your forearms. As they contract and relax, moving back and forth sometimes dozens of times per second, that pressure can slowly damage the nerves.

- The big problem with carpal tunnel syndrome and nociceptive pain in general can be how long it takes to go away. As the nerve fibers are damaged, their function is compromised, which can lead to chronic, sometimes debilitating pain.

- Some treatments for carpal tunnel syndrome involve putting the wrist into a splint. In some cases, surgery is necessary. The best way to deal with carpal tunnel is to avoid having it happen in the first place. Listen to the first signals of fatigue and pain from your wrists.

- Strokes sometimes cause other types of neuropathic pain. Your brain is usually able to distinguish regular touch signals from those that are caused by injury and should register as pain.

- In the spinal cord, small-diameter fibers (S-fibers) convey pain signals and larger axons (L-fibers) convey information about nondamaging touch sensations to transmission fibers (T-cells). The T-cells transmit the pain information from the spinal cord up to the brain.

- S-fibers and L-fibers are also connected to each other in an inhibitory fashion. This is called a gate-control model because when you receive a nondamaging touch, all your touch fibers are activated, but the L-fibers activate a gate that stops S-fibers from sending signals on to the brain.

- However, when damaging touch occurs, the S-fibers are more active than the L-fibers, so the L-fibers are not able to shut them down. The pain gate opens, and a pain signal is sent on to the brain.

- Unfortunately, this system sometimes malfunctions. The most common cause of its malfunction is the phantom limb pain experienced by amputees. After an amputation, the nerve fibers that used to connect the limb to the spinal cord are still in the spinal cord; sometimes, the S-fibers there get activated. With no L-fibers to shut the gate, the patient can feel intense, searing pain.

- This pain perception can be a big problem since there is little that can be done to treat it, other than vigorously rubbing the end of the part of the limb that is still present to activate what L-fibers remain.

- Much recent research has found that attention plays a big role in moderating pain at the cortical level. Doing something to take your mind off of your pain can be very effective. The converse is also true: Focusing your attention on even a small amount of pain seems to ramp up its intensity.

- One typical technique for studying pain perception involves having participants submerse their hands into ice-cold water and after a few seconds rate their pain on a scale from 1 to 10. Subjects who have taken analgesic drugs like aspirin and ibuprofen typically give a slightly reduced pain rating. So do subjects who are distracted by tasks like playing video games.

- Hypnosis has also been used in this way. Putting someone into a relaxed state and suggesting to them that they will not feel pain may not make them impervious to pain, but it will tend to reduce their pain ratings.

- Perhaps the most dramatic type of distraction—say, a high-stress, fear-inducing situation—can result in a total elimination of pain. It is very common for people to be injured quite seriously in a car accident without being aware of it. Police will often insist that you go to the hospital to be checked out after an accident even if you feel perfectly fine.

- Perhaps the most valuable aspect of attention-based techniques for reducing pain is the finding that they work in a greater-than-additive fashion in combination with drugs. That is, if an aspirin reduces pain ratings by 1 and a video game distracter reduces it by

1, then a combination of the aspirin and the video-game distracter reduces ratings by 3 or more.

- From a perceptual science perspective, these results tell us that pain is not delivered directly to some pain-sensor module that functions independently from the rest of the brain. Pain perception is indirect and influenced by a variety of other perceptual and cognitive systems.

- The medical community has actually been slow to fully embrace this idea. If you find yourself in a situation where you need to manage pain, I would urge you discuss these topics with your doctor.

- Another aspect of these findings worth emphasizing is that one thing pain sufferers should avoid if at all possible is lying in bed with no distractions from their suffering. Even moderate pain can get much worse if you focus your attention on it, especially for long periods. Keep your mind engaged with something other than the pain. It can lessen the need for drugs and ultimately speed the healing process.

- The most common treatments for pain involve pharmaceuticals. Certain chemicals influence pain receptors, both in the spinal cord and in the brain itself.

- The human pain-perception system is, to a large extent, self-regulating. If we experience pain but there is no large injury, the brain will naturally shift itself to be more pain tolerant. One of the most important mechanisms for this involves chemicals produced by the brain called endorphins.

- In the brain, endorphins block the transmission of signals that cause the perception of pain at the level of individual synapses. Many of the strongest pain-relieving drugs are chemicals whose molecules are very similar in shape to endorphins. Opium, heroin, morphine, and so forth are, in essence, artificial endorphins.

- They are also, as you almost certainly know, addictive, and a big part of that addiction has to do with the brain's natural tendency to modulate its level of pain perception. If there is pain and no injury, then pain perception is downregulated. If there is injury and no pain, then the opposite happens: Endorphin production is reduced. When the drugs are removed, the drug user experiences more pain—sometimes much, much more.

- A wide range of studies have examined the placebo effect. If you tell someone they are receiving a powerful, pain-relieving drug, often they will report reductions in pain even if the supposed drug is just a sugar pill. It is believed this effect is related to attentional pain-modulation issues.

- Another way to experience pain involves no personal injury at all: empathetic pain. You may have experienced this when you witnessed a loved being injured. You might expect this experience to cause figurative heartache or distress; in fact, many people experience literal nociceptive pain.

- Neuroscientists interested in pain have conducted some fascinating studies of this effect in recent years. Very specific areas of the cortex are activated in this context, and the greater the pain, the greater that activation.

- A lot of activation is seen in the touch-sensitive areas of the somatosensory cortex, located to the side of the top of the head, as well as in the temporal regions lower down on the side of the head.

- In fMRI studies, people looking at a picture of a stranger's injured hand are told the stranger has just slammed the hand in a car door. Some of those same areas of the brain are activated, but not the somatosensory cortex.

- If you feel strong emotional ties to someone, then when they experience pain, so do you—not just figurative pain but to some extent real, physical, measurable pain. As with all of the other senses, our perceptions of pain seem to be constructed and interpreted in a flexible way by our brain as a whole.

## Suggested Reading

Dworkin et al., "Pharmacologic Management of Neuropathic Pain."

Thernstrom, *The Pain Chronicles*.

## Questions to Consider

1. Many people regularly consume alcohol, a substance that, among other things, reduces our sensitivity to pain. Based on your knowledge of the biology of pain-sensory circuits, explain why drugs that reduce pain are associated with addiction.

2. There is good evidence that having a sympathetic person around when you are in pain makes the pain worse. Why do you suppose that is so?

# Pain—How It Works for You
## Lecture 12—Transcript

In high school and college, I was a pretty serious cross country and track and field runner. That was about 30 years and almost as many pounds ago, but I learned a lot of things about pain during those years. I had a coach who liked to shout slogans as we trained, running around the track faster than our bodies wanted to go; until they started to hurt, frankly. This coach would, of course, shout the usual, "No pain! No gain!" But that was too easy, almost cliché. He liked to be more creative with these slogans: "Pain is inevitable, suffering is optional!" Or, "If you can feel pain, then you know that you are not yet dead!" My favorite of his slogans was, "Pain is the sensation of weakness leaving the body!"

The whole idea of this ranting—at least I think what the idea was—was to help us push ourselves harder in this training; to get stronger and faster, and ultimately win more races. There was a philosophy there, however, which I think pervades our understanding of pain; specifically that pain is like an enemy. Pain is a headache; pain is a nagging injury that prevents you from doing something you want to do; pain is something bad to be overcome.

In the lecture today, I'll talk about some ways in which pain can go very wrong and be that enemy to be overcome; a disorder that needs to be corrected. But I wanted to start today by pointing out that our ability to feel pain is extremely valuable and it's important to our well-being. Pain provides a continuous monitoring system that provides us with information about when something is damaged or malfunctioning in our body. Yes, it's annoying if your knee hurts; but it's far better to limp on a strained tendon than to not know that it's injured until it completely fails and snaps loose. It's not a good thing to have a stomach ache, except that it might teach you about what to avoid eating in the future; what to avoid that's made you become ill. I've stubbed my toe too many times to count in my life. It's hurt on every occasion. It's also taught me, though, to walk more slowly and carefully, especially in the dark when I'm not wearing shoes. That lesson has been painful, but my feet will probably last a lot longer for it.

Perhaps the best evidence for the claim that pain is our friend is the example of what life is like for patients who are born without a sense of pain. People with congenital analgesia are typically born without the standard sensory cells that enable them to feel when they've injured themselves; say, stubbed a toe or when they have a stomach ache. This condition might sound like a dream to some people. No aches, no pains; how could that be bad? Hopefully it's clear to you why it is. Congenital analgesia patients don't mind stubbing their toe, so they keep doing it. They don't get stomach aches, so they don't develop eating habits that suit the characteristics of their digestive system. They don't have pain, but that means they don't get any of the benefits of it either. As you might imagine, congenital analgesia patients are usually injured. All of that injury typically leads to infections and complications. Most patients without pain die before they reach the age of 20.

Pain is good. Pain is our friend. Pain may be the sensation of weakness leaving the body; maybe not. But it's clear that pain is the sensation of your body helping you to modify your behavior to enable you to thrive.

In this lecture, I'll give you an overview of how our various systems of pain perception work. I'll talk about how your brain processes pain information, and how that helps to explain why distracting you from pain can reduce how much it hurts. I'll talk about pain empathy; how seeing others in pain can quite literally cause you to feel pain yourself, especially if you care about that person in pain. I'll finish the lecture today with a consideration of a really terrible situation that occurs in which the pain system breaks down. As it does, it sometimes gets stuck in the "on" position, plaguing a patient with a chronic pain that just won't go away.

Okay, let's get to the details of pain perception. There are 3 main types of human pain perception; 3 different systems that cause pain signals to be sent to the brain: nociceptive pain, inflammatory pain, and neuropathic pain. The first, and in many ways most basic, of these is nociceptive pain. We've talked about touch perception already; particularly pressure or temperature information that activates particular cells in the skin and sends that information on to the brain. The same basic principle applies for nociceptive pain. Extreme heat, extreme cold, or extreme pressure will activate those heat, cold, and pressure receptors. Some receptors also exist that seem to specifically encode the damage of the skin, especially when the skin is cut. Almost all touch receptors can, depending upon the stimulation, contribute to our pain perception. If almost any neuron is damaged or destroyed, the last thing it will do is fire off a very strong train of those action potentials we've discussed. The brain knows to interpret these as an indicator that the body is being damaged. You experience it as pain.

The second category of pain is inflammatory pain. When you exercise a lot and feel sore afterwards, it's inflammatory pain that you're feeling. If you stub your toe or fall and get banged up, there's an acute nociceptive pain that starts that; that's the first thing you feel. The aches and pains that follow for days after, however, are inflammatory pain. As your body works to repair damage to your muscles, skin, and other tissues, it sends a lot of extra blood and fluid to that area. In part, this is important because it's that blood that contains all the materials needed to do the repairs. The fact that the swelling and pressure on surrounding tissues causes pain is also important. It sends the pain signals to your brain, which can be annoying, but those signals serve as a reminder—sometimes a very continuous reminder—that you need to avoid using that body part while it's under repair. When you limp on a damaged knee, you're shifting the weight to the other uninjured leg, allowing the damaged one to heal properly.

Those congenital analgesia patients, the ones who can't feel pain, don't have these reminders. They can make what are initially small injuries linger for long periods of time, leading to other complications. Thank you, inflammatory pain.

The third major category of pain is called neuropathic pain. This can be a real problem for many people. It results from damage not to the muscles and other parts of the musculoskeletal system, but to the nervous system itself. Remember, those neurons are cells, too; they can get damaged. They can swell, and they can require repair. The most common example of neuropathic pain in our society is something called carpal tunnel syndrome. This usually impacts the wrists and results from holding your arms in a fixed posture for too long while using them. The most common situation, of course, is typing at a computer; but it can impact people who do lots of sewing, assembly line work, or use tools for long periods of the day. If your wrists are bent at one particular upward angle for long periods of time, it can put stress on the many nerve fibers that run from the arms into the hands. Many of the muscles that move your fingers are not in your hands, but in your forearms. As they contract and relax, moving back and forth sometimes dozens of times per second, that pressure can slowly damage the nerves.

The big problem with carpal tunnel syndrome and nociceptive pain in general can be how long it takes to go away. As the nerve fibers get damaged, their function is compromised, which can lead to chronic, sometimes debilitating pain. For instance, with carpal tunnel syndrome, once the tendons in this area of the hand swell and get larger, they may stay that way, continuing to press on the nerves and preventing the nerve damage from fully healing. Some treatments for carpal tunnel syndrome involve putting the wrist into a splint that prevents the movements that are ultimately responsible for the syndrome. These are often successful, but in some cases, surgeries are done. In that case, the surgeon will trim or even cut the ligament that presses on the nerves and causes that problem to continue. The best way to deal with carpal tunnel is to avoid having it happen in the first place. Avoid making too many repetitive wrist movements, and listen when your body gives you the initial, more subtle indications of fatigue and pain. By listening to those, you can prevent it from getting to that difficult, very bad point.

Strokes sometimes cause other types of neuropathic pain. I'll talk next about the gate control system that our pain perception system uses. It works very well, most of the time. But if a particular set of the axons in this system are damaged, it can result in chronic, neuropathic pain.

I mentioned that many of the touch sensitive cells in your skin participate in pain perception. Your brain—your nervous system in general—is able to distinguish regular touch signals from those that are caused by injury from those that should be registered as pain. The circuits in the spinal cord here are very complex, but a basic model of pain perception has been developed that seems to account for most experimental findings in this area.

In the spinal cord, there are small diameter fibers called S-fibers. These are the fibers that convey the pain signals. If I were to reach into your spinal cord and electrically stimulate one of these, you would not be very happy with me afterwards. These S-fibers synapse with transmission fibers, called T-cells. The T-cells transmit the pain information from the spinal cord up to the brain. Along with the S-fibers, there are larger axons, called L-fibers, which convey information about regular touch sensations; the non-damaging sensations that are not usually registered as pain. These L-fibers also connect to the T-cells—those transmission fibers—to convey their regular touch information to the brain.

The small pain fibers and the large touch fibers are both connected to the brain. They're also connected to each other in an inhibitory fashion. If you get a touch sensation, it may activate the large fibers and the small fibers, but the large fibers will stop the small fibers from sending their information on to the brain. It's called a gate control model because the large fibers activate a gate that stops the pain from being sent on to the brain.

Pretty much any time there's a strong stimulus delivered to the skin—say, clapping your hands together, kicking a ball, or even just jumping up and down on a dance floor—any time you get a strong stimulus, these pain fibers get active. "Ouch!" they say. "I'm in pain!" Fortunately, the large touch fibers are very active, too. They close the pain gate and say, "Oh take it easy. This is just regular, run of the mill sensation. Stop complaining!" Sometimes the stimulation gets too intense, however. Maybe it's a hammer hitting your hand instead of another clapping hand, or you fall down on that dance floor. Now the small pain fibers get more active; so active that the regular large touch fibers can't shut them down anymore. The pain gate opens, and voilà, a pain signal is sent on to the brain and you experience pain.

This gate-control-based system works very well. By moderating the gate control, you can still experience regular stimulation without feeling pain, but too much stimulation and you get a signal that's registered as pain, one that signals you to change your behavior. This is the normal function of the system; this is how it works when it's working well. Unfortunately, it sometimes malfunctions. The most common cause of its malfunction is experienced by amputees; people who have, due to accident or injury, lost a limb, say, an arm. After such an amputation, the arm is no longer there, but the nerve fibers that used to connect it to the spinal cord are still in the spinal cord.

Ideally, since none of these neurons in the spinal cord is connected to anything anymore, they stay quiet in that spinal cord; and they usually do. But for some reason, sometimes the small pain fibers there get activated. Even if they get activated a little, this can be a big problem, because there's no regular touch sensation coming from the large, regular touch sensors. Remember they're not connected to the skin anymore. If the small pain fibers are active, and there's no large fiber activation to shut that pain gate, then the patient feels pain; sometimes intense, searing pain. For these patients, one of the most frustrating things is that they're feeling pain in this limb that's no longer there; there's nothing they can do to get rid of the pain, they just feel it. Often these patients describe having a phantom limb. In Lecture 15, we'll talk about kinesthetic perception; the sense that we derive of the positions and postures of our body parts. This results from the many nerves that innervate our body parts. Almost all of them synapse with the spinal cord. Even if the limb is gone, there's often still a sense that it's still there, in a particular position, with a particular posture. The arm can sometimes feel hot and cold; it can get itchy; it can feel pain. In this pain perception situation, this can be a big problem since there's nothing that can be done to treat the pain at its site of origin.

Actually, there's one very simple thing that often works to some extent: vigorously rubbing the end of the part of the limb that's still present. There are still touch sensitive fibers there; those large fibers that are present in the end of the limb. By rubbing a lot, the stimulus can sometimes get large enough to close that pain gate again and provide some relief. Actually, this rubbing cure for pain is something you see people do a lot when they experience some acute impact injury, even people who haven't taken a course on the human senses. If you bang your arm on something, for instance, often our first instinct is to rub the spot that was hurt; it provides at least some very immediate relief. Hopefully you can understand why that is now. As you rub the injury site, you're ramping up the activity of those large regular touch sensitive fibers, and in so doing closing the pain gate, or at least closing it somewhat. In so doing, you reduce the sensation of pain.

Much recent research has found that attention plays a big role in moderating pain as well. This doesn't seem to have its impact at the level of this gate control system, but at a higher, more cortical level. If you're experiencing pain, especially chronic pain, it's clear that doing something to take your mind off of it can be very effective in reducing that pain. The converse is also true: If you're experiencing even a little bit of pain, then focusing your attention on it seems to be unfortunately effective in ramping up its intensity. Many dentists have taken to giving their patients, especially child patients, movies to watch or videogames to play while they undergo treatment.

Several well-designed experiments have found evidence that this doesn't just reduce complaining, it actually reduces the sensation of pain itself. One typical technique for studying pain perception involves having participants submerse their hands into ice-cold water. After a few seconds, this really begins to hurt. Participants are usually asked to put their hand in the water and then after some specified period of time rate their pain on a scale from 1 to 10, with 1 being almost no pain and 10 being the worst pain they've ever felt. This is how studies of the effectiveness of analgesic drugs like aspirin and ibuprofen have been done. If you've had a few pills like these, then after 20 seconds in that ice-cold water, you'll typically give a slightly reduced pain rating. Like drugs, distracting tasks like playing video games seems to work to reduce those pain sensations; they reduce the ratings that people give. Focusing your attention on the pain seems to do the opposite: to increase those ratings of pain. Hypnosis has also been used in this way. Putting someone into a relaxed state and then suggesting to them that they will not feel pain may not make them impervious to pain, but it will tend to reduce those pain ratings.

Perhaps the most dramatic type of distraction—say, a high stress, fear-inducing situation—can result in a total elimination of pain. It's very common for people to be injured quite seriously in a car accident without being aware of it. The terror and adrenaline of the experience is so intense in some cases that it turns off pain sensations for a while, even for many minutes or even an hour. Police will often insist that you go to the hospital to be checked out after an accident for this very reason. Even if you're completely confident that you're perfectly fine and uninjured, you're absolutely fine to go home, a few hours after the accident, you may awake to the full extent of your injuries, which may have grown much worse due to the delay in having them looked at.

Perhaps the most valuable thing about these attention-based techniques for reducing pain is the finding that they work really well in combination with drugs, and they work in a greater than additive fashion. That is, if an aspirin reduces pain ratings by an average of 1 and a video game distracter reduces it by 1, then a combination of the aspirin and the video game distracter would not reduce it just by $1 + 1 = 2$, but when you put them together, somehow it reduces them by 3 or more.

From a perceptual science perspective, these results are very interesting in that they tell us something important about pain perception. What we perceive as pain is not delivered directly to some pain sensor module that functions independently from the rest of the brain. Pain perception is indirect and influenced by a variety of other perceptual and cognitive systems. Hopefully for you, having considered all of the fascinating and complex interactions between the other senses—touch, pain, vision, all of them—having considered those, you won't find this surprising at all; but the medical community has actually been slow to fully embrace this idea. If you find yourself in a situation in which you have some pain to manage—after an injury or after some medical procedure—I would urge you discuss these topics with your doctor and then work with him or her to develop a plan to that makes use of them.

There's one other aspect of this attentional modulation of pain that's worth emphasizing. If you're in pain, maybe the worst thing to do is lie home in bed suffering. Even moderate pain can get so much worse if you focus your attention on it, especially for long periods. This can become a vicious cycle: Pain leads to inactivity, which leads to worse pain, which leads to even more inactivity. It might not be possible to go out and run around after experiencing some injury, but it's really important to keep your mind engaged by something other than the experience of the pain. It can lessen the need for drugs and ultimately speed the healing process.

Of course, the most common treatments for pain involve pharmaceuticals. We know a lot about how certain chemicals influence pain receptors, both in the spinal cord and in the brain itself. Remember from our discussion of that gate control theory of pain that the human pain perception system is, to a large extent, self-regulating. If we experience pain, but there's no large injury, the brain will naturally shift itself to be more pain tolerant.

One of the most important mechanisms for this involves chemicals produced by the brain called endorphins. When released into the brain, these endorphins block the transmission of signals that cause pain, or the perception of pain, by blocking the transmission of those signals at the level of individual synapses. Many of the strongest pain relieving drugs that doctors use are chemicals whose molecules are very similar in shape to endorphins. They flow into the brain and block transmission of pain just like the endorphins do. Drugs like opium, heroin, morphine, and things that are derived from those chemicals are, in essence, artificial endorphins. These drugs are, as you almost certainly know, addictive, and a big part of that addiction has to do with the brain's natural tendency to modulate its level of pain perception. If there's pain and no injury, then pain perception is down-regulated. If there's injury and no pain, then the opposite happens: Endorphin production is reduced and when the drugs are removed, the drug user experiences more pain; sometimes much, much more.

There's been a wide range of studies on what's known as the placebo effect in pain reduction. If you tell someone that they're receiving a powerful, pain-relieving drug, often they'll report reductions in pain, of their experience of that pain, even if the supposed drug wasn't a drug at all but just a sugar pill. It's believed that the effects of this are very related to those attentional pain modulation issues. It may be that they do exactly the same thing.

We've talked a lot today about experiencing pain when you yourself are injured or ill. There's another way to experience pain, however, that doesn't involve any personal injury at all: empathetic pain. I'd read about this for many years, but my first real experience with empathetic pain came when I took my infant kids to get their immunization shots for measles, mumps, and rubella; the dreaded MMR shots. They're typically given when a child's about a year old. Kids are so pudgy and cute at 1 year of age. They don't talk very well, but they communicate with you a lot; they move around all the time; they have a clearly defined personality; and they're really good at expressing their emotions.

This MMR vaccination is often the last one the child receives where they don't know what's coming. The nurse comes in with a little plastic basket with all the needles prepared; she says something nice and then blammo, sticks your sweet baby with a needle. I remember so clearly watching this, and feeling—literally feeling—as if the needle was sticking into me. I knew that it wasn't, of course, at some rational level; but there was this completely salient, palpable sense of pain. Not a figurative sensation of pain like maybe you'd get from reading a poem or something, but a literal experience of what could have been nociceptive pain. This, it turns out, is a very common experience. Many people report this, and not just with kids and vaccinations. If you see someone experience an injury, a painful injury, you may yourself experience pain. It's especially true if you have a close emotional bond with that person that you're witnessing undergo the pain.

Neuroscientists interested in pain have conducted some fascinating studies of this effect in recent years. If someone experiences pain, there are very specific areas of the cortex that are activated; and the greater the pain, the greater that activation. There's a lot of activation in the touch sensitive areas of the somatosensory cortex located to the side of the top of the head; there's also activation in more temporal regions, lower down on the side of the head. Imagine that you're in one of these studies and you lie in a scanner, and you look at a picture of someone's injured hand and are told they've just slammed their hand in a car door. The pictures they used in the study were very effective. When you look at the picture, even if you don't know the person, there's a tendency to wince a little bit. There's an empathetic pain response.

If you have someone in an fMRI scanner while they look at the picture and they hear that statement that the fingers were just slammed in a car door, some of those same areas of the brain are activated. The somatosensory cortex areas on the top are not activated. This makes sense: We're clearly aware of the difference between slamming our own hand in a car door and someone else slamming his or her hand. The temporal cortex brain regions, however, become very active; almost as active as if you were experiencing the pain yourself. Not everyone experiences that empathic pain, and some experience it more clearly than others. Participants in this study look at these photos and then also rate for each one their experience of that empathic pain. The higher their ratings, it turns out, the greater the activation in these brain regions. I have little doubt that when I watched my kids getting that injection that this temporal area of my brain lit up like the 4th of July. Thus, there seems to be a neural reality to this expression, "It hurts to watch." If you feel strong emotional ties to someone, then when they experience pain, so do you; not just figurative pain but, to some extent, real, physical, measurable pain.

In this lecture, we've considered a wide range of perspectives on pain perception. I've discussed several different types of pain perception: nociceptive pain perception, inflammatory pain perception, and neuropathic pain perception. We've also talked about empathetic pain perception. I've also described some of the details about how the spinal cord and brain implement those different pain perception processes. I've also suggested a variety of ways to avoid and reduce pain based on cognitive changes in your attention. As with all of the other senses, our perceptions of pain seem to be constructed and interpreted in a flexible way by our brain as a whole.

Hopefully you've learned some things about why pain perception is important and valuable. Pain may or may not be the sensation of weakness leaving your body, but I think it's clear that pain is, at least usually, your friend.

In our next lecture, we're going to consider how perception and action control relate to one another. In general, people understand that we gather information from the world around us and use that information to control our actions. For instance, if you're going to drive, you'd better get information from your sense of vision about the direction in which you're headed. If you're trying to pick something up, then you're going to need information about where and how big the target object is.

We use sensory information to control our actions; that's straightforward. More recent work has shown that the opposite is true as well: Our actions control our perceptions. That interplay of action and perception will be our next topic. I hope you'll join me.

# Perception in Action
## Lecture 13

S ensation and perception do not happen in a vacuum but in the context of an active, behaving body. We use the information we gather from the world around us to make decisions, plan actions, and implement those actions.

- People have been studying perception for hundreds of years. They have asked thousands of questions using a great many methods. However, until very recently, almost all experiments involved showing the study participant some sort of display and asking the participant to make conscious judgments about what he or she experienced.

- These studies are valuable because they tell us about how people use sensory inputs to construct experiences of the world around them. However, they do not tell us what perception is for—what specific purpose it serves.

- If we presume an evolutionary perspective—that our senses developed the way they did for the specific purpose of promoting our species's survival—then perception is not valuable until it helps us do something: find food, avoid predators, build things, and so forth. There is a great deal of evidence that this is exactly the case.

- If we want to understand our sensory systems, then we should consider how our senses work not just for use in judgment-based experiments but how they are used to control these real-world actions.

- One particular school of thought—and a large group of researchers—have built their careers on just this perspective. The most famous was a man named J. J. Gibson. When he began his career, many people were very invested in studying perception under unrealistic laboratory situations.

- Gibson grew concerned that anything discovered this way would not generalize to the real world. He thus developed the field of ecological perception and, more generally, ecological psychology, which does not study humans but their environments.

- Gibson wanted to identify the types of information humans unconsciously determined was important in their environments without much intervening mental processing, referred to as direct perception.

- If humans used such sensory information without ever being aware we were doing so, then the judgment researchers were using was insufficient or incomplete, a tiny subset of the things that our senses could do.

- Consider for a moment a frog that catches flies with its tongue. This might seem simple, the frog's vision and motor systems have to make a small prediction about what the fly's future distance and direction will be.

- Does the frog make conscious judgments about flies and distances and velocities? It is possible, but it seems unlikely. It is certainly not necessary for conscious perception to enter into this at all. Perhaps, suggested the ecological psychologists, most of human sensory processing is just like this, with direct links between certain sensations and actions.

- Consider the human baseball player—the outfielder. When the ball is hit hard toward the outfield, expert outfielders will immediately begin running right for the place where the ball will land. The ball's path is somewhat complex, but the player is not consciously performing mathematics.

- A researcher named Mike McBeath has shown that the outfielder runs so that the ball moves through his visual field in a straight, diagonal line. If the line curves one way, the player needs to speed up and turn. If it curves the other way, the player needs to slow down and turn the other way.

- The fielder follows this 2-dimensional control principle until the ball is directly overhead, at which point he reaches out and catches it. McBeath and his colleagues, after developing this, built a set of robots that can catch balls using just this method.

- Because the eyes themselves are spherical, outfielders actually run on a circular path that matches the curvature of the backs of their eyes, but the same principle applies. It is worth noting that actual outfielders have no idea that this is how they catch the ball. They describe their running and catching as instinctive or experience based.

- These findings, along with the brain-injured patients DF and RV mentioned in Lecture 4, have inspired some interesting research. (Remember, DF cannot consciously see things but can pick them up, while RV can see things but not grasp them.)

- In experiments where 2 black disks of the same size are placed on a white background, when you ask subjects which is larger, about half will choose the disk on the left and about half the disk on the right.

- However, if I surround the disk on the left with very small disks and the disk on the right with very large disks, it creates something called the Ebbinghaus illusion. The small disks will make that disk in the middle of them look much larger. The large disks will make the disk in the middle of those large disks look smaller.

- When the disks are the same size, the disk surrounded by little circles looks about 10% larger. When the disk surrounded by large circles is enlarged by about 10%, you have a situation where the 2 central disks are unequal in physical size but equal in perceived size.

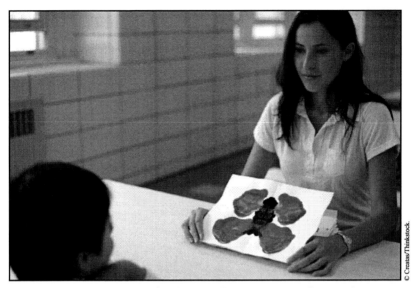

**The ecological psychologists felt that most laboratory tests of perception were highly artificial, not reflecting the way our senses function in the real world.**

- Note this still involves overt, conscious judgment, so tests like this one do not address the concerns of Gibson and the ecological psychologists.

- In the mid-1990s, a researcher named Mel Goodale shook up the perception world quite a bit by trying to assess the perception of such stimuli in a very different way. A few years earlier, other researchers had noted that the way in which we reach to grasp something is highly correlated with the size of our target.

- Goodale and his colleagues created one of these illusion displays in which the central disks were made of thin pieces of plastic so that participants could reach out and pick them up. Participants started by making the usual relative size judgments, with the same results. Then the participants reached out to pick the disks up, and the sizes of their maximum grip apertures were recorded and compared for these different displays.

- The analyses and interpretations of that reaching data are a little complex, but Goodale's key argument was that if the participants thought the disks were equal in size, their maximum grip apertures should be the same size. Yet they were not.

- Participants in these studies consciously perceive the displays as equal in size, but some part of their brains knew that one disk was bigger than the other, and their maximum grip apertures adjusted accordingly. It is a little unsettling to know that important things are going on in your head over which you have no awareness, let alone control.

- This finding has been replicated in a lot of different contexts. For example, if you stare at a set of stripes that are tilted to the right for a couple of minutes, you will fatigue the cells that encode edges at that particular orientation—one of those retinotopic maps.

- Just as colors and motion are encoded in an opponent process fashion, so is tilt perception. Neurons that encode tilt in a particular direction tend to inhibit neurons that encode tilt in the opposite direction.

- You can probably guess that if you stop looking at these stripes and switch to looking at a set of vertical stripes, because the first set of tilt cells are now very tired, the tilt cells for the other direction will start winning the tug of war, and as a result, the vertical stripes will appear tilted.

- If we were in a perception lab about 50 years ago, I might have asked you to make a judgment about whether the lines were tilted rightward or leftward. An ecological psychologist would now urge us to use a real-world action instead, perhaps reaching with your thumb and index finger to grasp the line while I measured the rotation of your wrist.

- The world looks one way to our conscious mind, but somewhere up in our head is an accurate representation, and it is that representation that controls our visually guided actions. If you remember DF and

RV, these results might not be that shocking to you, certainly not as shocking as they were to perception researchers who were fully invested in perceptual judgment methodology.

- There is a simple explanation for all of this based on that 2-visual-system theory: The ventral stream controls our conscious perception; it is influenced by illusions. The dorsal stream controls our visually guided actions; for some reason, it is not greatly influenced by illusions.

- This convergence of evidence from the domain of neurology (looking at brain-injured patients) and perception research (looking at uninjured brains) is really valuable because, just as there are limitations to studying brain-injured patients, there are limitations to perception research as well. But when these 2 very different types of experimental results point to the same conclusion, it starts to seem more and more likely that the conclusions they suggest are correct.

- Other models of brain organization have been suggested as well; for instance, the idea that there are not 2 but 3 streams of processing: one for conscious perception, one for action planning, and one for action control. As additional experiments are run, the story here has grown increasingly murky, rather than clearer.

- One of my own experiments in this area was conducted with an Ebbinghaus illusion display that varied the sizes of the 2 central disks. We asked people to select across all the different tasks which of the disks was larger.

- In some cases, we asked people to state verbally which was larger. When they did this, the usual illusion was produced, with the usual 10% difference in perceived size.

- We then asked participants to continue selecting which of the disks was larger but to stop telling us verbally and to grasp it instead. We tracked the formation of their maximum grip apertures and found a reduction in the impact of the illusion; that is, the illusion effected their conscious, verbal judgments but seemed not to effect their grasping.

- The strange thing we found, however, was that for the conscious judgments made just prior to the reach, the effect of the illusion was reduced as well. In other words, when they were looking at the same display but getting ready to reach for one of the disks, then the effect of the illusion was drastically reduced.

- Intending to reach for a target changes how you perceive it. Based on this, my colleagues and I have suggested the presence of 2 different modes of visual processing: one for observation and one for action. It may be that they do not happen in parallel all the time, until you are ready to perform a particular action.

## Suggested Reading

Aglioti, DeSouza, and Goodale, "Size-Contrast Illusions."

Milner and Goodale, *The Visual Brain in Action.*

## Questions to Consider

1. Some pictorial illusions that exert a strong influence on our conscious perception have a much smaller (or even no) effect on our visually guided action performance. It seems that some of our visual processing is almost immune to these illusions. Why would you build a brain this way? If our brain knows the correct size of some object, why would it not use that accurate information for everything, including our conscious perception?

2. When baseball players catch a fly ball, it seems clear that they do not calculate the precise parabolic path of the ball's motion. Instead, they rely on a straightforward relationship between the motion of the ball across their retina and an appropriate running behavior. Can you think of other visual tricks that you might use to walk through a doorway, pick up an object, or recognize your friend's face? Are there aspects of visually guided action where a trick seems unlikely to work?

# Perception in Action
## Lecture 13—Transcript

This lecture will focus on perception and action control. The last lecture concluded our focus on non-visual modalities of sensation and perception. We'll still talk about touch, taste, smell, and hearing, but often in the context of how they interact with each other and with vision.

The unit of lectures that we're starting now will consider how your sensory systems function within the context of your body and the surrounding environment. Sensation and perception don't happen in a vacuum, to a person simply sitting in a chair as the sensory world washes over her. Sensation and perception happen in the context of an active, behaving body. We use the information we gather from the world around us to do things: to make decisions, to plan actions, and to implement those actions.

In this lecture, I'll discuss perception and action control very directly. In the next 7 lectures, I'll discuss other aspects of this perception in context idea. I'll present information about perception and attention, considering how we focus our mental resources on some things and away from other things to maximize effective behaviors. We'll then move to kinesthetic perception, considering how touch and other related senses interact with our sense of our own body. We'll spend 2 lectures considering perceptual development. By studying how our sensory systems come on line and develop, we can not only understand infant and child perception, but better understand how our sensory systems function. Finally in this unit, we'll discuss perceptual learning. I've talked a lot in this course about how sensory systems make use of a great deal of perceptually intelligent inference to rapidly deliver information to you that's both richly detailed and accurate. In the perceptual learning lecture, we'll discuss some of the ways that your sensory systems get better at doing this through experience.

Okay, let's get to work on this lecture's topic: Perception in Action. People have been studying perception for hundreds of years. They've asked thousands of different questions, using a great many different methods. Almost all of those experiments, however, particularly until very recently, involved one particular characteristic: The experimenter would show the study participant some sort of display or series of displays and then ask the participant to say what they saw. The questions participants are asked are a little more subtle than just asking them to say what they saw, of course. Maybe they're asked which of 2 objects is farther away or which test patch looks green. But still, all of the questions ask people to make conscious judgments about what they experience.

Those studies are valuable, of course. They tell us about how people use sensory inputs to construct their experience of the world around them. We've been talking a lot about those studies in this course, and while the studies are still good, it should be said that they don't really tell us about what perception is for; what specific purpose it serves. If we presume an evolutionary perspective here—the idea that our sensory systems have evolved through some sort of selective adaptation process—if we presume that our senses developed the way they did for the specific purpose of promoting our survival and well-being, then perception isn't actually valuable until it helps us do something. Making overt, conscious reflections about the state of our surroundings is nice, but unless our senses help us to do things—to help us find food, avoid predators, get around in the world, to build things, and other similar activities—unless our sensory systems help with real actions, then they aren't really that important.

There's a lot of evidence, however, that our senses are really useful for doing all sorts of things. Indeed, I'll argue this today, there's evidence that our sensory systems are particularly adapted to help with just those sorts of behaviors. If we want to understand our sensory systems, then we should consider how our senses work not just for use in judgment-based experiments, but how they're used to control these real-world actions. We need to study perception without making the assumption that we're always consciously aware of our sensory functions and able to make conscious judgments about those sensory functions.

There's a particular school of thought—and a large group of researchers—who've built their careers on just this perspective. The most famous of these was a man named J. J. Gibson from Cornell University (where I earned my Ph.D., by the way). When he started doing psychological science research way back when—perception research in particular—people were very invested in studying perception in some very unrealistic laboratory situations. The stimuli that were used in these labs didn't look like the real world. They often involved very brief, flashing presentations of stimuli that consisted of just a few points of light or maybe very simple objects. Gibson grew concerned, as he looked at this research, that anything discovered in these very specific laboratory settings might not generalize to the real world. That is, he was worried that the theories developed in the lab wouldn't help us predict how people would see and behave anywhere outside that exact laboratory.

Gibson set out to fix this and in so doing developed the field that's become known as ecological perception; and more generally, in terms of the larger field, known as ecological psychology. Gibson spent a lot of time studying not people but the environment. What information was available in the environment that specified things that are important for performing everyday tasks? He thought that maybe if we could identify that information that maybe humans just pick up that information without a whole lot of intervening mental processing. This idea of direct information pick up and use without judgment or even necessarily awareness of it is often referred to as direct perception. It's possible that we use this information—this sensory information—without ever really knowing that we're doing it. If that's the case, then maybe using those judgment tasks that researchers use will similarly not generalize. Maybe all of that research has been insufficient or incomplete, sort of like it's focusing on a very tiny subset of the things that our senses can actually do.

Consider for a moment a frog that eats flies. It sits in the swamp most of the time and when a fly's nearby it shoots its tongue out, catches the fly, and eats it. This might seem very simple, but as with many visuomotor tasks, there's a lot to it. The frog has to know the location of the fly, both the distance to the fly and the direction between the frog's head and the fly. Flies also move very fast when they're flying by. If you were to shoot your tongue out at the current location of the fly, no matter how fast it was, by the time your tongue got there—even a few hundred milliseconds later—the fly would be gone; it would have moved on to some other location. In order to catch a rapidly moving fly (if you're a frog), you have to aim for where the fly is going to be in the near future. In essence, the frog's vision and motor systems have to make a small prediction about what the fly's future distance and direction will be.

In the visual system of a frog, there are neurons that respond to flies, and these neurons don't respond to much else. You can fool them with a small, fly-like object on a string, but in their natural environment, the only thing that frogs encounter that trigger action potentials in these receptors is the fly. The link between the stimulus and the particular action suggests that the frog does indeed control their tongue; that they launch their tongue in that future-oriented fashion, aiming ahead of the fly along its path of motion and succeeding catching flies. There's this very direct link between what they see on their retina and where their tongue goes.

Do you think the frog makes judgments about flies and distances and velocities as it does this? Does it consciously ponder these things in order to control the action? It's possible, but it seems unlikely. It's certainly not necessary for conscious perception to enter into this at all. It could, in fact, be that the experience of the frog is sort of like a reflexive response, like an eye-blink. When something is moving rapidly towards you—say I threw a pillow at your head—you would blink. You wouldn't ponder the size and distance of the pillow; your sensory systems would just register that there's something rapidly approaching you and send a command to the muscles that control the eyes saying to close them.

Perhaps, pondered the ecological psychologists, most of sensory processing is just like this, with direct links between certain sensations and actions that are very direct and unconscious. To the extent that they're right, then those conscious judgment studies might not tell us much of anything except maybe about how conscious perceptual judgments are formed.

Do humans have these vision-action linkages like frogs; things that don't run through a conscious perception stage but simply proceed directly from sensation to action? For a moment let's consider the human baseball player; the outfielder, to be specific. In a game of baseball, when the ball is hit hard toward the outfield, expert outfielders will immediately begin running. As they do, they'll head right for the place that the ball that will just hit is going to land. The physics of the path of a ball's flight are not incredibly complex, but they're somewhat complex. They require some mathematics about the nature of a parabolic trajectory; there are things about gravity that have to be included there in that calculation. If you know the velocity and direction of the ball, you can apply all this information about gravitational acceleration and wind resistance and calculate, using that parabolic trajectory, what the expected landing point will be.

Do baseball players do this? Do they instantly calculate the parabolic trajectory of a ball in flight as it's hit to determine where it will land? Many fantastic baseball players have never studied physics, and yet, within a few hundred milliseconds of the crack of that bat, these players are off and running, often at top speed, toward the location where the ball will land.

There's some very good evidence that baseball players don't need to do this whole physics problem, tracing the ball's parabolic trajectory through 3-dimensional space. First, there's a trick that a researcher named Mike McBeath figured out. The basic idea is that the fielder runs so that the ball moves through his visual field in a straight, diagonal line. If it starts to curve one way, then the baseball player needs to speed up and turn. If it starts to curve the other way, then the baseball player needs to slow down and maybe turn the other way. The fielder follows this very 2-dimensional control principle until the ball is suddenly directly overhead, at which point he just reaches out and catches it.

This control principle isn't just mathematically supported, it works in real life. McBeath and his colleagues, after developing this, actually built a set of robots that can catch balls using just this method. Do human outfielders use this? Perhaps the best piece of evidence that they do has to do with a consequence of using this system of control to figure out where to run and how fast to run. Because the eyes themselves are spherical—because the retina are spherical surfaces on the back of our eye—the outfielders shouldn't run in a straight path to the ball's eventual landing location. They should run actually on a circular path that matches the curvature of the backs of their eyes; and they do. The next time you watch a baseball game and a pop fly goes soaring out to the field, watch the fielder running to catch it. He won't be running in a straight line; he'll be running in a big circle that heads directly for the place where the ball's going to land.

It's worth noting that actual outfielders have no idea that this is how they catch the ball. There might be a few who've read McBeath's research papers on the topic—he's actually interviewed some people about it—but even then, the outfielders make it clear that they're not thinking about tracking the ball so that it moves in a linear path through their field of vision. Outfielders describe their running and catching as instinctive, or as things that happen very automatically based on years and years of experience.

J. J. Gibson would have loved this part of the finding. The sensory information comes in through the eyes and it's used to control running behavior. It does so without ever entering the realm of consciousness, let alone conscious judgment. The link from vision to action is direct. Using laboratory tasks in which you show people balls flying through the air and ask them to make judgments about them would shed no light on this at all. Gibson and the ecological psychologists argue that much of the most important aspects of perception might be very, very similar to this.

I want to talk about some research in an area that I've actually studied that's been inspired by this line of thinking, as well as by the work of those 2 brain-injured patients we discussed in Lecture 4, DF and RV. Remember, DF was the patient who has damage to her ventral stream, resulting in a large blind spot in which she can't consciously see things, but DF can still reach out and pick up objects that are placed in that blind spot. RV is the patient with the opposite set of damage and deficits. He has damage to his dorsal stream. RV can still consciously see and make judgments just fine; his problem comes when he has to control a visually-guided reach.

Let's start by talking about some old style perceptual judgment research. If you put 2 black disks in the middle of a white background, you can see that they appear to be the same size. If you ask someone to judge which of these 2 same-sized disks is larger, they'll choose the one on the left about half of the time and the one on the right the other half of the time. If I surround the disk on the left with very small disks and the disk on the right with very large disks, it creates something called the Ebbinghaus illusion. The small disks will make that disk in the middle of them look much larger. The large disks will make the disk in the middle of those large disks look smaller. If you were to ask someone to look at this display and tell you which one of these physically identical central disks is larger, almost everyone will pick the disk that's surrounded by the small disks.

The 2 central disks here are equal in physical size, but unequal in perceived size. This is caused by the sizes of those other disks surrounding them: The one surrounded by little disks looks bigger; the other, surrounded by the big disks, looks smaller. The disk surrounded by little circles looks larger by about 10% in this situation. If you increase the diameter of the other disk by about 10% and then ask people to pick then which one's larger, now they'll be back to this 50-50 split. In this case, we'd have a display in which the 2 central disks are unequal in physical size but equal in perceived size.

This is the way that this kind of illusion—or this illusion in particular, the Ebbinghaus illusion—has been studied for many decades. Many other illusions like it have been studied in the same way. You show a group of people a set of stimulus images and ask them to make judgments about them. Note that this all involves overt, conscious judgments. If we rely on this approach to studying perception, then we're inherently assuming that we have conscious access to all of the important parts of visual processing. To the extent that we don't—that some of the most important aspects of perception are not accessible to conscious judgment—then this technique will be flawed. This is the central argument of those ecological psychologists, like J. J. Gibson.

In the mid-1990s, a researcher named Mel Goodale shook up the perception world quite a bit, actually, by trying to assess the perception of stimuli like these that I'm describing in a very different way. Some work published just a few years before Goodale undertook his studies had noted that the way in which we reach to grasp something is very highly correlated with the size of that target (it's actual size in this case, I should say; not a manipulated image of its size).

To study this, very accurate position trackers are attached to the thumb and index finger. As someone reaches to pick up a target, the positions of the fingers are recorded. If you calculate the distance between those 2 fingers, you can calculate what's called the grip aperture; the size of the hand opening you make as you're reaching to pick up something. For instance, if you reach for some object with this pincer grasp, with the index and thumb, you typically start with the 2 fingers right next to each other. As your hand moves toward the target, you open the fingers up, wider and wider until, until about halfway through the reaching action you reach a point of maximum grip aperture. At that point, you begin closing your fingers down until you make contact with the target at the end of the reach.

Studies of this action have found that the maximum grip aperture is much larger than the target object, but is very highly correlated with its size. That is, if I asked you to reach for 2 targets, and one was just 1 millimeter larger than the other, as you reached for the larger target, you would consistently produce a maximum grip aperture that's about 1.5 millimeters larger than the grip aperture we produced when reaching for the smaller target. The result here is that if I know as you're making this reach how far apart your thumb and index finger are at that point of maximum grip aperture, then I can know how big your visual system—at least the part that controls the hand—thinks that the object is, the thing you're reaching for.

With this technique in hand, let's go back to that illusion display. Goodale and his colleagues created one of these illusion displays in which the central disks were made of thin pieces of plastic so that participants could reach out and pick them up. For these studies, participants started by making the usual relative size judgments that have always been made with these figures; the overt, conscious judgments. The results replicated the basic effect of the illusion just as all of the earlier research had; there was nothing really new there. People still judged the sizes of the 2 disks differently, the same way that they had before. Then the participants in these studies reached out to pick those disks up. As they did, the sizes of their maximum grip apertures were recorded and compared for these different displays. The analyses and interpretations of that reaching data are a little complex, but let me go straight to Goodale's key argument about this

Consider that display in which the 2 targets were unequal in physical size but equal in perceived size. That is, participants looked at this display—this exact display—and judged that those 2 disks appeared equal in size. If that's the case, then we would presume—quite reasonably, I think—that when they reach for these supposedly equal-sized disks, they should produce the same maximum grip apertures at the midpoint of their grasping actions. They don't. Participants in these studies consciously perceive the displays as equal in size, but somewhere up there in their heads, some part of their brain knows that they aren't equal. Some part knows that one of the disks is bigger than the other, and it's that part of the brain that controls that grip aperture.

This is a strange idea to most people; the idea that we don't use our conscious perception to control our actions, and that perceiving doesn't necessarily involve conscious judgments. It's a little unsettling to know that there are things going on in your head that are really important over which you have no awareness, let alone control.

This might have been a one-time thing—maybe the illusion resistant action control only works with this particular display—but a variety of other similar evidence has since been obtained; it's not just about this display, this finding has been replicated in a lot of different contexts. Let's consider one of them now. If you stare at a set of stripes that are tilted to the right for a couple of minutes, you'll fatigue the cells that encode edges at that particular orientation. As you stare at the tilted stripes—if you keep staring at them for an extended period of time—what you're doing is fatiguing one of those retinotopic maps that we discussed in the 2nd and 3rd lectures of the course. Just as colors and motion are encoded in an opponent process fashion, so is tilt perception. Neurons that encode tilt in a particular direction tend to inhibit neurons that encode tilt in the opposite direction.

As you stare at tilted stripes, one set of cells is winning the orientation perception tug of war that's resulting in this perception of tilt in a particular direction, but in so doing it is getting fatigued. The cells that encode tilt in the opposite direction conversely are losing the tug of war, but they're getting a nice rest. You can probably guess what will happen, based on the lecture about color perception and the discussion about opponent processing. If you stop looking at these stripes tilted in one direction and switch to looking at a set of vertical stripes, you'll be giving the 2 sets of tilt receptors equal amount of input. Because the tilt cells in one direction are now very tired, the tilt cells for the other direction will start winning the battle; and as a result, even though the stripes are perfectly vertical, you'll see them as tilted in that opposite direction.

That's the usual method to study a motion-after-effect illusion. If we were in a perception lab about 50 years ago, I might have asked you to make a judgment about whether the lines were tilted rightward or leftward; maybe asked you questions about how much. How could we study this using not a conscious judgment method but one of these action-based assessments?

An ecological psychologist would certainly urge us to use one of these real-world actions; something other than this conscious judgment. It might be that the visual processing that guides our actions functions very differently than that which guides our conscious perceptions.

As you reach with your thumb and index finger to grasp a long, thin, rectangular object by its ends, you orient your hand to match the orientation of the target. As with the maximum grip aperture, the rotation of the wrist during that reach is highly correlated with the orientation of the target for which you're reaching, even well before your hand makes contact with it at the end of the reach. With the maximum grip aperture, I can know halfway through the reach how big you think a target is. With a measure of hand orientation, I can similarly know halfway through the reach what you think the orientation of the target is (the one for which you're reaching).

If you fatigue the tilt cells in one direction, it has a large and salient effect on perceptual judgment. It has little to no effect on the reaching action. As with the Ebbinghaus illusion, it seems that our actions are resistant to pictorial illusions. The world looks one way to our conscious mind, but somewhere up in our head, there's an accurate representation; and it's that representation that controls our visually-guided actions.

If you remember DF and RV, these results might not be that shocking to you; certainly not as shocking as they were to perception researchers who were fully invested in this perceptual judgment methodology. There's a simple explanation for all of this based on that 2 visual system theory: One stream, the ventral stream, controls our conscious perception; it's influenced by illusions. The other stream, the dorsal stream, controls our visually-guided actions; for some reason, it's not greatly influenced by illusions.

This convergence of evidence from the domain of neurology (looking at brain-injured patients) and perception research (looking at uninjured brains) is really valuable. There are limitations to the approach of studying brain-injured patients; remember, for instance, my kitchen blender examples from Lectures 3 and 4. There are also limitations of perception research as well. But when these 2 very different types of experimental results point to the same conclusion, it starts to seem more and more likely that the conclusions they suggest are correct.

Other related models of brain organization have been suggested as well; for instance, the idea that there are not 2 but 3 streams of processing: one for conscious perception, one for action planning, and one for action control. As additional experiments are run, the story here has grown increasingly murky rather than clear.

I can't resist telling you about one of my own experiments in this area. My students and I conducted this with the display involving the Ebbinghaus illusion. We varied the sizes of those 2 central disks; the ones that are made to look larger and smaller by the large and small inducing element disks. We asked people to select across all the different tasks which of the 2 disks were larger. In some cases, we asked people to simply state verbally which disk was larger; the disk on the right or the disk on the left. When they did this, with this verbal response task, the usual illusion was produced with the usual 10% difference in perceived size.

We then asked participants to continue selecting which of the 2 disks was larger, but to stop telling us verbally. For this second task, participants were to figure out which disk was bigger or perceive which one was bigger, and then reach out and grasp it. As with the other studies, we tracked the formation of that maximum grip aperture and found a reduction in the impact of the illusion on that; that is, the illusion effected their conscious, verbal judgments but seemed not to effect their grasping. When people reached, the effect of the illusion was significantly reduced.

That's so far nothing really new; that's just a replication of a previous study, that Goodale study I talked about. The strange thing we found, however, was that for the judgments (the relative size judgments; the conscious judgments) made just prior to the reach—that is, the selections made when preparing to reach for one of those 2 disk targets—for these selections, the effect of the illusion was reduced as well. This is a strange finding, so let me try to say it again. If you're looking at the Ebbinghaus illusion display with no intention to reach for it, there's a strong effect of the Ebbinghaus illusion. If you're looking at that same display but getting ready to reach for one of the 2 disks, then the effect of the illusion is drastically reduced.

Intending to reach for a target changes how you perceive it, for your own action control but for your conscious judgments as well. Based on this, my colleagues and I have suggested the presence of 2 different modes of visual processing: one for observation and one for action. It may be that the 2 different types of visual processing don't happen in parallel all the time. Perhaps when you get ready to perform a particular action, your visual system switches into a mode of processing that will serve to best guide that behavior.

As I mentioned, studies in this area are continuing. There are some real mysteries here about how the brain is organized. I love pondering the solutions to these puzzles.

What's certainly clear at this stage is that J.J. Gibson's idea that studying perception and action together was right. We do make perceptual judgments and do so in a consistent, reliable manner. I don't think many would argue that we should abandon the type of research that involves those judgments, but action seems to clearly mediate how our perceptual systems work. Studying perception only while people sit in a lab looking at invented stimuli would clearly be a mistake. By studying how perception and action go together, a much more complete and accurate understanding of the human sensory processes emerges.

What's emerged from modern research on perception and action is an understanding of a complex, dynamic human brain that's embedded within a dynamic and complex body. Understanding human perception will inherently require understanding action at the same time. Our sensory systems seem to be organized in a way to specifically control the action systems that we have. By understanding how we coordinate actions, we may ultimately gain insights into vision and our senses in general that we might not be able to get in any other way.

In our next lecture, we'll be considering how our focus of attention similarly interacts with your senses. In some cases, focusing on one thing—and away from everything else—can affect your perception even more dramatically than choosing to perform a particular action. The next lecture will have some magic tricks in it. I hope you'll come to the show.

# Attention and Perception
## Lecture 14

W hat is most amazing about the senses is how much information we obtain about the environment, how quickly we get it, and how detailed and rich it is. All this is possible because our senses our inferential. We experience much more information than we take in.

- Many people think of the senses as passive receivers of sensory information—the brain is like a camera, the ears are like a tape recorder, and so on.

- Touch is perhaps the only clear exception to this notion. We choose to reach out and actively touch something.

- The surprising thing for many people is that selectivity applies not just to touch but to all the senses, especially vision. The brain is forever choosing to process part of the visual input—certain regions and even certain properties of it—and not other aspects of it.

- Attention enables us to allocate our finite mental resources effectively. This is a good thing, but by the same token it can lead to big problems in certain situations. We greatly overestimate in general how much we actually do perceive.

- *Attention* is one of those words that has a general meaning outside of psychological and perceptual science, but in these areas it has specific meanings. Attention often seems to work as a spotlight, highlighting certain aspects of visual input and not others.

- In other ways, attention seems to serve as perceptual glue, pulling together different aspects of a stimulus into perceptual objects.

- Attention is necessary to perceive things. When you choose to touch something, you pick up information about it. Unless you engage in that active behavior, there is no sensation of touch in the hands. Vision works, in many respects, in the same fashion.

- Most of us have the impression we perceive the world around us in great detail, all the time. A wealth of evidence suggests this is not the case.

- When you enter a new room for the first time, you scan the room, you take in a lot of information through quick glances, but then your visual system makes a big assumption: It assumes that if anything changes, it will move as it does so. Conversely, if nothing moves, then nothing has changed.

- This is a generally good assumption, and humans are very good at perceiving motion, especially with peripheral vision. This assumption also frees up mental resources; you do not need to keep reprocessing the visual input areas where nothing changes, leaving the brain free to focus on a select few things.

- A major theme of this course has been how we greatly underestimate how much of what we actually perceive versus what our brains infer. If you are watching this lecture on video, you may have noticed a few changes to my appearance and the appearance of the studio over the past minute or 2.

- Each time the camera changed, several things changed: My jacket and tie changed several times. The podium changed into a vase, a plant, and changed location. Sometimes a mug appeared in my hands and then disappeared a moment later. The posters behind me changed.

- If you noticed all of them, then you have a remarkable sensory system. As many as half of viewers do not notice any changes at all.

- On the sets of most movie productions, a person is specifically assigned to manage continuity. Still, there are many famous continuity errors in classic films, even though most viewers never notice them.

- We believe that it is different in the real world, that we would notice such continuity errors in a room if we closed our eyes, opened them, and something had changed in the meantime. But a good deal of evidence suggests that you would not.

- Professors Dan Simons and Dan Levin tested whether they could make big changes in the real world without people noticing them. An experimenter would approach someone and ask him or her for directions. While this conversation was happening, 2 other experimenters would walk up carrying a door and would walk between the experimenter and the unwitting subject.

- While the door was between them for a few seconds, the experimenter would switch places with one of the door carriers. The person asking directions was now a different person. Only about half the subjects noticed the switch.

- Even when the experimenter said at the end, "This was a psychology study. Did you notice anything strange just now?" most people said they did not.

- Other variations on this person-switch experiment encountered similar results, even if the new person is a different height, has a different hairstyle, is wearing different clothes, and in some cases even had a distinctly different voice.

- The next time you are at a restaurant, after you have ordered your food, take a moment to recall what your server looked and sounded like. Many people will have trouble recalling.

- There are some changes people do seem to notice. If the experimenter was a man and switch is made to a woman, subjects always catch this. Significant age differences are almost always noticed, as are differences in race. We are not completely incapable of noticing change, but we are much worse at it than we think we are.

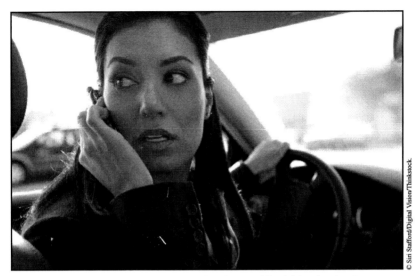

**Recent statistics reveal that talking on the phone while driving is about as dangerous as driving while intoxicated.**

- These phenomena are often referred to as inattentional blindness. In the absence of specifically looking for something, we seem unable to see it. These phenomena are not just a laboratory curiosity; they have telling implications outside the lab.

- A variety of studies have demonstrated that talking on a cell phone or texting while driving drastically increases your chances of being in an accident. Statistically, the risk is as large as if one is legally intoxicated.

- When you devote your attention to the phone, you become blind to any unexpected changes on the road. You will fail to notice even big, important things in the environment.

- In many states, there are laws against using handheld cell phones or sending text messages while driving. But hands-free cell phones can be a problem as well. Listening and thinking intently about what the person on the other end of the line is saying significantly elevates the risk of car accidents.

- In terms of sensory processing, attention has at least 2 very different meanings. It can function as perceptual glue, or it can function as a spotlight.

- Imagine that I show you an image with many distracters and a single target, such as finding a green horizontal line as quickly as possible among many green vertical lines. This is a fairly easy task because of the horizontal line's novel orientation.

- If I were to ask you to find a green horizontal line again but this time there were red horizontal lines along with the green vertical line distracters, that would be harder. Attention researches call this a conjunction search.

- Most people have the sense that they have to look at all of the distracters and dismiss them one at a time until they happen on the target. That is not the case, but you do have to allocate some attention to each target. As you do, you seem to be able to combine the information about these different features.

- Attention is what enables you to combine the different features of a stimulus. You can scan for color or orientation, but to scan for both at once requires attention.

- Attention acts like a spotlight when you fixate on one particular place in an image. In an experiment, I might ask you to gaze at an image in general and push a button whenever you see a small flash of light appear somewhere in the image. Let's presume that you would respond in about 500 milliseconds.

- If I asked you to keep your eyes aimed at the middle of the display but to focus your attention off to the left side and do the same button task, your response time would be faster when the light flashed on the left side of the image, say 450 milliseconds.

- Attention also enhances your ability to differentiate tiny changes in color, brightness, orientation, or almost any other aspect of sensory input. Focusing attention makes you better at sensory processing in almost every way. If you focus your attention on one tiny spot, the enhancements in processing will be greater.

- But there is a cost as well. If you focus your attention on something, it means you are focusing your attention away from things almost everywhere else. In the button-press example, when you focus your attention on the left, your response will be faster on the left, but it will be slower on the right.

- This is a useful property of our sensory systems. It enables us to take our finite mental resources and focus them on the things that matter most to us. There are some things we seem to process automatically in terms of the perceptual spotlight and perceptual glue as well.

- The best examples can be seen in terms of auditory perception. Imagine wearing headphones playing different audio tracks into each of your ears.

- You could focus your attention on one or the other, and the perceptual spotlight would help you process the information on that side faster and with greater sensory resolution. It is like metaphorically turning up the volume on that ear.

- Imagine that I asked you to pay attention to the right ear and you heard "Give me liberty, or please shut the door." In the left ear at the same time, you heard "When you leave, give me death." If I asked you to repeat the words from the right ear, you would almost certainly make a mistake.

- Your attention would most likely focus on the famous quote "Give me liberty, or give me death," no matter how you tried to pay attention to the right ear. Similarly, if you started with the left ear, your attention would deliver you the sensible sentence "When you leave, please shut the door."

- Your attention is focused on one ear or the other at the start, but there is still processing that takes place outside of intentional focus. Your attention directs some of your resources, but some mental processing takes place for all incoming sensory information, especially for particularly meaningful stimuli.

- This is why you notice someone saying your name even among dozens of different conversations taking place at a noisy cocktail party. To have one particular conversation in this environment, you might have to focus your attention, but the familiar sound of your name will be processed outside your attentional focus. Scientists even call this the cocktail party effect.

## Suggested Reading

Chabris and Simons, *The Invisible Gorilla.*

Tipper and Behrmann, "Object-Centered Not Scene-Based Visual Neglect."

## Questions to Consider

1. I am aware of the world around me, or so I think. Many studies suggest that unless I focus my attention on something, I have not perceived it. Yet I am still aware of a complex, continuous world around me. How can both of these things be true?

2. We usually aim our eyes at the thing that is the focus of our attention. It has been repeatedly demonstrated, however, that we have the ability to focus our attention away from our direction of gaze. Can you think of situations where you do this in your everyday life?

# Attention and Perception
## Lecture 14—Transcript

Hello. Throughout this course, I've argued that your sensory systems are amazing but inferential. The amazing part has to do with just how much information we obtain about the environment, and how quickly we get it; also with how impressively detailed and rich that information is. The inferential part explains in part how we achieve this. We take in some information about the environment around us, but we experience much more than we take in. We fill in missing information, and infer the presence of information that's very likely to be there.

This lecture is about attention and perception, and it's about ways in which your sensory systems change the way they function on a moment to moment basis as you direct your attention towards certain things and away from others. Many people think of our senses as passive receivers of sensory information. For vision, we think of our brain as somewhat like a camera, taking in sequences of images. For hearing, the common metaphor is of a tape recorder; sound comes in, and our ears record it and process that sound. For the other senses as well, we often think of them as receiving energy patterns from the environment and then inferring meaning from them. In terms of how we think about our senses, touch is perhaps the only clear exception to this notion of passively receiving stimuli. When we reach out and actively touch something, we choose to touch some surface or object and choose not to touch others. We're thus selective in terms of what information we pick up with our sense of touch. The surprising thing for many people is that this selectivity turns out to be true not just for touch, but for all of the senses, especially vision. Our brain is forever choosing to process part of the visual input; certain regions and even certain properties of it. As our brain chooses to process certain parts of our visual input, it chooses not to process other aspects of it. To some extent, it completely ignores them; almost like not making contact with them at all.

In this lecture, I want to explore how visual attention works in the human visual system. I'll talk about how attention enables us to allocate our finite mental resources effectively. This is a good thing, but by the same token I'll explain that it can lead to big problems in certain situations. I'll argue that we greatly overestimate, just in general, how much we actually do perceive. I'll talk about our ability to detect changes, and our inability to detect them in certain types of situations. I'll then describe how attention functions. "Attention" is one of those words that has a general meaning outside of psychological and perceptual science. Researchers in this area, however, have derived several separate, more specific meanings of this word "attention." For instance, attention often seems to work as a spotlight, highlighting certain aspects of the visual input and not illuminating others. In other ways, however, attention seems to serve as perceptual glue, pulling together different aspects of a stimulus into perceptual objects. I'll finish this lecture by discussion the meanings behind these glue and spotlight metaphors.

Let's begin with a consideration of how attention is necessary in order to perceive things. I suggested a metaphor a few moments ago that vision works like touch. When you chose to reach out and feel something with your fingers, you pick up information about that thing. Unless you engage in that active touching behavior, there's no sensation of touch in the hands. Vision works, in many respects, in the same fashion, although most people never realize it. Most of us have the impression that we perceive the world around us in great detail, all the time. If something interesting impinges on our senses then of course it must impact our perception, right? A wealth of evidence suggests that this is not the case.

Most people greatly overestimate the amount of information that our senses process at any given time. When we walk into a new room or open our eyes and look around us for the first time, we scan the room, we move our gaze around, and with that high-resolution fovea that we've discussed we take in a lot of information through these scanning glances and use it to form a mental representation of what's out there. At that point, after these few seconds, our visual system makes a big assumption. Specially, it assumes that if anything changes in the surrounding environment, then as that change occurs it will move. Conversely if nothing moves, then things are assumed to be exactly as they were when I first looked around the room.

This is a good assumption usually, and a very useful way to approach the task of perception. For one thing, the assumption is almost always true. When the things around us change, they typically do move. Second, we're very good at perceiving a motion, especially with our peripheral vision. Away from the fovea, remember, we're not so good at perceiving fine details or color, but we're very good at perceiving motion; and when there is motion, this peripheral vision processes the information very quickly. It sends signals to our visual system, even to our subcortical visual processing systems, telling them to generate an eye movement; to look at this area where the motion has happened. Once our eyes look at that area, we can see what's changed, and maybe even see it continuing to change.

The other reason the assumption is good is that it frees up a great deal of mental resources. We don't need to continually reprocess the visual input in those areas where there isn't change. That leaves our brain free to focus its work on a select few things where we do need to be processing carefully.

As I've said, in general, we overestimate the amount of information that we're actually perceiving; that is, we greatly underestimate the amount of stuff that we perceive that's really inferred. This has been a major theme of this course, in many ways since the first lecture of the course in which we identified the blind spot in your retina and noted that your visual system fills in that blank spot. Even at the level of the receptors, fundamental things like where you can see are inferred. We don't realize it's happening. With apparent motion, we talked about how we see motion, we perceive motion; but we really can't see it directly. We see one object in one location, we see it vanish; we see another object that looks very much like it in another location and, voilà, we infer the motion. Even the timing of that motion is filled in by our visual system, right? You can't see the vision until it's over, but we have a sense that we see the motion before the object arrives at the second location.

Vision isn't the only sense for which this occurs. In hearing, we use the context of a sentence to be able to guess what's coming next in the stream of speech input. This works so well that if I delete one of the sounds, as long as I cover it with something else like a cough sound, you'll perceive the sound as actually having been there. Again, you're perceiving the sound, perceiving things in general, even though you aren't sensing those things. They just aren't present in your sensory input.

You may have noticed a few changes to my appearance and the appearance of the studio behind me over the past minute or 2. Every time I switched from one camera to another, several things changed. If you noticed all of them, then you have a remarkable sensory system. Many people—as many as 50%—typically don't notice any at all. My jacket and tie changed several times; the podium changed into a vase, a plant, and changed location; sometimes a mug appeared in my hands and then disappeared a moment later; the posters behind me changed as well.

On the sets of most movie productions, there's a person specifically assigned to manage continuity. He or she is usually called the script supervisor, and among the principle jobs of this person is to make sure that things don't dramatically change from shot to shot. Still, there are many famous continuity errors in classic films. You might watch an actor talking with someone while sipping a drink, for instance. At one moment her glass will be 2/3 full; a second later, her glass will be nearly empty; a few seconds later, it might be full again. Another common mistake is if an actor is smoking. As different takes of a scene are spliced together, the cigarette might seem abruptly to grow longer and shorter, even over the span of just a few seconds. In the *Wizard of Oz*, there's one of my favorite of these. There's a scene right near the beginning in which Dorothy walks along a fence and falls into the pigpen. As she does, she gets covered in mud. Bert Lahr comes to her rescue and lifts her up and out of the pigpen; he also somehow magically cleans her clothes, which are perfectly mud-free from that moment on in the movie. We think we would notice these things, but we usually don't.

You might be thinking, "We miss changes in videos and movies, but big deal. In the real world—in the room I'm sitting in right now, for instance—I'm perceiving things very clearly and precisely." For instance, if you were to close your eyes and think about the room around you, it seems that you could call to mind a great deal of detail. You would notice if something in the real world changed like this, wouldn't you? A good deal of evidence suggests that you would not.

There's a now somewhat-classic study in which Dan Simons and Dan Levin tested whether they could make big changes in the real world without people noticing them. In the typical situation, an experimenter would approach someone and ask him or her for directions. "Can you tell me, sir, how to find the ice-skating rink?" Most people would be nice and start to give directions. "You head down the street here and make a left, and you walk about 3 blocks and turn right." While this conversation was happening between the 2 people, 2 other experimenters would walk up carrying a door. They would somewhat rudely interrupt saying, "Excuse me, excuse me," as they walked between the first experimenter and the unsuspecting study participant. While the door was held up in between the 2 people, the study participant wouldn't be able to see the first experimenter, the one to whom they were giving the directions; they couldn't see them just for a few seconds. During that time, the original experimenter would switch places with one of the door carriers. As the door continued moving past, this would leave a new experimenter standing there. Essentially, the person asking directions was now a different person than he was just a few seconds before.

Some people, about half, do notice this; but a surprising number of people do not. They just continue on giving directions and then start to say goodbye. Even when the experimenter asks at the end, "Excuse me, this is a psychology study, did you notice anything strange just now?" most people don't say that they did. If they do, the most common response is, "Yes, I did notice something; those 2 people carrying that door were very rude."

In another version of the study, students would arrive at a building to pick up some forms. As they showed up, they had to walk down a hallway to a counter where there was an experimenter waiting. The experimenter would talk to the student for a moment and then start looking around for the form that they were supposed to give the student. "Oh," the experimenter would say, "I'm sorry, where did I leave that?" At that point, the experimenter would duck down behind the counter, seemingly to look for the form on some shelf that was down there behind the barrier. A moment later—a second later—a different person would stand up. Again, a surprisingly small percentage of people notice this change. They don't realize that their conversation has switched; that they're now talking to a different person than they were talking to before. This happens even if the person is a different height, has a different hairstyle, if he or she is wearing different clothes, and in some cases even has a very distinctly different voice.

Next time you're at a restaurant, after you've ordered your food and you're waiting for it to arrive, take a moment and think: What did your waiter look like? What was he wearing? Did he have glasses on? What did his hair look like? Some people won't have any problem answering these questions, but many—especially if they're engaged in some conversation or thinking about something else—will have trouble answering those questions. Try asking the people at the restaurant with you; many of them won't be able to answer correctly.

There are some changes people do seem to notice. If a person who was a man suddenly changes into a woman, people catch that every time. If one person is a college student and the other a 50-year-old man, then most students catch the change. If the 2 people are from different racial groups, people tend to notice that as well. It's not that we're completely incapable of noticing change, but we're much worse at it than we think we are.

Taken together, these phenomena are often referred to as inattentional blindness. That is, in the absence of specifically looking for something, we seem to be unable to see it, almost like we're blind. Inattentional blindness isn't just laboratory curiosity; it has some very telling implications outside the lab. One of the most serious has to do with people talking on cell phones or texting while driving. A variety of studies have demonstrated that when you're talking on a cell phone, you're at an increased risk of being in an accident; and the increase isn't a small one. In fact, the increased accident risk is as large as if one is legally intoxicated while they're driving. Driving while talking on your cell phone is essentially like committing a DUI in many ways.

Many people who wouldn't dream of getting behind the wheel while drunk use their cell phones all the time. Why? The best explanation is this inattentional blindness. When you devote your attention to the phone— to sending a text message, to dialing, to even talking on it—and when you direct your attention away from the road, you become blind to any unexpected changes. If a person runs in front of your car, or if the car in front of you suddenly hits the brakes, you're likely to fail to notice it. Just like the changes in my outfits, just like the change in the identity of the person to whom you're speaking, you'll fail to notice even big, important things in the environment around you. The really bad part is that people don't realize that they're blind to these things while they're engaged in using the cell phone. It's the overestimation of our perceptual abilities that's really responsible for all of the accidents.

Several states have clued into this fact and taken steps to reduce the use of cell phones in cars. In many states, there are actually laws against using hand-held cell phones or sending text messages while driving. As I was driving through a highway construction zone just this week I noticed big signs that stated, "Orange cones, no phones," to try to drive home this message. Part of the problem, of course, comes from those moments when you direct your eyes away from the road and to the phone. In that case, you really are blind to changes because your eyes aren't looking in the right direction.

Hopefully based on the material in this lecture, you realize that this isn't the whole problem. Even if your eyes are on the road—even if you're looking right at that car that hits its brakes in front of you—if your attention is elsewhere, there's a greatly increased chance that you won't notice the thing that happens in front of you. So hand-held cell phones are a problem, but so are hands-free cell phones. Even if you aren't holding the actual phone unit, if your attention is on the call—if you're listening intently and thinking intently about what the person on the other end of the line is saying—then there's a potential problem. Even with hands-free phones, there's a significantly elevated risk of car accidents.

This might be one of the most important things that I tell you in this course. If you must talk on your phone when you drive, please be careful. Be extra vigilant about the cars and people around you. Realize that as you're on that phone call, you're driving with a visual system—a perceptual system in general—that's compromised in its abilities to perform. Of course, if you can avoid using the phone while driving, that would be best of all.

I've talked about attention and described how important it is to your perception. I've argued that without attention, in-depth perception is essentially impossible. I want to spend a little time now talking about how attention functions. "Attention" is a single world in our language, but in terms of our sensory processing, "attention" has at least 2 very different meanings.

Attention can function as perceptual glue, and attention can function as a spotlight. Let me describe the meaning of the glue metaphor first.

Imagine that I show you an image with many distracters and one target. For instance, imagine that I ask you to find a green horizontal line as fast as you can in an image in which there are many green vertical lines. A task like this would be very easy for you; in fact, no matter how many of those vertical lines were present in the image as distracters, you would find the horizontal line almost instantly. In the language of researchers in this area, the horizontal line would just pop out of the display. Attention really isn't needed here to process the distracters; to sort out the horizontal lines and look for the line that has the novel orientation. You're able to rule out all of the distracters in a parallel processing fashion, processing them all at once.

If I give you a very similar task, it will be much harder. Imagine I ask you to find a green horizontal line again, but this time, along with the green vertical line distracters, there are also red horizontal lines and green vertical lines; that is, you're looking for a green horizontal line just like before, but there are lots of other lines that are green and lots of other lines that are horizontal. There's only one target, however: a line that is both green and horizontal. Attention researches call this a conjunction search, since you're looking for a target that's defined by a conjunction of 2 features; in this case green color and horizontal orientation. This task is much harder. Most people have the sense that they have to look at all of the distracters and dismiss them one at a time, until you happen upon the target one. You don't have to fixate your eyes, necessarily, on each one of the distracters, but you do have to allocate some attention to each target. As you do, you seem to be able to combine the information about these different features.

People who study this have come to think of attention as the thing that's necessary in order to combine different features of a stimulus. You can scan the entire environment around you in terms of color all at the same time; you can scan the entire image in terms of orientation all at once; but if you want to glue these 2 features together, that requires attention. Perhaps the best evidence for this is what happens when you change the number of distracters. If there's only 1 target and 1 distracter, you're very fast at finding the target; 2 distracters and you're slower; 10 distracters, slower still. There's a direct relation between the number of distracters and your reaction time in this target search test. This is exactly what you'd expect if a finite attention resource was needed to examine each item as you searched for a target.

Attention can be thought of as perceptual glue. It can also be thought of as a perceptual spotlight. Imagine that you look at one particular place in an image and you fixate that spot, but don't particularly focus your attention in anywhere in particular. A task I might ask you to do for some perception experiment might be to respond by pressing a button whenever you see a small flash of light appear somewhere in the image. You'd be able to do that task, of course. Whenever a spot of light flashed on the image you would perceive it, and after a few hundred milliseconds you would press the button. Let's presume that you would respond in about 500 milliseconds; this would be our baseline for this task. Imagine that I asked you to keep your eyes aimed at the middle of the display, but to focus your attention off to one side; say, the left side. If I then ask you to do that button-press task just like before, your focus of attention would change your response time for this type of task. If I flashed the light where you were focusing your attention, you would respond faster; say, 450 milliseconds instead of 500 milliseconds for that button press. Focusing attention makes you faster. Attention also enhances your ability to differentiate tiny changes in color, brightness, orientation; almost any other aspect of sensory input. Focusing attention makes you better at sensory processing in almost every way. It's almost like you're shining a spotlight on the image in just the spot where you're attending. This is where the spotlight metaphor comes from; and like a spotlight, the smaller an area on which you focus that spotlight, the brighter it becomes. If you focus your attention on one tiny spot, the enhancements in processing will be greater. If you diffuse your attention over a wider area, there will still be enhancements, but they'll be much smaller.

In general, then, focusing your attention makes you a better senser and perceiver in almost every way. But there's a cost here as well. If you focus your attention on something, it means that you must be focusing your attention away from the things almost everywhere else. For instance, in our button-press example, I suggested that you'd respond faster by about 50 milliseconds when you focused your attention on the left. What about the right? If you focus your attention on the left, then you'll be faster on the left but you'll be slower on the right. In the same way that you're a better perceiver where you focus your attention, you'll be worse everywhere else. This is a useful property of our sensory systems, however. It enables us to take the finite mental resources that we have at our disposal and focus them on the things that matter most to us.

When I discussed inattentional blindness, I mentioned that there are some changes that we seem to notice even when we aren't specifically paying attention to them; a change in the race or sex of a person, for instance. There are some things that we seem to process automatically in terms of the perceptual spotlight and perceptual glue as well. The best examples can be seen in terms of auditory perception. Imagine that you wore some headphones and listened to different audio tracks being played in the 2 different ears. Even though this would sound a little strange, you could certainly focus your attention on the sounds in one ear or the other, just like focusing your attention on one location on a computer screen or another. I should note that the perceptual spotlight would function the same way here. When your attention is focused on your left ear, you'd process the information there faster and with greater sensory resolution. It's, again, as if there's a spotlight focused on a particular aspect of your sensory input. In this case, the metaphor is more like turning up the volume on that ear for which your attention is focused and turning the volume down for the other ear.

Imagine that I asked you to listen to the sounds coming into your right ear and to repeat whatever words you hear there. In that right ear you would hear the following sentence: "Give me liberty, or please shut the door." (An odd sentence, I know, but it will make more sense in a moment.) In the left ear, at the same time, you would hear a different sentence: "When you leave, give me death." If I asked you to repeat the words in the right ear, you'd almost certainly make a mistake. You'd do well in the first part of the sentence ("Give me liberty or") but then you'd slip over to the left ear and finish the famous Patrick Henry quote ("Give me liberty, or give me death"). You'd similarly make an error in the other direction. If you started with the left ear ("When you leave") you'd likely switch to the right ear and finish the very sensible sentence "Please shut the door." What's going on here?

Your attention is focused on one ear or the other, certainly at the start, but there's still apparently processing that takes place outside of that realm of intentional focus. Your brain is still processing the information in the other ear, and if the context of the sentence fits very well it results in an involuntary shift in your focus of attention. Even though your attention directs some of your resources at a particular target (in this case, a target ear), there's still some mental processing that takes place for all incoming sensory information, especially for particularly meaningful stimuli like, in this case, a famous quotation.

One of the best examples of this occurs with something that's probably extremely familiar to you: your name. If you're at a noisy cocktail party, there might be dozens of different conversations happening at the same time all around you. The sounds of all of them will be falling on your ears at the same time. In order for you to have one particular conversation, you might have to focus your attention fairly intently on the person in front of you. We can do this, of course, but a funny thing happens if someone somewhere else in the room, among those dozens of other conversations, says your name: You hear it. Often it sounds very loud and clear above the din of the other sounds. You might even experience an irresistible urge to look for who it was that said your name. Psychologists call this the cocktail party effect.

You can try this out next time you're in one of these crowded situations. Pick a friend who's some distance away and say his or her name. You might have to do it a few times, but even if you say it at a moderate conversational level, you'll find that the person looks your way.

Again, what seems clear is that even though we miss a lot of things if we aren't paying attention to them, we still do some processing outside of our attentional focus, mostly for stimuli that are very familiar or very salient.

In this lecture, we've discussed how attention influences our sensory processing. I've argued that perception only happens with attention. If we don't direct our attention at something, it's almost as if we're blind, deaf, and generally unable to perceive anything. It's important to keep this in mind as we make our way through the world using our senses. Even though were away of many things, we don't perceive nearly as much as we think we do.

In our next lecture, we'll explore something called kinesthetic perception. Kinesthesis provides us with information about where our body and our body parts are located. In a sense, the next lecture will provide a nice counterpoint to this one. Here, we talked about things that we think we perceive but actually do not. With kinesthetic perception, I'll be telling you about a remarkable range of sensory information that we clearly process, but without any awareness at all. I hope you'll join me then.

# Kinesthetic Perception
## Lecture 15

Kinesthetic perception is often left off standard lists of the human senses, at best shoehorned in with the sense of touch, but as you will see, it is a combination of several other senses, along with receptors devoted specifically to kinesthesis.

- Imagine that you are standing in front of an elevator with your hands at your sides. You plan to go up a few floors, so you reach out to press the "up" button. Which muscle does your body activate first?

- If you think it through, you will realize you have to bring your arm forward and up first. But for every action, there is an equal and opposite reaction. The movement of your arm generates a push back and down in the rest of your body.

- Your body must generate a counteractive force to keep you upright as you move your arm. Therefore, the first muscle to contract is not in your arm or shoulder but in your hips.

- Like many issues in perception and action control, the body just seems to take care this automatically. But that does not mean it happens without complex and precise processing behind it.

- Like other issues in human sensory processing, it was not apparent how complex motor control was until we tried to build robots to do things humans do every day. Reproducing the simplest human behaviors can be remarkably difficult.

- We do not yet fully understand human perception, but it is clear that kinesthetic perception is one of the key pieces to this puzzle.

- Kinesthetic perception is classically considered as consisting of 2 separate components: vestibular perception and proprioception.

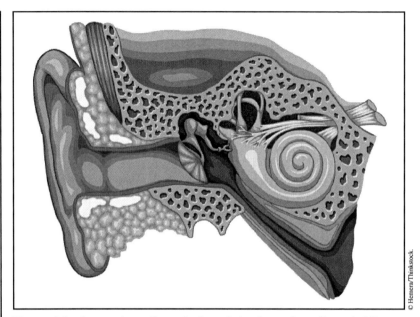

**The semicircular canals are the arch-shaped structures above the end of the snail-shaped cochlea.**

- Vestibular perception is about perceiving the current position, orientation, and movement of your whole body. Proprioception is about perceiving the position of individual body parts based on touch receptors and actions of the motor system.

- Our vestibular senses are based heavily on the 3 semicircular canals of the inner ear, just above the cochlea. One is oriented vertically, one horizontally, and one in depth.

- Each is filled with fluid that can flow back and forth inside the tubes. The inside of each tube is also covered with tiny hairs, each attached to its own neuronal receptor. When the fluid flows past a hair cell, it causes it to bend, in turn causing the associated receptor to send off a train of action potentials.

- The fluid flows in response to the movements of your head. The inertia of the fluid makes it want to stay still; the motion of the head causes the flow in the opposite direction inside the tube. By encoding the relative motion inside all 3 canals, it is possible to encode all 3 directions of head rotation at the same time and for your brain to reconstruct the rotation of your head, even when your eyes are closed.

- This is your vestibular system. When it is functioning well, it tells you how you move and when you move. It keeps you from falling over, determining when you are leaning forward, back, left, or right. But it does not work independently most of the time.

- Your sensory systems are good at using any information available to maintain their sense of location relative to the room around you. If you close your eyes and let someone spin you in an office chair at a consistent speed, in the absence of other cues, you will quickly lose your sense of orientation.

- This is because while the vestibular system responds very well when you start moving, once you are moving at a constant velocity, it essentially stops responding. Within a few seconds, the fluid inside the tubes is spinning in the same direction as the tube and at the same velocity. The vestibular system responds to acceleration, not the movement itself.

- Under normal circumstances, vision would come to the rescue. The semicircular canals tell you when movement has started and how much acceleration is involved, and your eyes track the amount of overall motion.

- An interesting motion illusion you can get in a dark room capitalizes on this link. You will need a pitch-black room with a single small source of light, like a dim LED alarm clock.

- Stand in the dark across the room from the alarm clock and simply look at the clock. Notice that the numbers periodically seem to move up or down, or left or right, and then back to the starting position.

- This is because you are moving. We rely on visual information to maintain an upright posture. Vestibular information is not quite as accurate; we tend to wobble a little without realizing it.

- The other aspect of kinesthetic perception is proprioception, the sense of where your individual body parts are located. Some of that information can come in through your eyes, but if you are in the dark or looking at something else, you need another source of information.

- A good test of the limits of your proprioception can be done by holding one hand above your head and spreading your fingers apart. With the other hand, alternate between touching the tip of your nose and each of the fingers above your head—first with your eyes open, then with your eyes closed. You will find it harder with your eyes closed.

- Part of your proprioceptive perception is derived from information obtained when you move a body part. We discussed how the motor system sends 2 copies of each motor command to the brain—one to the muscles themselves and another to the visual cortex. This enables your visual system to know when the environment is moving as opposed to just your eyes.

- A similar system seems to function for proprioception. If you wiggle the fingers on your raised hand during the closed-eye finger-touch test, you should notice that the task becomes easier again. The finger motions are now available as additional information.

- There are many different types of receptors involved in proprioception. Specialized neurons are present in the muscles and the tendons that sense tension as well as the angles of each of the joins. The skin itself also contains stretch receptors that can be used to infer how much a particular part of your body is extended, such as a limb.

- This wiggling finger demonstration makes clear, however, that the motor commands we generate also play an important role in proprioception. All of this information is fed into an enormous network of neurons in the cerebellum, at the top of the spinal cord. It makes up about 10% of the overall brain volume in humans and contains more neurons than the rest of the brain put together.

- Damage to the cerebellum is associated with many different types of deficits, particularly motor coordination, balance, and timing of actions. Proprioception seems to be accomplished by the circuits located in this part of the brain.

- An element of mystery surrounds cerebellar function, but there are several leading theories. Most center on an internal model of the body that is maintained and used to plan actions. This model cannot be seen or touched; it is a neural activation–based representation of all of your body parts and their relations to one another, as well as their current positions.

- Humans generate action intentions in the motor cortex, but essentially all of the signals pass through the cerebellum on their way to the spinal cord and beyond. As they do, the plans seem to be refined and implemented on the basis of this internal model.

- This is where, as in the example at the start of the lecture, your brain anticipates the counterforce needed to keep you upright when you press that elevator button. It seems that the cerebellum simulates the action, looks for any problems, fixes the action, simulates it again, and so on until things work out the right way. Then the signals are actually sent on to the muscle and the real action commences.

- Evidence for this simulation process is based on characterizations of how people perform certain kinds of motor tasks. In one such set of studies, participants sat in the dark in front of a table onto which target objects were placed. They were instructed to pick up the blue object whenever the lights came on.

- The basic finding was that the farther away that blue object was located, the longer it took people to start their reach. There is no inherent reason for this unless they needed to simulate the movement before performing it.

- We do not usually visualize these kinds of actions explicitly, although there are a few domains in which it seems to be used very explicitly, such as in track-and-field competitions. High jumpers, for example, do an odd little dance before they begin to run toward the high bar. They mentally simulate their jump before they try to perform it. A wealth of evidence suggests that this improves their performance.

- There may be many reasons that this influences performance, including a simple boost of confidence. However, given our understanding of how the human brain implements sensory-guided actions, there is reason to imagine that the cerebellum and proprioception are also influenced by this explicit mental simulation.

- In the early days of perception research, people presumed that proprioception was either a simple extension of touch perception or something that was not interesting or important. It has become clear that the opposite is the case.

- Nowhere is this more apparent than when studying patients who have lost their sense of proprioception. Ian Waterman is one such patient. He can move but cannot sense the effects of his movements. Lying with his eyes closed, he reports that he cannot sense where his body is or even that it exists below his neck.

- Waterman has become a bit of a celebrity based on his absolute refusal to give in to his disorder. He refused a wheelchair and spent years fighting his illness, determined to relearn to control his body.

- In the process, he discovered that if he focuses his vision and his attention on the body parts involved in performing the task, then vividly and repeatedly imagines (that is, mentally simulates) how he is going to accomplish the goal of his task, he can control his body.

- Waterman practices this technique in an amazingly tenacious and disciplined fashion. He trained himself to stand and walk with the rigor of an Olympic athlete, spending hours and hours per day, day in and day out, until he achieved success and has won back most of the control he had lost, although he will never be able to perform these tasks without intense concentration.

- After a few minutes of pondering this, I do not think any of us should ever take our proprioception for granted again.

## Suggested Reading

Dolins and Mitchell, *Spatial Cognition, Spatial Perception.*

Stewart, Gapenne, and Di Paolo, *Enaction.*

## Questions to Consider

1. In this lecture, I described the importance of kinesthetic perception for performing everyday actions, such as reaching and walking. Are there any tasks for which kinesthetic perception might not be important?

2. If a surgeon is performing a delicate operation on someone's body, he or she will look intently at the areas on which incisions are being made. Can you think of a reason that kinesthetic perception would still be useful (and important) in this situation, even though there is visual information available about the position of the arm, hand, and scalpel?

# Kinesthetic Perception
## Lecture 15—Transcript

This lecture will consider kinesthetic perception. It's one of the human senses that's often left off the standard list of 5 senses. If one had to pick a category, kinesthetic perception would probably go most closely with the sense of touch, but, as you'll see, it's a combination of several of the other senses, along with some receptors devoted specifically to kinesthesis.

To start to illustrate that, I want you to imagine that you're standing in front of an elevator with your hands down at your sides. You're planning to go up a few floors, and so you're going to reach out and press the elevator button to call it. Which muscle do you think your body activates first in order to make that button-pressing action happen? If you think it through, you're going to have to raise your arm up as you reach out to press that button. You'll swing the arm forward and up. As Isaac Newton taught us, for every action, there's an equal and opposite reaction. That's not just true for moving planets and rockets; it's true for your body as well. As you swing your arm forward, it will move forward, but in so doing it will generate a push back in the other direction; it will push the rest of your body back a little. You won't realize this because you'll stay perfectly upright, or pretty close to it. Before that push can shift your body back, your muscles will generate a counteractive force forward to prevent it from happening. The first muscle to actually contract—the first thing your body does when you reach forward—is not your finger, it's not your arm, it's not even your shoulder; the first muscle to move is in your hips.

Like many issue in perception and action control, this is one of those control issues that our body just seems to take care of for us automatically. It's reminiscent in a way of when you reach to grasp something and your fingers form into a shape that matches the grasping target almost perfectly. It happens without conscious effort, but that doesn't mean it happens without some complex and precise processing behind it.

Also like other issues in human sensory processing, it wasn't really apparent to people just how complex motor control was until they tried to build robots to do the things that humans do every day. Every once in a while, you'll see a new high-tech robot on the news that can walk across a room while holding up a tray of drinks, or something like that. As you watch this robot making tiny, slow, awkward steps you might think, "Woo hoo. How many millions of dollars did you need for that?" As easy as it is for us, however, to do these sorts of tasks, controlling even simple behaviors can be remarkably difficult.

How do we do it? How does the human brain accomplish complex motor control? While we continue to struggle to fully understand and duplicate our human system, it's clear that kinesthetic perception—the topic of today's lecture—is one of the key pieces to this puzzle.

Kinesthetic perception is classically considered as consisting of 2 separate components: vestibular perception and proprioception. Vestibular perception is about perceiving the current position, orientation, and movement of your whole body. Proprioception is about perceiving the position of individual body parts based on touch receptors and actions of the motor system. Let's consider these 2 things in turn.

Our vestibular senses are based heavily on a set of semicircular canals located in the inner ear, just above the cochlea we discussed in the lecture on auditory perception. There are 3 of these semicircular canals: one is oriented vertically, one horizontally, and one in depth. Each semicircular canal is filled with fluid that can flow back and forth through the inside of these tubes. The inside of each tube is also covered with tiny hairs, each one attached to its own neuronal receptor. When the fluid flows past one of these hair cells, it causes it to bend one way or the other. This causes the associated neuronal receptor to send off a train of those action potentials that are then sent on to the brain.

What makes the fluid flow back and forth? Movement of your head. For the canal oriented from front to back, rotation of the head in a forward direction causes the fluid to flow backward. Backward motion causes the fluid to flow forward. The inertia of the fluid makes it want to stay still; the motion of the head is what causes the flow in the opposite direction inside that tube.

A physical analogy might help here, at least a little bit. Imagine you have a hula hoop with some tiny plastic balls inside of it. If you hold the hula hoop still, the balls will roll to the bottom and they'll stay there. Imagine you could even mark the spot on the hula hoop where the balls are located. If you then rotate the hula hoop abruptly in one direction, the balls will move in the opposite direction, relative to that rotation. If there were tiny hair cells inside the hula hoop, then those balls would have caused them to bend as they rolled past.

That's what happens inside these semicircular canals. For the canal that's oriented from front to back, front to back rotation is encoded. Side to side motion doesn't impact this canal, but the side to side canal is greatly impacted by side to side motion. By encoding the relative motion inside all 3 of these canals, it's possible to encode all 3 directions of rotation at the same time and, based on the responses of the receptors there, for your brain to reconstruct what that rotation is.

If you close your eyes and sit in a chair that spins around, this semicircular canal system will help you to tell how you're moving, or at least how you rotate. This is your vestibular system. When it's functioning well, it tells you how you move, and certainly when you move; it tells the when you move part very accurately. If you're standing in the dark, the thing that keeps you from falling over is this vestibular system; it's the thing that tells you when you're leaning forward, back, left, or right.

As great as this vestibular system is, it doesn't work all by itself most of the time; in fact, it's not very good at working all by itself. If you sit in that chair that spins, like an office chair, and close your eyes while someone spins you slowly around, you'll very quickly become disoriented. (I'm presuming—to make this work—by the way, there can't be any landmarks created by sound sources, like an air conditioner in the corner. Your sensory systems are very crafty at using pretty much any information that's available to maintain their sense of where they are located relative to the room around you.)

After you've spun around a few times—presuming there aren't any of these landmarks—even if that rotation is slow, you won't know which way is which any longer. If you try to point in the direction of the door, you'll only be able to guess. The reason for this is that while the vestibular system responds very well when you start moving, once you're moving at a constant velocity, it stops; it essentially stops responding. Within a few seconds, all of that fluid that's inside the tubes has accelerated to be spinning in the same direction as the tube, at the same velocity. None of the hair cells are bent over because the fluid's not moving, and so the system stops responding.

The vestibular system responds to acceleration, not to velocity or actual amount of movement; just to acceleration. In order to encode the total amount of body movement, we need some other information. In this situation, under normal circumstances, it's vision that comes to our rescue. As you rotate to the right, for instance, the world rotates left relative to you. As you tip forward, the world rotates backward relative to you. Under normal circumstances, it's the visual change that helps track the amount of overall movement we experience. The eyes and the inner ears work together. The semicircular canals tell you when any movement has started and how much acceleration is involved, and your eyes track the amount of overall motion.

There's an interesting motion illusion that you can actually get in a dark room that capitalizes on this link between the visual and vestibular information. To achieve this effect, you need a completely pitch black room with a single small source of light that doesn't spread to illuminate the rest of the room itself. If you have a large, dark bedroom with a small, dim LED alarm clock you have an ideal setup for this. Stand in the dark—maybe from all the way across the room from the alarm clock—and simply look at the clock. As you do, you'll notice that the numbers on this clock periodically seem to move up or down, or left or right, and then back to the starting position. The clock is completely stationary; why should it appear to move? It appears to move because you're moving. We rely on visual information to maintain an upright posture. If the lights are turned off, we have only the vestibular information to rely on. Since that vestibular information isn't quite as accurate, we tend to wobble a little without realizing it. This causes the projection of the alarm clock to move a little bit on the backs of our retina. If you're stationary—which you think you are—and the retinal projection is changing, your visual system will make the most logical inference that it can: It must be the alarm clock that's moving. That's what you perceive.

There are some very impressive virtual reality rides in amusement parks that capitalize on this visual vestibular interaction as well. They typically involve large-screen videos of movement; say, an iMax movie screen that fills up your field of view showing the view from the cockpit of a jet fighter. You watch this movie from a theater seat that has the capacity to move up, down, left, and right and to rotate a bit in synchrony with the video presentation. The seats can't move more than a few feet in any direction—in terms of rotation, really just a few inches—but when they're combined with the video, it can make you feel in a very compelling fashion as if you're making enormously large shifts in your body's position.

Imagine that the video shows your plane rolling to the left, all the way over until it's right side up again—a "barrel roll" in air force pilot lingo. Under normal circumstances, as you experience a barrel roll, your semicircular canals would activate sharply as the roll started, but then they would become quiet during the rest of the roll. The visual information conveys that information. In the virtual reality situation, the seats tilt sharply in one direction, and slowly come to a stop, so that your semicircular canals don't send another sharp signal indicating that the rolling motion has stopped. The overall impression of this, if all of this works correctly, is that you have rolled over. Based on the visual and vestibular sensory inputs, your perceptual system infers that this is the most likely cause.

Often, people who experience one of these virtual reality rides experience motion sickness, either during or after the ride. For many people, whenever the visual and vestibular systems produce conflicting information, nausea results. If your eyes say you're rolling over but your vestibular system does not, you may get motion sick. This is the cause of seasickness on boats as well. If you're inside the cabin of a boat and the sea is rocking back and forth, your vestibular system is getting information about the rocking motion, but if you're downstairs surrounded by the furniture of the cabin and the walls and you're not looking out at the water, the visual inputs are for a stationary room. Often if someone is very seasick, an experienced sailor will tell them to look at the horizon. "The horizon is your friend." This is good advice from a kinesthetic perception perspective. If you're looking at the horizon, then any time the boat rocks downward, the horizon will move exactly the same amount upward, and vice versa. This will eliminate the conflict between the visual and vestibular inputs and hopefully help your nausea to subside.

There's an even simpler way to eliminate a visual-vestibular conflict, however, one that many people discover on airplane flights. The cabin of a typical jetliner is another situation in which there's a completely stationary visual input even as the airplane tilts and bounces around from time to time. The easy solution to eliminate the visual-vestibular conflict is to simply close your eyes. It may feel very counterintuitive to close your eyes when you're feeling very nauseous, but after a few minutes the nausea will typically be greatly reduced or even vanish.

Okay, so you hopefully have a good understanding of the working of the vestibular system, both how it works independently and how it interacts with your visual system. This is one part of kinesthetic perception, but it's about how your body as a whole is moving. The other aspect of kinesthetic perception is proprioception, the sense of where your individual body parts are located. Some of that information can come in through your eyes—you can look out and see where your body parts are—but if you're either in the dark or looking at something else, you have to have some other way of knowing where the parts of your body are located.

A good test of the limits of your proprioception can be done by holding one hand up above your head and spreading your fingers apart. With the other hand, alternate between touching the tip of your nose and then one of your fingers. Work your way through each one of the fingers on this upraised hand: the nose then the thumb, the nose then the index finger, the nose then the middle finger, and so on. First, try it with your eyes open so you have both the non-visual proprioceptive information and the visual. Next, I want you to close your eyes and try again. This time, keep your fingers and hand as still as possible as you do it.

You'll find that this time it's much harder. You have the proprioceptive information, but you don't have the visual information to guide you. Part of your proprioceptive perception is derived from information obtained when you move a body part. In the lecture on motion perception, we talked about how your motor system sends 2 copies of each motor command, one that moves your eyes to the muscles themselves, and another copy to the visual cortex. This efference copy enables your visual system to know when the environment is moving as opposed to just your eyes moving within a stationary environment. A similar system seems to function for proprioception.

Let's do that finger touch test again. Close your eyes again, but this time as you do it, wiggle the fingers on the raised hand as you do. You should notice that the task is much easier when these fresh efference copies of the finger movements are available to your motor system

There are many different types of receptors involved in proprioception. Specialized neurons are present in the muscles and the tendons of our bodies that sense the tension of those muscles and tendons, as well as the angles of each of the joins. The skin itself also contains stretch receptors that can be used to infer how much a particular part of your body is extended, such as a limb. This wiggling finger demonstration makes clear, however, that the motor commands we generate to move our body parts also play a very important role in proprioception.

All of this information from these many different sources is fed into an enormous network of neurons in a part of the brain called the cerebellum. This part of the nervous system sits at the base of the brain, at the top of the spinal cord. It's often referred to as the hindbrain because of its location here at the back end, and also because it looks somewhat like a small version of the brain tucked underneath the big brain. Even though the cerebellum only makes up about 10% of the overall brain volume in humans, it contains more neurons than the rest of the brain put together. Damage to the cerebellum is associated with many different types of deficits, but motor coordination, including balance and the timing of actions, seems very linked to this important little structure. Proprioception, in particular, seems to be accomplished by the circuits located right in this part of the brain.

There's an element of mystery as to just how this enormously complex part of the brain functions, but there are several leading theories that account for most of the known data on this topic. Most of those theories center around the idea of something called an internal model of the body that's maintained and used to plan actions. This model of the body is not something you could see or touch, but is a neural activation based representation of all of your body parts and their relations to one another, as well as their current positions. Humans generate action intentions in the motor cortex up here, but essentially all of the signals pass through this cerebellum on their way to the spinal cord and the muscles beyond. As they do, the plans seem to be refined and actually implemented on the basis of this internal model that's maintained in the cerebellum.

At the start of the lecture, I talked about how, prior to engaging in a reach forward to press an elevator button, the hips are engaged to compensate for the backwards push that will be generated by the forward movement of the arm. The cerebellum and its internal model are the place where this kind of calculation is done. It seems that the cerebellum simulates the action, looks for any problems, fixes the action, simulates it again, and so on until things work out the right way. At that point, the signals are actually sent on to the muscle and the real action commences.

There's some evidence for this simulation process based on characterizations of how people perform certain kinds of motor tasks. In one such set of studies, participants sat in the dark in front of a table surface onto which target objects would be placed. The instructions were really simple: They just sat there in the dark, and whenever the lights came on, they should reach out and pick up the blue object, wherever that blue object was located. One of the most basic findings that emerged from this is the farther away that blue object is located, the longer it takes people to start their reach. Note that it's obvious that people should take longer to complete the reach, since the hand has to move farther to get to where the object is located; but there's no inherent reason that people should need to wait longer before they start the movement unless they need to simulate the movement prior to starting actually performing it. The longer the actual movement takes, then the longer the simulation will require, and the longer the delay before the reach will begin. Findings such as this—and there are a lot of very similar studies that have tapped into that—are very consistent with this internal model approach.

If you ask people to start with their hands upside down on the table in this study where the lights come on and you reach for the blue object, they require even more time; more time, again, not to move, but just to start moving. This suggests that flipping the hand over requires an extra step in the simulation as well.

A wide range of research suggests that action planning requires this type of simulation in order to be implemented properly. We don't usually visualize actions explicitly; certainly we wouldn't in these simple reaching tasks I'm describing. The simulation I'm describing here proceeds very quickly and unconsciously, based on a wide source of proprioceptive and visual information. While this simulation is usually unconscious, there are a few domains in which it seems to be used very explicitly, very consciously, as people engage in mental simulation.

If you watch Olympic track and field, the high jumpers can be a really interesting test case here. Essentially, every one of the best jumpers in the world will stand at their starting position and do an odd little dance before they begin to run toward the high bar. They bob their heads, wiggle their arms, and twist their body just slightly, all the while staring fixedly at that high bar that they're about to try to jump over. These athletes are mentally simulating their jump before they actually try to perform it. There's a wealth of evidence to suggest that this works; better, more consistent performance results for almost any athlete that tries visualizing it before they actually try to perform it. Many athletes report imagining successful performances of their particular actions as part of their game (whatever that might be) or as part of their preparation before games. There may be many reasons that this influences performance, including maybe just a simple boost of confidence that comes with imagining success. However, given our understanding of how the human brain implements sensory-guided actions, using simulation prior to performance, there's reason to imagine that the cerebellum and proprioception are also influenced by this explicit mental simulation.

I mentioned early on in the lecture that proprioception is often not considered as one of the 5 basic senses: see, hear, touch, taste, and smell. When those lists were developed in the early days of perception research, people presumed that proprioception was either a simple extension of touch perception or perhaps something that just wasn't that interesting or important to include. It's become very clear that proprioception is extremely important, however. Nowhere is this more apparent than when studying patients who've lost their sense of proprioception. Ian Waterman is one such patient who, at the age of 19, was struck by a very rare disease that destroyed the nerves in his body that send information from the body back to the spinal cord and the brain.

His motor neurons—the neurons that actually stimulate the movements of the muscles—were spared. After the disease had run its course, Waterman was left with the ability to move (sort of) but without the ability to sense the effects of those movements. If he lay with his eyes closed, he reported not having any sense where his body was or even that his body was there anywhere below his neck.

This is a bit frightening even to consider, I think. Essentially all of the very few patients who've had this disorder are completely incapacitated by it. They can't walk, stand, they can't even sit up. They can't control their arm movements to feed or change themselves. Their limbs will often flail about, but uncontrollably. They are, for all intents and purposes, functionally paralyzed.

Waterman, however, has become a bit of a celebrity based upon his absolute refusal to give in to this. He refused a wheel chair and spent years fighting his illness, determined to re-learn to control his body. After several months of effort, for instance, he managed to teach himself to sit up. More important than that simple achievement of sitting up was the discovery he made while he was trying to do it; a discovery that's very relevant given the material covered in this lecture so far.

Two key factors are central to how Waterman tackles one of his deficits when he's addressing it. First, he focuses his vision and his attention on the body parts involved in performing the task, whatever that is. For sitting up, these were the leg and stomach muscles. Second, he vividly and repeatedly imagines—mentally simulates—how he's going to accomplish the goal of his task. The other thing that Waterman does it to practice in an amazingly tenacious and disciplined fashion. He trained himself to stand and walk with the rigor of an Olympic athlete, spending hours and hours per day, day in and day out, until he achieved success; he's able to walk now. Ultimately, Waterman has won back most of the things that he'd lost. He's developed a distinctive, somewhat shuffling kind of a gait that enables him to keep an eye on his feet and legs as he moves forward, but he can walk. He can talk and even manage to gesture, in some cases only with a peripheral view of his hands. If you were to meet this guy and just talk with him, until he told you about the disorder you might go for quite a long time without figuring out that there's anything wrong here at all.

All of this said, there's a part of proprioception that Waterman will never regain: the ability to do all of these everyday motor tasks without intense concentration. We often walk while talking, dialing the phone, looking for friends, and even while chewing gum. Waterman can walk, but what used to be accomplished automatically is now a very taxing, consciously directed task. After a few minutes of pondering this, I don't think any of us should ever take our proprioception for granted again.

In this lecture, we've considered many aspects of kinesthetic perception. I've described how our vestibular sense works both alone and in concert with our visual sense; how it works to track the movements of our head and the body attached to it. We've also discussed the immensely complex process of motor coordination and how proprioception helps to make it possible.

In the next lecture, we will consider perceptual development. We'll be looking at some very cute babies and talking about the sensory tasks that they can, and in some cases can't, accomplish. As we do this, I want you to better understand infants, but also to develop a better understanding of adult perception. In some cases, by studying how a system develops—how the pieces of it come online in parts—we can obtain insights that just can't be obtained if you only study the adult state of the system. The babies and I will look forward to seeing you next time.

# Seeing, Remembering, Inferring Infants
## Lecture 16

Infants see things differently than adults do, and infant perception changes over the course of the first few years of life. Researchers, including me, who study this topic not only want to better understand infants; they also want a better understanding of adult perception.

- Studying infant development is similar in some ways to studying brain-injured patients. If children can do many things but still fail to accomplish some perceptual task, it suggests that some aspect of the sensory system is not yet functioning at full capacity.

- The limitations of this logic are also similar. Even if we get a clear dissociation in performance between different stages of brain development, a combination of areas may be developing together, providing a mistaken impression that one particular component is responsible for the change in performance.

- Perceptual development as a field has made great progress in the past few decades. As late as the 1960s, textbooks in pediatric ophthalmology stated that human infants are born more or less blind, their eyes only perceiving a blooming and buzzing confusion.

- It was believed that infants are born as blank slates, requiring a great deal of associative learning before they could ever do something we might refer to as perception. There is now a wealth of evidence suggesting this is incorrect.

- Infants cannot see and reason as well as adults, but they come into the world able to see, hear, smell, taste, and feel, and their reasoning is more impressive than one might imagine. What they cannot do, of course, is communicate their perceptions in great detail.

- The most important technical innovation in the field of infant perception research was the video camera, which provided an inexpensive method for recording and analyzing infant behavior. Infants' eye motions make it clear that they can make a great deal of sense of the world around them.

- When adults look at things, they make 2 very different types of eye movements: saccadic movements and smooth tracking. When you scan a stationary stimulus, your eyes move in discrete rapid jumps, called saccades. You can and do make smooth eye movements, but only when you are tracking a moving, directly visible target.

- Human infants are born with the ability to make saccades but not smooth tracking movements. Infants do not follow you with their eyes the way adults do. If you move a colorful object around in front of a newborn, he or she will look toward it with delayed, darting eye movements, not smooth ones.

- If we move the same object back and forth in front of a slightly older infant, say a 5 week old, we see the same pattern of eye movement, although the infant tends to look at the object and follow it better than when he or she was first born—the eye movements are faster, more accurate, and gradually more predictive, jumping ahead of the moving object in its path. Still, there is no smooth tracking.

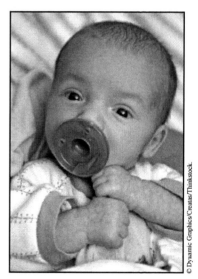

Babies are born with an innate preference for looking at faces.

© Dynamic Graphics/Creatas/Thinkstock.

- Right around 2 months of age, infants make their first smooth tracking eye movements. Once their eyes are locked on a target, they follow it, keeping the target in the center of the field of view without any abrupt shift in eye position.

- For most infants, the onset of smooth tracking happens abruptly, sometimes from one day to the next, sometime between 6 and 8 weeks after birth. Beyond this point, baby eye movements look very adult like, although there is evidence that smooth tracking continues to improve over the next 2 years.

- Infants have some preference for looking at things that are interesting. The more complex some stimulus is, the more infants will be drawn to it. If you show an infant an image with a grey patch on one side and a black-and-white stripe pattern on the other, the infant will consistently look in the direction of the stripes.

- Stimuli like these, developed by Davida Teller, are carefully printed such that the average brightness of the gray and the striped patch are identical. In fact, in some cases, the stripes are so thin, an adult cannot tell the difference between the gray and striped patches, but the baby still shows a preference.

- Infants are born relatively nearsighted. The eyes of a newborn are actually not spherical like an adult's but a bit foreshortened. In general, young infants can see best only out to about 2 feet away and lack the ability to make out the very fine details.

- Infants have a fovea, but their visual receptors are not nearly as densely packed. Their eyes thus deliver a much lower-resolution scan of the environment to the brain. If the stimuli we are testing have fine details in them, the infants might not be able to see the things we think we are showing them.

- Even with this low-resolution, nearsighted vision, babies still have some decided preferences. One of their favorite things to look at is a human face. Compared to a plain circle of light, they will track a projected image of a human face moving across a screen over twice as far.

- Were they attracted to the face or to the complexity of the face image versus the oval? Infants follow a face with scrambled features about twice as far as they follow a plain oval, but still not as far as they follow a normal face.

- Studies have explored what it is about faces that newborns prefer. In general, newborns (as young as a few minutes old) have a preference for anything that is oval shaped with more internal features in the top half than the bottom half.

- Infants can hear a little in the womb, their sense of touch is active, and there is evidence for taste activity during the final stages of development. In terms of vision, however, developing infants live and grow in the dark. Any visual preferences must somehow be genetic.

- Can newborn infants encode sensory information in their brains? I believe they can, based on an experimental technique called habituation, which also shows that they have functioning memories. Habituation allows researchers to ask all sorts of other questions about what infants can and cannot see, hear, touch, taste, and smell.

- Imagine I showed you something you had never seen before, something brightly colored and perceptually interesting. You would look for a while and eventually look away. If I took the stimulus away for a while, then showed it again, you would look again.

- As soon as you realized it was the same thing, you would probably look away again. If I kept doing this over and over, you would get pretty bored with this object, only glancing to confirm it was the same. This is a rough description of the habituation procedure.

- We can perform this procedure with any infant, even a newborn. Suppose I showed a baby a jar of cayenne pepper. The colors on the jar were bright; the bottle was shiny. After about 32 seconds, however, she looked away.

- We took the jar away for 15 seconds, then brought it back. She looked again. Each time we repeat this, depending on the object and the infant, the looking times might be different, but on repeated presentations of any stimulus, an infant will look at the object less and less.

- For this to be true, babies must have certain innate abilities: The baby must be able to see. She must be able to control her gaze. Most importantly, she must have a functioning memory.

- In the 1960s, when this was first discovered, it came as a big surprise to many. Most of us cannot recall any memories before we were 4 or 5 years old. How could this baby be remembering things already?

- Even though we cannot make and later retrieve long-term conscious memories of events, it seems that we can encode and use our sensory experiences in a short-term fashion, as required for this habituation task.

- How else can we use habituation studies to better understand perceptual development? Using multiple static stimuli (such as different-looking jars), researchers have determined that babies have a preference for and can recognize novelty.

- An increase in looking time is called dishabituation, and it provides the most frequently used tool to test when children can tell the difference—and when they cannot—between 2 stimuli. Studies like this have shown that even very young children can see the world around them in color.

- Another classic perceptual development study suggests that young infants, like adults, make inferences about the world around them based on sensory input.

**Figure 16.1**

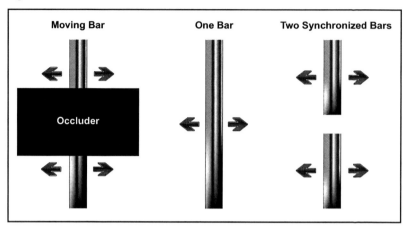

In the occluder experiment described in the lecture, even babies a few months old are surprised to see 2 bars when the occluder is taken away. Certain suppositions about the world seem hard-wired into our brains.

- Infants were shown an approximately vertical rod moving back and forth behind a stationary piece of wood. The infants could see the top and bottom sections of the rod as it passed behind the wooden occluder (See Figure 16.1).

- Adults typically described the moving part as a single rod, but it could also have been 2 small rods moving in synchrony.

- Four-month-old babies presented with this display stared at it for 30 seconds or more, then looked away. A curtain was drawn across the display, then removed. They looked again for a shorter time—showing habituation. The experimenters repeated this until the infants' looking time had dropped by at least 50% versus the first 3 presentations.

- When the curtains opened again, the central occluder was gone. The infants viewed one of 2 different displays—a single rod or 2 separate pieces moving in synchrony.

- If the infants perceived the habituation display like adults do—as a single, connected rod—then they should look longer at the split rod, which would be more surprising. They did. Infants, like adults, seem to use their senses to infer the details of the world around them.

## Suggested Reading

Gopnik, Meltzoff, and Kuhl, *The Scientist in the Crib.*

Kellman and Arterberry, *The Cradle of Knowledge.*

## Questions to Consider

1. If I show my 3-month-old baby a sign with the word *cookie* on it, she will look at it for a while and then look away. If I keep showing her the same sign over and over, she will look for shorter and shorter times before looking away. If I change to showing her a sign that says *bottle*, she might look longer. If I find this consistently, does that mean that she can read? What does it mean?

2. Infants seem to recognize their mother's voice, orienting their looks toward her within the first few minutes of life. If a particular story is read to them each day, they will orient toward the sound of it as well, even if it is read by a different person. Does that mean that infants remember things from when they were in the womb? What do they understand about the story? What is it that they remember?

# Seeing, Remembering, Inferring Infants
## Lecture 16—Transcript

This lecture is the first of 2 that will explore perceptual development. I want to tell you about how infants see things—and in some cases don't see things—and about how infant perception changes over the course of the first few years of life. My goal, like many of the people who study this topic, is not only to better understand infants, but also to provide a better understanding of adult perception. In some cases, by studying how a system develops—by how it comes online in parts—can provide insights that just can't be obtained if you only study the adult state of a system.

In a weird way, studying infant development can make use of logic that's similar to that of studying brain-injured patients. I told you about the case of a man who lost the ability to recognize faces after suffering damage to his right inferotemporal cortex. Studying him doesn't tell us exactly how we recognize faces in a normally functioning brain, but it does provide a clue that there's a particular system of the brain—perhaps a modular system— that's dedicated to that face-perception process. We saw a similar type of finding with DF and RV, suggesting that there are systems devoted to conscious perception and visually-guided action control. With babies, this can proceed in a similar fashion. If kids can do many things but still fail to be able to accomplish some perceptual task, it suggests that there might be some aspect of their sensory system that's devoted specifically to that task, one that isn't yet functioning at full capacity.

I should say that the limitations of this logic also come over from the work with the brain-injured patients. Even if we get a clear dissociation in performance, for instance, between different stages of brain development, it might be analogous to that blender situation we studied, where a combination of areas are developing together and only providing a mistaken impression that one particular component of the brain is responsible for the kid's change in performance.

Regardless, studying infant development can provide great clues about the underlying structure and organization of general, adult sensory processing. Let's consider some of them now.

Perceptual development as a field has made great progress in the last few decades. As late as the 1960s, if you were to have taken a class in pediatric ophthalmology, your textbook would have stated that human infants are born blind. Their eyes, according to this claim, are somewhat functional and connected to the brain, but infants are unable to make any sense of the "blooming and buzzing confusion" of the flood of sensory input. Infants, for instance, might see the color red and a cup-like shape, but it was presumed that they needed to learn to associate these 2 sensory features before they could ever see a red cup. In essence, it was believed that infants are born as blank slates, requiring a great deal of associative learning before they could ever do something that we might refer to as perception.

There's a tremendous wealth of evidence suggesting that this is incorrect. Infants can't see and reason about the world as well as adults when they're born, but they come into the world able to see, hear, smell, taste, and feel, and able to reason about the world in some pretty impressive ways. Infants can't tell you what they're thinking and perceiving, of course. To be frank, I think that's one of the biggest reasons that people presumed that infants aren't born with the great perceptual intelligence that they have. The most important technical innovation in the field of infant perception research wasn't an fMRI or anything nearly so expensive; it was the video camera. Video cameras provide an inexpensive method for recording and then immediately playing back their behaviors for analysis. Even better, you can play those behaviors back in slow motion, enabling a careful analysis of just what infants are doing.

One behavior in particular—looking—makes it clear that infants are able to make a great deal of sense about the world around them. Let's consider how infants direct their eye movements and how that ability develops over the first few months of life. Once we have this in hand, we can use it as a tool to infer how infants reason about the things that we show them.

When adults look at things—as they scan the environment around them— they make 2 very different types of eye movements. These are called saccadic eye movements and smooth tracking. If you scan a stationary stimulus—say the room in front of you—it might feel as if your eyes are moving smoothly from one side to the other, the way maybe a camera might pan across a room, but they aren't; you're physically incapable of this. When you scan a stationary stimulus, your eyes move in discrete rapid jumps, called saccades. In between those jumps, your eyes remain relatively still. You can and do make smooth eye movements, but only when you're following a moving target. In this situation, your eyes do move smoothly from place to place; they move without any abrupt shifts in position. Again, you can only do this when there's a directly visible target right in front of you that you're tracking with your eyes. This type of eye movement is called smooth tracking.

Human infants are born with the ability to make those saccadic tracking movements, but without the ability to smoothly track targets. This again might be one of the reasons that doctors used to believe that infants are born blind. When you move around in front of newborn infant, they don't follow you with their eyes the way a sighted adult person inevitably will. It almost looks as if the baby can't see you.

If you shake a colorful, noisemaking object in front of an infant—even a newborn—she'll look in the direction of the object. If you then move it to the left, center, and right sides, her eyes will tend to shift to the left, the center, and the right sides after a short delay. If you're being a skeptical scientist— and I hope that you are—you might be thinking that infants don't have to be able to see to follow the target. It's making noise, after all. You know a lot about sound source localization now from the first auditory perception lecture, so you could even say how the baby might know to turn her head left or right. To be really careful, I'd have to use an object that doesn't make any noise. Let me assure you that even with a silent, colorful, moving object, even a newborn infant will turn in that direction. Again, it only happens after a short delay.

If we watch an infant looking at a moving object display in slow motion, the saccadic aspect of her visual tracking becomes very apparent. The infant might be looking directly at the object but as it drifts to the side, she keeps looking straight ahead, right at where the object was a few moments ago before it moved away. Then, after a delay, the eyes shift abruptly to look at the new location. Of course, if the object keeps moving, she'll lag behind it again, always looking at where the object was rather than where it is, or where it will be in the future. The eyes jump, jump, and jump again.

If we move an object back and forth in front of a slightly older infant, say around 5 weeks of age, we'll see the same basic pattern of eye movement. The infant tends to look at the object and to follow it better than when she was first born. The eye movements are faster and more accurate. They also tend to be more and more predictive; that is, the eyes will jump slightly ahead of the moving object's current position so that the infant's able to see more of the object as it moves through her field of view. Still, however, there's no hint of smooth tracking behavior at this age of 5 weeks. At this age, the brain systems that control that smooth tracking behavior are still not active enough for these types of eye movements to be made.

Right around 2 months of age, kids make their first smooth tracking movements. A good demonstration of this can come from shaking an object to get an infant's attention and gaze to be directed at the object. At that point, if you stop shaking the object and then smoothly move it past the infant, the eyes will follow. A slow motion video of this makes the eye movements very clear. Once the eyes are locked on to the target, they follow it, keeping the target in the center of the field of view without ever making any abrupt shift in eye position to do that. For most infants, the onset of smooth tracking happens very abruptly, sometimes from one day to the next, sometime between 6 and 8 weeks after they're born.

Beyond 2 or 3 months of age, baby eye movements look very adult-like, with a mix of both smooth tracking and saccadic eye movements. There's some evidence that the smooth tracking continues to improve and become more frequent through as much as 2 years of development, but most of the changes are complete by the end of the 3rd month.

Infants are not only not blind, they have the ability to control their eye movements to follow interesting-looking things. A point to note here is that infants have some preference for what things are interesting. In general, the more complex some stimulus is, the more infants will be drawn to it. A standard method is available that enables a test of just how well infants can see. With adults and even older children, we usually test visual acuity by showing people an eye chart and asking them to tell us what they see. Infants can't tell us, of course, but we can infer what they can see based on where they look.

If you show an infant a grey patch on one side of an image and a black and white stripe pattern on the other side of the image, the infant will very consistently look in the direction of the stripes. Stimuli like these, developed by a very famous developmental scientist named Davida Teller, are very carefully printed such that the average brightness of the gray and the striped patch are identical. That is, if the infant is looking at the striped patch, it isn't because it's brighter or darker, it's because the infants' eyes are sensitive to the striped pattern that's present on that side.

If you make the stripes thinner, they'll be harder to see. Indeed, if you make the stripes thin enough, even an adult won't be able to tell which side is striped and which is gray. If you've ever looked at a photograph in the newspaper from a distance, it looks like a smooth, continuous image. If you look very close, however, you can see that the photo is created with many very tiny black dots. The varying density of the dots blurs together at a distance once it moves beyond the limits of your visual acuity. The same thing is true with the infants. The question is: How small do those stripes have to get before the infants can't see the individual parts anymore?

Infants are born relatively nearsighted. The eyes of a newborn are actually not spherical like an adult's, but a bit foreshortened. In general, young infants can see best only out to about 2 feet away. Young infants also lack the ability to make out the very fine details of their visual input. They have a fovea just like an adult, but the visual receptors there are not nearly as densely packed as they are for an adult. Infants' eyes thus deliver a much lower resolution scan of the environment to the brain.

While infants can certainly see, they don't see all that well. When we're trying to understand how they make sense of the world around them, we need to keep that in mind. If the stimuli we're testing have very tiny, fine details in them, then the infants might not be able to even see the things that we think we're showing them.

Even with this low resolution, nearsighted view of the world, kids still have some very decided preferences, and not just for stripes. One of their favorite things to look at is another human face. In one classic series of studies, newborns were held on their backs, looking up at a semicircular projection screen. Onto that screen, an oval-shaped spot of light was projected directly in front of them. Not surprisingly, the infants looked at it. The experimenters then slowly moved the light to the side, off to the left or right of the center of the projection screen. Again, not surprisingly, the infants followed it. The primary measure in this study was how far the infants would follow the projected light before they looked away, usually back to the center point of the screen. With a plain stimulus, they would follow the light with about 20 degrees of head rotation before the snapped back to the center. If the stimulus was, instead of just being a plain spot of light, a picture of a face, now they would follow it almost 50 degrees to the side.

Those newborns were very attracted to that face image. Or were they? Perhaps it wasn't the face per se but the fact that it was a more detailed, complex image. (If that occurred to you before I mentioned it, then good job being a skeptical listener.) The experimenters had this same concern, and so they included another stimulus: a face in which the face parts—the nose, the mouth, the eyes, the eyebrows—were all scrambled up in different positions. The stimulus was thus just as complex as the face, but not anything you would look at and recognize as a face.

The complexity does seem to matter; the infants followed the scrambled face out to about 40 degrees to the side, rather than just the 20 degrees they followed with the plain oval of light. However, they still followed the actual face pattern further, significantly farther.

Later studies have explored just what it is about faces that newborns prefer using this and some related methods. By the time they're a couple of months old, infants prefer photos of faces. As newborns, they have preferences for something face-like, but it's actually not a face per se. In general, newborn infants have a preference for anything that is oval-shaped with more internal features in the top half than the bottom half.

That might not seem so impressive; it seems pretty easy to distinguish between an oval with some stuff in the top half and an actual face. Infants who can't do that may seem quite perceptually limited. You should keep in mind, however, that these are newborns. These are children who, in some cases, are only a few minutes old when they participate in the study. They've only been around long enough for doctors and nurses to do a quick check and make sure that they've come through the birth process okay, without any health concerns that need treatment. For the infants to have these preferences, they have to be essentially inborn, congenitally specified. Infants can hear a little in the womb, their sense of touch is active, and there's evidence that infants can even experience taste sensations during the final stages of pregnancy. In terms of vision, however, developing infants live and grow in the dark. There's no time for them to have learned this visual preference. It must be somehow specified right in their genetic structure. That's pretty fascinating, I think, and a long way from the idea that infants are born as blind, blank slates.

Infants can see and have some preferences, even at the moment that they're born. Can they make use of that information in any meaningful way? Can they encode sensory information in their brains? I'll argue in the next few minutes that they absolutely can based on an experimental technique called habituation. In addition to showing that infants have a functioning memory, this habituation technique provides an important tool to ask all sorts of other questions about what infants can and can't see, hear, touch, taste, and smell.

Imagine that I showed you something that you'd never seen before; something brightly colored and perceptually interesting. You'd look at it for a while. Eventually, you'd look away. If I then took my novel stimulus away for a while and after some delay showed it to you again, you'd look again. You might look for a while, but as soon as you realized it was the same thing, you'd probably look away again. If I kept doing this over and over, you'd get pretty bored with this object; this thing I kept showing you. Only after maybe a quick glance just to verify it was the same thing, you'd be off again, looking for something else that might be of interest.

What I've just given you is a rough description of a habituation procedure, one that I could perform with any infant, even a newborn. Suppose I showed a baby a jar of cayenne pepper. (Let's imagine this isn't, by the way, a taste experiment. Just looking here; no tasting.) The colors on the jar are bright; the bottle was shiny. It was attractive and held her gaze for a while. After about 32 seconds, however, she looked away. After she looked away, we took the cayenne pepper away for a few seconds, say about 15 seconds. If we then brought the bottle back into view, the infant would look again. The 2nd time, the infant might look for about 14 seconds. Again, we took the bottle away for a delay of about 15 seconds, and then we showed it to her again. On the 3rd trial, the infant might look for about 6 seconds. In a 4th and 5th repetition of this procedure, the infant might look for about 3 seconds and then maybe again for about 3 seconds.

Depending on the objects and the infant, the exact looking times might vary quite a bit, actually. If it's a really fascinating, moving, talking, singing electronic toy, the infant might look the first time for several minutes before looking away. If, on the other hand, the object were a plain, blue block then perhaps only a couple of seconds of looking time would be obtained. The habituation trend, however, occurs for essentially every infant and every object that you might use. On repeated presentations of any stimulus, an infant will look at it progressively less and less.

Think for a moment about what an infant must be able to do to accomplish this task. Think about what abilities you'd have to build into a robot baby in order for it to perform this way. First, the baby would have to be able to see. If she can't visually encode the properties of the object, then there's no way that this could occur. Second, she must be able to control her gaze. We know that babies can do this already from other demonstrations that we've talked about right in this lecture; but if the child's not exerting some choice about where to look, when to look at the object, and when to look away, then this is sort of a non-starter. Third, and this is the big one here, the infant must have a functioning memory. She must be able to look at the object during the other later presentations and connect it with some stored memory of the experience of seeing it in the past. Only then can she recognize that this is the same thing she's been looking at for a while, and then move on to try to find something novel.

In the 1960s, when this was first discovered, it came as a big surprise to many. If you think back to your earliest memory, the first thing that you can remember happening during your childhood, you'll probably come up with something that happened when you were 4 or 5 years old. Occasionally, someone has a memory from earlier, maybe when they were 3; but only then if the memory was usually about something a bit traumatic, like an accident or getting lost at the mall.

All of our experience suggests that memory, as a cognitive process, doesn't really kick in until a few years of age, not a few months. How could this baby be remembering things already? I think it's actually unlikely that this baby will have a conscious, long-term memory of this experience. (It's actually my daughter who participated in this, and now she's several years of age. I can verify that she does not, in fact, remember me making a video of it.) Even though we don't have the ability to make and later retrieve long-term conscious memories of events, it seems that we can encode and use our sensory experiences in a short-term fashion, such as is needed for this habituation task.

What could we do with this habituation technique? It's, I think, interesting all by itself; but how can we use it to better understand perceptual development? Consider again that baby looking at the cayenne pepper. Actually, she's not looking at it very much. After about 6 presentations of a simple, stationary stimulus like a jar of cayenne pepper, an infant might only look at it for a few moments before looking away again. What would happen if I took the jar of cayenne pepper away for 15 seconds and then, for the next trial, showed her a jar of celery salt? If I do exactly that, the infant would probably look for about 6 seconds. That's substantially more than the 2 or 3 seconds that she was looking at the cayenne pepper; more than twice as long, actually. If that happens consistently—and it does—I can conclude something else about the baby's perception: I can conclude that she can tell the difference between what I was showing her before and what I'm showing her after.

Young children, in general, have a preference for novelty. If you give them a choice of playing with an old toy, with which they've had extensive time to play, and a new toy that they've never seen before now, the new toy will be chosen essentially every time.

With this comparison to celery salt, I have evidence that the baby can tell that this is something new. If she couldn't tell the difference, then from her perspective, it would be just like another presentation of that same jar of cayenne pepper. This increase in looking time is called dishabituation and it provides the most frequently-used tool to test when children can tell the difference—and when they can't tell the difference—between 2 stimuli. Can she read the words on the bottles? Probably not. The jars are the same approximate shape, but the color of the celery salt and cayenne pepper are very different. Studies like this have shown that even very young children can see the world around them in color.

So kids can see, they can control their eye movements, and they can remember things. Let me tell you about one more classic perceptual development study that uses all 3 of these tools to suggest that young infants, like adults, do more than just encode their sensory inputs; evidence that infants, like adults, make inferences about the world around them based upon their sensory inputs and then they perceive those inferences. (Audio customers should consult their guidebooks for figures detailing the perception of partially occluded objects.)

In a classic study performed by Phil Kellman and Elizabeth Spelke in the 1980s, infants viewed an approximately vertical rod moving back and forth behind a stationary piece of wood. The piece of wood blocked their view of the middle of this rod that was oscillating back and forth. The infants could see the top half of the rod moving back and forth, and the bottom half of the rod, also moving back and forth. The kids could not see the middle of the display, which was blocked by a stationary, wooden occluder.

When adults view this display, they typically describe it as a single rod moving back and forth behind an occluder. It could certainly be constructed this way—that could be what's present in the display—but it could also be that there are 2 small rods, one at the top and one at the bottom, which happen to be moving in synchrony. Both of those perceptions would be valid. Adults consistently describe it as a single rod because they infer that connection between the 2.

When they were presented with this display, the babies—who were 4 months of age—looked right at it. The rod was black, presented against a white, dotted background, so it was easy for the kids to see. As it moved back and forth, the kids stared at it for 30 seconds or more in some cases. Eventually, as with any stimulus, the kids looked away. The experimenters drew a curtain across the display, waited for a few seconds, and then showed it to the infants again. The infants looked again, but for a shorter duration; they were habituated. The experimenters repeated this until the infants were clearly habituated to the display; until their looking time had dropped by at least 50% in comparison with the first 3 presentation trials. At that point, the experimenters declared the infants "officially bored" and drew the curtains one last time. When the curtains opened again, the central occlude—that piece of wood that blocked the infants' view of the middle of the rod—was gone. The infants viewed one of 2 different displays. Either they would see a single, connected rod oscillating back and forth or they would see 2 separate pieces with a clear gap in the middle oscillating back and forth.

The general idea here is that infants tend to look at novel displays; at things that are more different from the thing that they've viewed in the past. If the infants perceived the habituation display like adults do, as a single, connected rod, then they should look longer at the split rod; and they do. It seems that 4-month-olds, like adults, perceptually complete the moving rod behind the occluder. They infer that the rod continues behind the occluder, even though they can't see it. Infants, like adults, seem to use their senses to infer the details of the world around them; to fill in some details that they can't see. This tendency to make educated guesses about the environment—things that go beyond the sensory input—seems to be present very early on in life.

In this lecture, we've talked about some early infant sensory abilities: infants can see, control their eye movements, and use their sensory input to make inferences about things that they can't directly see. Infants also come into the world with certain sensory preferences; things that must be inborn. Children learn a lot about the sensory world around them over the first few months of life, but they certainly don't start as blank slates.

In the next lecture, we'll consider the other sensory modalities of infants, as well as how infants then use information gained from the senses to control their actions. I look forward to telling you about that and more next time.

# How Infants Sense and Act On Their World
## Lecture 17

I n the late 1990s, researchers began studying humans' earliest hearing and memory abilities not in newborns but in utero. During the last month of the pregnancy, pregnant mothers were given a particular Dr. Seuss book and asked to read it aloud several times each day, conveying their voice into the womb.

- The developing infant lives within a fluid environment, nestled underneath several substantial layers of muscle and tissues. As such, sound—particularly high-pitched sound—is muffled and filtered. A microphone placed into the womb confirms that the mother's voice sounds like the teacher's voice in an old Charlie Brown cartoon.

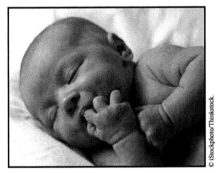

- After the baby is born and confirmed healthy, the experimenters place tiny headphones on the baby and give her a

**Researchers used infants' suckling instinct to study memory development.**

special pacifier with a pressure sensor inside of it that records the baby's rate and intensity of sucking (colloquially referred to as a suck-o-meter).

- The suck-o-meter was hooked up to a computer that could play recorded sounds. In one version of the procedure, the computer was programmed to play the sound of the mother reading that particular Dr. Seuss story whenever the baby sucked the nipple at a rate of once per second.

- The babies would trigger the story by accident but were able figure out what they did and to adjust their sucking rate to keep it going. They seem able to learn how their behaviors connect to their environment.

- Having this type of operant control over the environment around us is reinforcing to infants and to humans in general. The most important thing to note here is that the baby is in control of the sound and able to make a choice about how long that sound keeps playing.

- The experimenters were interested in whether or not the baby would recognize the sounds whether or not she would take action to hear them.

- There is good evidence that the babies did recognize and like this sound. If the sound of someone else reading the story was played, the babies would still like that and keep sucking, but they would not do so as long.

- The babies also sucked more for their mother reading the familiar story they had heard in the womb than for their mother reading a different Dr. Seuss story. The infants were able to recognize the story itself, even though they do not speak a language yet.

- As we discussed, infants are born with some visual sensory abilities and the ability to make memories, as well as the ability to make sensory inferences. Now we must address how well infants' nonvisual senses develop and how they connect their sensory abilities to early action control.

- The Dr. Seuss experiment and other research suggest that infants' other senses are similarly developed and active during their prenatal development. Newborns' taste preferences, for example, are influenced by the maternal diet, and fetuses experience touch through pushing on the womb and the mother pushing back.

- As with studies of adult sensory processing, however, the visual modality dominates infant sensory research. This is somewhat ironic, since it seems to be the last to develop, given the lack of prenatal visual input.

- Shortly after an infant is born, a pediatrician will test his or her reflexes, including cheek pressure (the rooting reflex) and the ability to suck. Together, these 2 reflexes promote feeding behaviors.

- Infants are also born with a grasp reflex. If you press an infant's palm with your finger, the baby will close his or her hand around it. It is thought this was important for survival in our evolutionary past, reducing the odds that a mother would drop her infant.

- Other reflexes seem to have little or no immediate value to the infant, which makes them even more interesting. For example, if you extend the arms of a newborn, the hands tend to close; if you place the arms close to the body with the elbows bent, the hands tend to open. There is no physical connection, just a reflexive link.

- To reach for things, you typically move your arm away from your body and close your hand around your target. The foundation of that motion seems to be organized at birth.

- Another basic motor program is the stepping reflex. When you support an infant in a standing position on a hard, level surface, the newborn's feet press down, but only for a few moments before one leg moves forward. Children do not typically walk until they are about 12 months old, but the motor program to walk is in place at 1 day old.

- Our visual motor reflex has been extraordinarily influential in the field of perceptual development research. This complex reflex involves some in-depth information about one's own body.

- In the early 1970s, researcher Andrew Meltzoff had talked with many mothers who described their very young children imitating their facial expressions. Metlzoff and his colleagues developed a method to see if imitation was real and how it worked.

- Meltzoff made 30-second video clips of himself engaging in actions that babies might imitate—smiling, opening and closing his mouth, sticking out his tongue, frowning, and hand opening and closing. He then showed these clips to babies within a few minutes after they were born.

- A video camera recorded the face and hand movements of the infants for later coding. Research assistants who had not been present for the data collection looked at the babies' movements and had to guess which clips the babies were watching. The coders were right about 40% of the time.

- That might not sound very accurate or impressive, but given the context, what is important about the 40% accuracy is that it is twice as big as what you would expect by chance. The study indicates that newborns are capable of imitating facial expressions.

- Consider what our DNA has to build into a baby to be able to accomplish this facial imitation task: The babies must be able to see and must be able to control facial movements; smiling alone requires the selective contraction of 19 different muscles.

- The babies must be able to recognize faces as well. Finally, and most impressively, the babies must be able to draw a connection between the face they are seeing and their own faces. Imitation must be built in to the nervous system.

- We do not know what the experience of this study was like for the infants—whether they were aware of their actions, for instance. But if behavior this complex can be built in, then perhaps other complex or even more complex behavior can exist as early as the day we are born.

- Infants seem to use some depth cues from a very early age but do not master other cues until about 7 months of age, as demonstrated by their reaching behavior.

- Children begin to reach at 4 months of age. Almost right away, they reach for objects or parts of objects that are nearest. Stereopsis seems to come online very early.

- Infants are not nearly as good at using pictorial cues, however; 5- and 6-month-old children do not use linear perspective, relative size, familiar size, or texture density to guide their reaches, although 7-month-old children do.

- As with adults, some fascinating evidence indicates perception and action control are coordinated in complex ways. Studies used a visual cliff, where infants are placed on one side of a table surface on which a clear checkerboard pattern is present.

- On the other half of the table, there is a drop off of several feet, covered in invisible glass. Anyone with working depth perception would expect to fall if they walked (or crawled) off this cliff.

- At 6 months, babies do not hesitate to crawl off the cliff when their mothers call them. At 7 months, with more crawling experience, they steadfastly refuse.

- A few months later, those same babies as new walkers will walk straight up to that edge, as if in this new action situation the baby has to start over in terms of learning about the surrounding world. They do not generalize knowledge from crawling to walking.

- We talk about different modules of the brain as seeming to look at the world separately from one another. With this type of action and perception study, we have an analogous story to tell.

Goldin-Meadow, *The Resilience of Language.*

McMurray and Aslin, "Infants Are Sensitive to Within-Category Variation in Speech Perception."

## Questions to Consider

1. Infants lack the ability to smoothly track objects with their eyes until about 7 weeks of age. They can move their eyes to track things, but they do so with abrupt, saccadic eye movements. Does that mean that the world looks jumpy to them?

2. Newborns have some reflexes that seem to serve as foundations for learning to perform certain actions as adults. We discussed the stepping reflex—the foundation for walking—and the way that the hand tends to close as the arm is extended—the foundation for grasping. If you were going to build a baby, what other reflexive behavioral foundations would you include?

# How Infants Sense and Act On Their World
## Lecture 17—Transcript

In the late 1990s, several fascinating studies were begun that explored humans' earliest hearing and memory abilities. To complete the studies, the researchers didn't recruit parents of young infants; they actually recruited pregnant mothers to participate. During the last month of the pregnancy, the mothers were given a particular Dr. Seuss book and asked to read it aloud several times each day. As the mothers read, the sounds of their voices were conveyed into the womb. The developing infant in the womb lives within a fluid environment at that point, nestled underneath several substantial layers of muscle and other tissues. As such, the sound was muffled and very filtered. In particular, the high-pitched sounds are mostly blocked. If a recording microphone is placed into the womb, when the mother speaks you can hear the sound, but it sounds very unusual. I usually describe it as sounding like the parents in those old Charlie Brown cartoons; sort of a "Wa wahhh, wa wahhh, wa wah wah wahhh."

The developing infant—technically the developing fetus at that point—is exposed to the sound of a Dr. Seuss story, at least this filtered version of a Dr. Seuss story, several times each day for several weeks prior to being born. After the baby is born, and after initially they're checked just to make sure that they're healthy, the experimenters arrive. They place tiny headphones on the baby and give her a special nipple to suck on; it's a non-nutritive nipple, just sort of a plastic pacifier basically, with a special pressure sensor inside of it. It records the baby's rate and intensity of sucking. This is often colloquially referred to as a "suck-o-meter."

The suck-o-meter was hooked up to a computer that could play recorded sounds. In one version of the procedure, the computer was programmed to play the sound of the mother reading that particular Dr. Seuss story whenever the baby sucked the nipple at a rate of once per second. Too much faster, and the sound would stop. It would also stop playing the story if the baby slowed or stopped sucking the nipple complete. The infant is in charge of when the story gets played. It's worth noting, it's just interesting at this point to note, that the baby seems able to learn to control something with the rate of their sucking. It's interesting that they can do that at all.

Babies are born with a sucking reflex, so when the nipple is placed into the baby's mouth, she'll start to suck on it regardless. At some point, as she's doing this, she'll happen to trigger the computer to play that sound, just by accident that first time. As she sucks at varying rates, the sound will go off again, just by accident in the future. The baby will keep doing this, just sucking at varying rates, and every once in a while the sound will go on again. As this happens a few times, there are many, many things that could be causing that sound to turn on. Maybe it's the kicking of the baby's legs; maybe the turning of her head; maybe, it's worth noting, nothing at all. Maybe it's just some random event that happens while the baby's just lying there, listening to things that are happening around her and sucking on the nipple. There's no reason that necessarily there's a connection there; these babies don't know that they're in an experiment. As the baby's placed in this situation, however, over the course of several minutes she discovers this relation between the sucking rate and the sound. As she does, she modifies her behavior and makes the sound turn on again and again, to the point where it'll be playing rather continuously.

Having this type of operant control over the environment around us is very reinforcing to infants and to humans in general. There's no food being given as a reward for this once-per-second sucking; there's no explicit positive reinforcement like that in this situation. The only thing that's driving the infant's behavior is the simple pleasure of knowing that something that you're doing, some behavior that you're causing, has an impact on the surrounding environment.

The exact mechanisms of this type of learning have been the topic of much research, and they're complex to fully describe. For the moment, the most important thing to note here is just that the baby is in control of the sound, able to make a choice about how long that story sound keeps playing. The experimenters in this story memory experiment were interested in whether or not the baby would recognize the sounds—recognize the thing that they'd heard when they were still in the womb—and suck in order to hear them. There's good evidence that the babies did recognize and like this sound, in particular the sounds of their mother's voice reading that familiar story. If the sound of someone else reading the story—someone other than their mother—was played, the babies would still suck to hear the sounds, they still liked that, but they wouldn't keep it on as long as for the sound of their own mother reading the story. This tells us that the babies can recognize the sound of their mother's voice.

The babies also sucked more for their mother reading the familiar story, the one that they'd heard in the womb, than for the sound of their mother's voice reading a different Dr. Seuss story. Remember, half of the mothers recruited for this experiment read *The Cat in the Hat*; half read a different story, *Green Eggs and Ham*. This is important from a skeptical scientist perspective. If the experimenters hadn't designed it this way, then maybe newborns just like some particular Dr. Seuss story more than others. That's not the case here, right? It's possible to conclude that, because half of the infants listened to one story more than the other; half to the other story more than the other. Which one of those 2 stories they preferred was a function of which one was read to them when they were in the womb.

The fact that the infants sucked longer for the familiar story tells us something pretty cool: The infants are able to recognize the story itself. They don't know the words, they don't know the meaning necessarily of the story—in fact, we can be pretty confident they don't—but the meter, the rhyme; something about that particular story seems to have been encoded in the memories of these infants during that prenatal development phase. That memory came out of the womb with the babies, where it was able to influence their behavior.

This lecture is the second that considers perceptual development. In the previous discussion, I described some of the basics of this area of research. Infants can definitely see, they can definitely control their eye movements, and choose what to look at and when to look away. Infants are born with some sensory abilities already in place as well, and some preferences that we've talked about; for instance, preference for faces. I argued that this is a remarkable thing given that infants exist totally in the dark up until the moment that they're born. Lastly in that lecture, I talked about the notion that infants, like adults, don't just perceive things that their senses directly deliver to them. In that occluded object experiment, the infants looking habituation and dishabituation clearly indicated that they infer the presence of something that they can't see. That inferential aspect of human perception seems, therefore, like the preference for faces, to be something that's ingrained in our sensory systems very early, perhaps even in our DNA.

In this lecture, I want to build on those ideas. How well do infants' other, non-visual senses develop? How do infants connect sensory abilities to early action control? Finally, how does the development of action abilities—like reaching, grasping, crawling; things like that—how do those action abilities influence infants' sensory and perceptual abilities?

The study I described here at the beginning of this lecture makes it pretty clear that infants are able to hear from the moment they're born; indeed, that infants are able to hear for some time before they are born. Other research suggests that infants' senses are similarly developed and active during their prenatal development.

For instance, there've been many studies identifying a relation between what moms eat during the pregnancy and the newborn's flavor preferences. Most newborns are not big fans of garlic, for instance. They'll make a "yucky face" expression if a drop of garlic solution is placed on their tongues. They'll even turn away from a cotton swab that just has a strong garlic odor on it. If a mother eats a diet rich in garlic during pregnancy, however, most of this initial preference, or rather lack of preference, for garlic goes away. Some carefully controlled studies have even used garlic pills, such that the mother herself doesn't experience the garlic flavor herself. Still, the garlic gets into the mother's bloodstream and makes its way to the fetus, where it experiences and impacts the development of preferences.

The fetal sense of touch also seems to function well before birth. There have been experiments performed on this topic, but most moms do a little version of them a lot during the last few months of pregnancy. They often do this when the baby starts to kick and push on the inside of the womb. If you push back from the outside, the fetus will often respond to this with more kicking and pushing. In a sense, this little game is the earliest social interaction that most infants have, and it makes clear that the infants can feel that pressure; that their sense of touch is functioning.

Let's see: taste, smell, touch, and hearing. That's all 4 of the non-visual modalities; they're all working right there in the womb, and certainly when the baby's born. As with studies of adult sensory processing, most of the experiments done with infants have been conducted using visual stimuli, however. This modality, as I've mentioned, dominates our research, and to some extent our primate brains seem to be dominated by vision. With infants, this is a little ironic. Of all of the senses, vision seems to be the last and slowest to develop, given the lack of visual input during that dark stage of prenatal development.

I want to spend a little time here talking about what action abilities infants seem to have when they're born. Ultimately, I want to discuss how action and perception interact in early development; but let's start with the action abilities that are already present at birth.

Shortly after an infant's born, a pediatrician usually visits and tests for the presence of a set of infant reflexes. If an infant's developing normally, then he or she should have all of these reflexes present, even right after they're born. If those reflexes aren't present, it can indicate that there's some problem with the development of the nervous system; some problem that will require treatment. Many of these reflexes are very straightforward. For instance, if an infant feels pressure—even light pressure—on one of her cheeks, she'll tend to turn her head in that direction. This is called the "rooting reflex." If something is placed in her mouth, an infant will reflexively suck on it. Together, these 2 reflexes promote feeding behaviors. If the breast is placed next to the infant's face, the reflexes work to turn the head in the right direction where hopefully contact is made with the mouth and feeding begins.

One filmmaker recorded a fascinating sequence of events with one particular newborn over the course of the first 30 minutes of that baby's life; the first 30 minutes after she was born. After some basic medical checkups to verify that the baby was okay, the newborn was placed on her mother's belly and essentially just left there independently. The baby did what you might imagine after she was placed there—she squirmed around, she flopped her head up and down a bit—but at first glance she didn't seem to be doing much of anything; certainly not going anywhere. Over the course of that half hour, though—those 30 minutes—the baby managed to very slowly pull herself up to the mother's breast and begin to feed. These basic reflexes of the infant seem capable of promoting survival in a very successful way, even very shortly after birth.

Infants are also born with a grasp reflex. If you press an infant's palm, say with your finger, the baby will squeeze her hand closed around it. Many of the muscles in the newborn body are very weak and flexible. For instance, the neck muscles are typically too weak to really even hold the head up for more than a few seconds. The forearm muscles that control that grip, however, are very strong; strong enough to support the infant's weight if you put your fingers in both of her palms and gently lift upward. Pediatricians typically do just that during that initial physical exam to make sure that the grasp reflex is present and functioning normally.

It's thought that this grasp reflex may have been important for promoting the survival of infants in our evolutionary past. Infants are carried around a lot, even now. If the infant can hold on while he or she's being carried around, the likelihood of ever being dropped is reduced; and that's a good thing. Similarly, the rooting and sucking reflex seem to promote the survival and health of the infant.

There are other reflexes, however, which seem to have little or no immediate value to the infant. From a scientific perspective—from a developmental science perspective or a sensory science perspective; from a perspective of wanting to understand where adult perception and action control come from—these non-functional reflexes are, in many ways, the most interesting. For instance, there's an initial reflexive synergy between the position of the arm and the posture of the hand. If you extend the arms of a newborn— if you just pull them away from her body—the hands tend to close. If you place the arms back close to the body with the elbows bent, the hands tend to open again. If you do this repeatedly, it sometimes seems as if there's some direct connection between these 2; almost like there must be some tendon or muscle that causes the hand to close as you pull the arms outward. There isn't a physical connection; there isn't some particular tendon or muscle connection that makes it happen. There's a connection; however, it's in the developing nervous system, in the brain.

When you reach for things, you typically move your arm away from your body and close a hand around the target of your reach as you do. As adults—or even as slightly older children—we're able to control the arm and the hand relatively independently. The foundation of that control, however, doesn't seem to be an independent arm and hand controller. Instead, infants seem to be born with an initial synergy to reach out and close the hand. Our neural control of this action at that level seems to be built from that foundation.

Another hint that this is how our visual and motor systems are organized at birth, with many of our basic motor programs in place, comes from something called the stepping reflex. To demonstrate the stepping reflex, you support an infant in a standing position on a hard, level surface. The feet of the newborn press down on that surface, but only for a few moments. After you do this, the infant will lift one of the legs and move it forward a bit before placing it back on the table surface. At that point, the other leg lifts up and moves forward. Children don't typically walk until they're about 12 months of age. They don't even crawl until about 6 months. Yet, in the 1st day after being born, a full year before they'll need it, babies seem to have the basic motor program to enable them to walk. It may be that many of the basic systems that we use to perceive and act on the world around us are built-in in this fashion, encoded right in our DNA.

Let me tell you about one more of these reflexes; it's a visual motor reflex this time that combines the sense of vision with the motor system that makes actions happen. This particular reflex has been extraordinarily influential in the field of perceptual development research. Up until now, I've talked about very simple reflexes, at least relatively simple reflexes; things like grasping, sucking, moving the legs in a stepping pattern, and things like that. This next one is substantially more complex. It involves vision, it involves complex action control, and it involves some pretty in-depth information about one's own body. The reflex is imitation.

This study that I want to describe to you was conducted in the early 1970s by a researcher named Andrew Meltzoff when he was at Hampshire College. (As a small college alum myself, I'm a big fan of the idea that you don't have to be at some giant research institution to make breakthroughs like this.) Meltzoff had talked with many mothers who described their child, even their very young child, as imitating facial expressions. Almost anyone who's spent time around a baby will have this experience. You smile at the baby and she smiles back; you open your mouth and so does she. Stick your tongue out at the baby, and you'll get a tongue stuck out at you. This is interesting and fun, but is it real? It might be that we're actually imitating the babies. Maybe the baby makes a face, or starts to make a face, and we unconsciously match it. Meltzoff and his colleagues developed a method to test to see if this is how imitation works.

In the key experiment, they recruited pregnant mothers to participate in the study; actually, for their babies to participate. When the mother went into labor, Meltzoff would get a call and head for the hospital. When the baby was born, the doctors and nurses would do those initial checkups to make sure the baby was healthy, and then the parents would get to spend a little time with their new family member. Then the study would take place—not for very long, just for about 3 minutes—after which the baby would be returned to the parents.

Meltzoff recorded 5 30-second video clips of himself engaging in particular actions that babies might imitate. For one of the 30-second video clips on smiling, he repeatedly smiled and returned to a neutral expression, and smiled again, and neutral expression, and so on. In the mouth-opening clip, for 30 seconds he opened and closed his mouth repeatedly. He did a 3rd where he stuck his tongue out and put it back in repeatedly. He frowned for 30 seconds and then went back to a neutral expression. The final clip was actually not of the face but of a hand opening and closing. Meltzoff made this set of video tapes and then randomized the order in which those 5 clips were presented. He had videotapes with 2 ½ minutes of video on them with these 5 30-second clips all scrambled up; different babies, all different orders. For the experiment itself, he placed the newborn close to a video screen where the baby could watch this 2 ½-minute video. While the video was playing and the baby was watching it—or certainly the baby was pointed at it—a video camera recorded the face and hand movements of the infants for later coding.

Meltzoff then brought these video recordings of the babies back to his lab for coding. Research assistants who hadn't been present for the data collection, and who thus couldn't know the order in which those different facial expression clips were presented, took a look at these videos. The task these coders had was very simple: For every 30 seconds of the baby video recordings, guess which one of the video clips the baby had been watching.

The coders got the answer right about 40% of the time. That might not sound very accurate or impressive, but consider the context in which they were made. For one thing, the infants probably weren't actually imitating in every one of these cases. Just because you see a funny face doesn't mean you have to imitate it. Some of the infants might have been drifting off to sleep for all we know; being born can be a very tiring thing. Also, infants probably aren't perfect imitators. Just because they can imitate doesn't mean that they're all ready to be big screen actors. What's important about the 40% accuracy number is that it's twice as big as what you would expect by chance. If the babies weren't imitating at all—for instance, say they couldn't see—then you would expect the coders to still guess the right expression about 20% of the time. The odds of getting 40% correct just by accident, however, is vanishingly small; almost impossible given the number of babies that were used. The study clearly indicates that newborns—kids who are literally just a few minutes old—are capable of imitating facial expressions.

Let's pause for a moment and ponder how impressive that is. Consider what you'd have to build into a baby to get her to be able to accomplish this facial imitation task. First, the baby must be able to see. We know this already, but it's worth highlighting again since it wasn't commonly believed in the early 1970s when this study was run. Second, the babies must be able to control their facial movements in some very systematic fashion. Smiling requires the selective contraction of 19 different muscles in the face. Sticking out the tongue requires even more complex contractions and relaxations of very specific muscles in your face and neck. These are newborns; they haven't had time to practice these things. It must somehow be programmed into their nervous system from the beginning. Third, the infants must know something about faces. They must be drawn to look at them; we've talked already about how they have this particular preference.

The last part, though—the last thing they're going to need to be able to do this imitation—is the most impressive; it's hard to fathom, really. These newborns must be able to draw a connection between the face that they're seeing and their own face. These infants, even at a few minutes of age, had actually already seen a few faces; they'd seen their parents' faces, they'd seen the faces of the doctors and nurses (although the bottom parts of those faces were typically covered with surgical masks). That said, the babies had only seen that very small number of faces for a very brief period of time. More importantly, however, the infants had never seen their own face; never, not for a second. There certainly wasn't time for the baby to practice in the mirror here; to learn associations between certain patterns of muscle contractions and certain resulting facial expressions. None of that. Imitation just has to be built in to the nervous system. There's no other way for this experiment to have worked.

We don't know what the experience of this study is like for the infants. We know that they imitate and that this means they must have some impressive visual motor systems in place when they're born, and presumably they have these systems in the womb for at least a little time before they're born. We don't know, for instance, if the infants know that they're imitating. We don't even know if the infants realize that they have a face, let alone how to control it. The infants might not be aware of what they're doing, but the imitation is an inherently complex system with visual components, motor components, and some even more impressive systems for putting those 2 things together. If something this complex can be built in, then it might be that there are other things this complex, or maybe even more so, and that these things might be there, too, even as early as the day that the baby's born.

How about depth perception? Do infants come into the world perceiving depth like adults do? The answer here is that infants seem to use some depth cues—some very much like adults—from a very early age; but for others, they don't seem to master them until they're about 7 months of age.

The technique that's been most useful in this area is based on reaching. At about 4 months of age, children start to reach out and grab things. Almost right away, they have a preference to reach for the part of an object, or the object, that's closest to them. If there's a rectangular object, for instance, that's presented at a slightly tilted orientation such that one side is closer than the other, the infants will tend to aim most of their reaches toward that closer side.

This is interesting by itself, but it provides a great tool for exploring early depth perception. What depth cues can tell an infant which side is closer, and what cues can't? Stereopsis seems to come online very early; earlier even than this reaching method can assess it, so certainly it's there at 4 months. If you let an infant look at almost any nearby display with 2 eyes, they'll perceive the closer side in a very adult-like fashion. For those pictorial cues to depth, however, infants aren't nearly as good. If you put a patch over one eye so that they don't have stereopsis or any of other binocular cues that we've discussed, there are still a lot of ways to indicate that one side of an object is closer than the other. For instance, if you use linear perspective or relative size; if you're using relative size, then the side of a rectangle that's closer will project a larger retinal image size than the one that's further away.

Five-month-olds, even most 6-month-olds, don't seem to care about this at all; at least they don't see to use this information to guide their reaches. At 7 months, something seems to shift in terms of infant perception such that they make use of a very wide range of those pictorial cues; relative size, familiar size, linear perspective, even things like texture density. Remember, texture density is that cue you see when you look at a repeating texture like a brick walkway as it recedes into the distance. The farther away some part of that walkway is, the smaller and more dense those texture elements become, at least at the level of a retinal projection. A 7-month-old infant seems to use that information when they reach for part of a display, figuring out which one of the 2 sides of the display is closer.

As with adults, there's some fascinating evidence that perception and action control are coordinated in complex ways. My favorite example of this is from another set of studies on what's called the visual cliff. In these studies, infants are placed on one side of a table surface on which a clear checkerboard pattern is present. On the other half of the table, there's a drop off of several feet. If one were to crawl over this edge, you'd expect to fall. I should note that in almost every study of this, there's an invisible, very sturdy sheet of glass placed over that drop-off for safety. If the infant does decide to crawl over the edge, she won't actually fall. Also, it should be said that the glass is carefully lit from the bottom and not at all from the top to make sure that it's invisible; that is, the infant won't look at the glass and see her reflection looking back.

Do infants know about depth as it relates to these visually specified cliffs? When they first start to crawl, right around 6 months of age, the answer is no. These procedures usually involve someone standing on the far side of that cliff on the other side of that sheet of glass, beyond where that apparent drop off is. This person, usually the mom, holds some attractive toy and calls to the baby; she asks the child to crawl over toward her. At 6 months, when the baby is a novice crawler, she'll happily do just that, usually without much hesitation; she'll simply crawl off what appears to be a cliff. Fast forward a few weeks, however, after the infant has a little more crawling experience. With that experience under her belt (or under her dipey, I suppose) the baby will now steadfastly refuse to crawl over that cliff. She might reach over and touch the surface that's there, but she won't try to crawl off the edge where there's an apparent drop off. No matter how much the mother implores her to come across, the baby will just sit on that shallow side of the cliff. The baby has, presumably through experience, learned the relation between a visual cliff and crawling over it. Specifically, it seems that the infant doesn't want to fall down.

The really fascinating thing about this study happens a few months later when the baby starts to walk. She'll stand up, usually with the support of nearby things at first, and start to move around on 2 feet. A novice walker in essentially every case is very experienced at getting around in the world, not on 2 feet but on the hands and knees as a crawler. Nonetheless, if you place the novice walker in this visual cliff study, a really strange thing happens: She won't crawl off the edge, but she'll walk right over. It's as if, given this new action situation—this standing and walking—the baby has to start over in terms of learning about the surrounding world. It's really surprising that babies don't generalize the knowledge that they gathered when crawling to walking. We talk about different modules of the brain—different parts of the visual system—as seeming to look at the world very separately from one another. It makes sense in some situations to say that you only have one conscious experience of the world, but for different parts of perception you look at the world with several very different, somewhat separate, visual systems.

With this type of action and perception study, we have an analogous story to tell. It's as if the baby stands up, and even though she's been looking at and interacting with the world for a full year, it's as if she's seeing it for the first time. She starts from scratch to learn the demands and characteristics of this new way of getting around.

In this lecture, we've considered infant sensory development in more detail. We've seen that all 5 senses are functioning at the time a baby's born and to some extent even sooner. We've also seen that these senses are, right from the beginning, linked to memory and to the action systems that enable infants to interact with and move around the world. All of these things are true in adulthood, but it seems that the connections are specified even at the beginning of development.

In these 2 lectures on perceptual development, I've talked about all of the amazing things that seem to be built in from the beginning of life outside the womb. In other lectures, I'll consider what I'll call perceptual learning, which is in many ways the opposite of this. I'll discuss how the sensory systems learn to sense new things, how they learn to use new sources of information, and learn to process that information in new ways.

In the next lecture, however, we're going to have some fun. Let's talk about illusions and magic. I hope to see you then.

# Illusions and Magic
## Lecture 18

S tudying illusions can be fun, but it can also be educational. By looking at illusions and applying your knowledge about how the senses function, you can better understand not just what you are seeing but why you see it. In fact, some researchers have built their entire careers around this pursuit.

- Often the visual system takes in sensations and makes inferences about the state of the surrounding environment that go beyond those sensations. This characteristic is present in many of the perception experiments we have discussed in the course.

- In many ways, creating a good visual illusion is like running a small-scale experiment with exactly one participant: the artist. The next step is to show that display to others to see if they see it in the same way.

- The illusions can point us to principles of human sensation and perception, but the opposite often happens as well. If we have a good understanding of sensory processing, that can provide clues about how to make a great illusion.

- One of the most famous illusions, the Kanizsa triangle, was created by Italian researcher and artist Gaetano Kanizsa. Most people describe it as a white triangle in front of 3 disks with another triangle outline located behind it.

- In fact, it is composed of 3 incomplete circles and 3 V-shapes—no white triangle, no outline, no background. Our visual system likes to parse visual input into as few simple parts as possible, so it sees 5 regular pieces instead of 6 somewhat irregular ones.

- Perception scientists refer to this desire for simplicity as *Prägnanz*, German for "pithiness." It is one of a large number of principles that seem to be applied as we parse continuous visual input into discrete, separate objects.

- Continuation is another of those principles, also present in the Kanizsa triangle. If 2 clear, high-contrast edges are separate but aligned, the visual system assumes they are 2 parts of the same object with the middle occluded.

- With the Kanizsa triangle, you group pieces of the image together based not on their actual connection but on your perceptual knowledge of how things tend to group together in the world.

- The background of the image—the white space onto which the black figure parts are applied—is exactly the same color outside the figure as in its center, but most people do not see it that way. So powerful is our inference about the composition of this figure that it feeds down to the areas of visual cortex that encode brightness.

- Evidence indicates that the same parts of your brain that respond to real edges respond to these illusory edges as well.

- We have discussed how energy and information from the world flow in through the senses via transduction and how patterns of neural impulses are processed through the sensory systems, where more and more complex perceptions result. This is called bottom-up processing.

- Your response to the Kanizsa triangle, however, is an example of top-down processing, where higher-level perceptual inferences influence how you process incoming sensory information.

- There are many examples of top-down processing with the other senses as well. If you hear the sentence, "On election day we go to the polls and … " the word "vote" is very likely to be the last word in that sentence, and your auditory system responds as if it is there. This is called the phonemic restoration effect.

- In the café wall illusion, a black-and-white rectangle pattern was installed on the front wall of a café in Bristol, England. A pair of researchers noticed that the tiles did not look horizontally level.

- Instead of being a checkerboard, the squares were misaligned by half a step. The rows thus appeared to be alternating wedges when they were actually straight lines.

- Why do we see this illusion? Imagine for a moment that you are looking at a horizontal brightness edge in some image—black below and white above. An equal amount of brightness is present on the left and right.

- Tilt the edge a little clockwise, and now there is more brightness on the right than on the left. At the level of the simple receptors within your retina and lateral geniculate nucleus, this is how tilt is determined: based on the distribution of brightness.

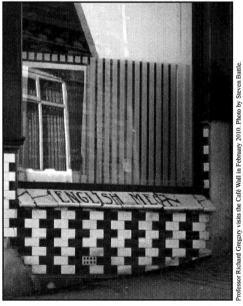

- On the café wall, in some areas there is more white on one side and more black on the other.

**The café in Bristol, England, where the café wall illusion was first noticed.**

When the visual cortex receives that input, it concludes that there is probably a tilted edge there causing the bias in left-versus-right-side brightness. Thus you perceive tilt.

- One of my favorite motion illusions shows what you might see from the perspective of someone driving a motorcycle down a long, straight road. The trees speed past—or do they? In fact, the movie is a loop of 3 still images: 2 of a country drive and 1 of a plain gray background.

- Usually, when something in the environment changes, it moves and calls your attention to it. During the shift from the second photo to the blank image, everything changes. When the movie shifts from the blank image back to the first photo, everything changes again.

- Even though the blank lasts only a few hundred milliseconds, that is plenty of time for your visual system to forget what was seen in the very recent past. The result is a perception that every image is different.

- A related effect is motion-induced blindness. This illusion is generated by 4 colored dots: A green flashing dot in the center and 3 yellow dots a short distance away. They are rendered on a grid of blue plus shapes that can be rotated around the viewing screen.

- As the grid of blue plus symbols begins to rotate, subjects fix their attention on the flashing green dot. Then something strange happens: The yellow dots seem to vanish. Usually when this happens, especially the first time, people feel an irresistible urge to look at where one of those yellow dots was located.

- When the subject looks, the yellow dot comes back. When the subject looks back at the green dot, the yellow dot disappears again. In fact, any saccadic eye movement makes the yellow dots reappear.

- The explanation is directly related to the motorcycle motion illusion. Here, the motion of the blue plus symbols is wiping out your perception of something that is actually in the stimulus. Your visual system's best guess is that they have moved in front of the yellow dots.

- In the domain of depth perception, motion-based cues are dominant. For example, magic tricks are, in essence, behavioral illusions. Many of the best involve well-practiced sleight of hand. The key is diversion of the audience's attention at the proper moment.

- If you interact with a street magician, you will notice that they never stop talking—asking you where you are from, what you are doing here in town, what your favorite color is, and so on. The magician probably does not care about your answers. He or she just wants you to use your finite attention resources elsewhere.

- This is also the reason that magicians typically refuse to do a trick more than once. The first time you watch an event, you are much easier to manipulate than the second time, especially if you are looking around for the cause of the trick on that second run through.

- The famous magician Harry Blackstone tells the story of one of his favorite tricks—making a goat appear out of thin air right in the middle of the stage. The effect was striking and entertaining, but the thing he liked best about it was how amazingly simple it was.

- Harry Blackstone would always wear a black tuxedo with a big black cape over it. As he was getting ready to walk on stage, he would pick his goat up under one arm and drape the cape over it. He would carry a white handkerchief in the other hand and wave it dramatically.

- When he arrived at center stage, he made a dramatic flourish and then just put the goat down on the stage. People would "ooh" and "ahh" at this every time. All Blackstone needed to do was keep their attention away from his arm (and the goat), and magic ensued.

- Staring at a color image builds up a retinotopic map in color-responsive cells. If you do so with a negative of a normal-color image, you can use the color adaptation aftereffect to produce the normal image on a blank white page or wall.

- Note that these small tugs-of-war are taking place at every location on your retina, not just in the visual cortex as a whole.

- Another illusion you are likely to have encountered is the portrait whose eyes seem to follow you. One variation is the paper dragon illusion. The dragon seems to follow you with its eyes and even its head.

- The key to this illusion is a misperception of the 3-dimensional structure of the paper dragon display, much like with the Ames room. We presume that the nose of the dragon is closer to us than the body; that is, we assume this is a convex object.

- In fact, the opposite is true: The paper dragon display is, in essence, inside out; it is convex. The closest thing to us is the thing that seems farthest away and vice versa.

- As you shift your point of view, your visual system is constantly trying to derive its structure and determine its shape given the pattern of motion that is present on your retina, but the motion information conflicts with the perception of the static form of the dragon. Ergo, your brain believes the dragon is moving.

## Suggested Reading

Macknik, Martinez-Conde, and Blakeslee, *Sleights of Mind*.

Seckel, *Optical Illusions*.

1. Illusions are fascinating, but our senses give us good information about the world around us most of the time. If we pursue an understanding of how the visual system functions by studying illusions, how might our theories of the senses be affected?

2. Most magicians make a point of never performing the same trick more than once for a particular audience. Given your understanding of how magicians work their magic on the human sensory systems, why do you suppose that is so?

# Illusions and Magic
## Lecture 18—Transcript

Hello, and welcome to Lecture 18 of the course. In this lecture, we'll be looking at some of my favorite visual illusions. This should be fun, but my hope is that it will be educational as well. By exploring why we see certain illusions, we'll be able to reinforce and further develop things that you've already learned in this course about the senses. You know a lot about human sensation, perception, and action at this point; 17 lectures worth, at least! By looking at the illusions and then applying this knowledge that you have about how the senses function, we can understand not just what you see, but why you see it.

There's a long and impressive history of exploring the human senses by creating illusions like the ones we'll look at. Some researchers have built their entire careers around this pursuit. The basic workflow involves creating some image, looking at it, and then pondering what that means. Every once in a while, someone engaged in this task finds something that looks strange; really strange; a little off from what was physically created. When this happens, when the perception doesn't seem to match the image that was created, something's happening that should be familiar to you. The sensations consist of the lines and colors of an image. Often our visual system takes in sensations and based on them makes inferences about the state of the surrounding environment that go beyond those sensations. Our inherently inferential perception is what results.

This characteristic is present in many of the perception experiments that we've discussed in the course. It's also true for these illusions. In many ways, creating a good visual illusion is like running a small-scale experiment with exactly one participant: the artist. Of course, the next step—it's very important from a scientific perspective—is to show that display to others to see if they see it in the same way. For good practitioners of this scientific art, that almost always turns out to be true.

I should also say that these illusion artists are not blindly, randomly drawing pictures and making images in their search for these illusions. Often the very theories of sensation and perception that we've been discussing here are the things that lead to those illusion displays. The illusions can point us to principles of human sensation and perception, but the opposite often happens as well. If we have a good understanding of our sensory processing, then that can provide clues about how to make something that looks pretty cool.

One of the most famous illusions out there is the Kanizsa triangle, created by the Italian researcher and artist Gaetano Kanizsa. Most people describe it as a white triangle in front of 3 disks with another triangle outline located behind it. It's important to note that this is not what's present in that figure. There are 3 Pac-man shapes; round, but with an angular indent in each one of them. Similarly, there's no outline triangle in the background; in fact, there's no background. This is a fully 2-dimensional printed image. There are 3 "V" shapes that are oriented and placed at 3 different places in the image.

Our visual system seems to like to parse our visual input into as few simple parts as possible. This could be—in fact, is—3 Pac-man shapes and 3 "V" shapes; that's 6 unusual shapes to keep track of. It could also be a front and back triangle with black discs at the vertices of the front triangle. That parsing of the image involves fewer pieces—5 pieces instead of 6—and all of those component shapes are simpler and regular. Perception scientists refer to this inherent desire that our senses seem to have for simplicity and regularity as Pragnanz, after the German word for "pithiness." It's one of a large number of principles that seem to be applied as we parse our continuous visual input—the continuous pattern of light that projects onto our retina—into discrete, separate objects.

Actually, another one of those principles is present in this image as well: good continuation. If 2 clear, high-contrast edges are separate but aligned with one another—as they are, say, with this ruler—then they're likely to be produced by 2 parts of the same object, with the middle of that object occluded by something else. If I hold this in my closed hands, you can see the 2 ends of it and you see that those edges align. It could be that there's one object back here, or it could be that I have 2 separate, accidentally aligned parts of an object, or 2 separate, aligned objects. Maybe they're just accidentally aligned. But it's more likely that these well-aligned edges are part of a single object. Your visual system knows this, and it perceives the display as such.

With the Kanizsa triangle, you group pieces of that image together, based not on their actual connection, but based on your perceptual knowledge of how things tend to group together in the world. This is a powerful process of perceptual grouping; so powerful that it creates the most striking feature of this Kanizsa display: illusory contours.

The background of the image—the white space onto which the black figure parts are applied—is exactly the same color outside the figure as in its center, but most people don't see it that way. The central, inferred triangle seems to be a brighter shade of white. The borders of this interior illusory triangle are visually apparent. You can see the edges in between the Pac men shapes, along the border of the "V" shapes. There's no contour here. If you use your hands to block the view of the black figure parts around one of these edges, you'll clearly see the edge vanish. The contours are really illusory contours. So powerful is our inference about the composition of this figure that it feeds down to the areas of visual cortex that encode brightness. There's actually evidence that the same parts of your brain that respond to real edges respond to these illusory edges as well.

There's another idea stimulated by this work with these illusions. We've primarily discussed how energy and information from the world flows in through the senses via transduction and then how the patterns of neural impulses are processed up through the sensory systems, where more and more complex perceptions result. This is called bottom-up processing. There is, however, another type of information flow—and corresponding neural connections to go with it—called top-down processing. In some cases, your higher-level perceptual inferences influence how you process incoming sensory information. In this situation, your expectation that there's an edge located at one particular part of a Kanizsa triangle figure impacts the receptors that encode real images.

There are many examples of this top-down processing with the other senses as well. If you hear the sentence, "On election day we go to the polls and vote," The word "vote" is very likely to be the last word in that sentence. If I were to edit it out of a recording of someone speaking the sentence, your auditory system would still respond just a bit as if the word "vote" was present. If I recorded a cough sound to cover that gap in the recording where the word "vote" had been located, you probably wouldn't notice that the word was missing at all. "On election day we go to the polls and [cough]." This is a top-down process, what we call the phonemic restoration effect.

Let's look at another illusion, this time the café wall illusion. I've also put an image of this one in the guidebook so you can follow along and try it with some friends. A black and white rectangle pattern was installed on the front wall of a café in Bristol, England, near the lab of 2 researchers who were the first to report this illusion, actually. As these researchers looked at the newly installed wall of the café, it looked off; it just didn't look level. It looked as if the masons who'd installed that wall had mismeasured things horribly. The pattern on the café wall didn't consist of a perfectly aligned checkerboard; the black and white squares were misaligned by a half step. Every other row of tiles was shifted a few inches to the left relative to the other rows. If we shift every other row of the bricks over by just a little, the horizontal lines of the café's bricks suddenly change. They no longer look level, but instead appear to be tilted. The rows appear to be alternating wedge shapes, every other one oriented with the narrow end to the left and to the right. They're not tilted, of course, not in reality; the horizontal lines are still perfectly horizontal, but an illusion of tilt is created.

In a sense, this reminds me of that motion aftereffect illusion that we discussed. In that case, there was perceived motion, but nothing was moving anywhere; nothing seemed to be getting anywhere. There was a strange sense of seeing things both moving and yet stationary at the same time. With the café wall illusion, something analogous results. The rows of bricks seem to form into these tilted wedge patterns, yet if you look closely at any individual part of any particular edge, it doesn't seem tilted. Somehow an overall impression of tilt is created by a set of lines that are, individually, perfectly level.

Why do we see this illusion? There's a very complex, technical explanation for this that's grounded in the particular response properties of cells in the lateral geniculate nucleus and the primary visual cortex, but let me try to give you a more straightforward, general explanation. Imagine for a moment that you're looking at a horizontal brightness edge in some image, for which there's black on the bottom and white on the top. As you perceive this, there's an equal amount of this brightness—the brightness that's present in the image—on the left and right sides. If you were to tilt this edge a little bit clockwise such that the top, white part of the image moves to the right, now there will be more brightness on the right side than on the left. Alternatively, if I tilt the other way, now the top, white part of the image will shift over to the other side, and the bottom, black part of the image will shift in the opposite direction.

This is what would happen with a real tilt of a black and white region boundary. The brightness distribution would shift. At the level of the simple receptors within your retina and lateral geniculate nucleus as well, this is how they determine tilt: based on the distribution of lightness.

In the café wall, there are parts of the image in which there's more white on one side and more black on the other. When the visual cortex looks at that pattern of sensory response, especially as it's present throughout a whole row of the retinal input, it concludes that there's probably a tilted edge present there, and that this tilted edge is causing the bias in encoded left-versus-right-side brightness. Since this is the most likely cause of the sensory response pattern, it's what you perceive. Voilà! The café wall illusion. I like to highlight this particular illusion because it's one that wasn't intentionally created at all. Someone who was interested in the senses and knew a little about them just went out for a cup of coffee. As she looked around and thought about her perceptions of the surrounding environment, she happened to look at this particular wall. Now, based on dozens of studies on related displays, we've learned a lot about visual processing and visual processing in general, not just about café walls.

Let's talk about one of my favorite motion illusions. A video of this illusion shows what you might see from the perspective of someone driving a motorcycle down a long, straight road. The trees speed past as the cycle speeds through the countryside; or do they? If one looks closely in this video—at particular trees in the moving image, for instance—you'll notice something strange. The motorcycle isn't getting anywhere. This movie only has 3 images in it, and those 3 images are shown over and over and over again, but somehow they result in a perception of continuous forward motion. What's going on here?

The first 2 images in the illusion display are what you might see in an actual movie of driving through the countryside. There's one image taken from one location, and then another image, taken a few moments later from a position that's slightly ahead of where the 1st one was. This is what you see when you move forward in general. The key trick is that 3rd image in this movie, which contains only a plain, gray background. You probably notice it flashing past and flickering in the movie. After it appears for a few hundred milliseconds, the first image is shown again and the cycle repeats. The resulting perception is not of a repeating pair of photos, but that's all that's there in that stimulus.

In Lecture 14, on attention and perception, I talked about how we don't actually perceive as many details about the world as we think we do. When we're faced with a new stimulus—say, when we walk into a room—we look around and form a mental representation of what's around us. We move that high resolution fovea that we have around the room to pick up information about the fine details and colors of nearby objects and surfaces. Once we have that information, our visual system makes a big assumption: Unless we see something move, we can assume that it's the same as when it was when looked at just a few moments ago.

Our peripheral vision is very good at detecting that motion, and things don't typically change without making some sort of movement as they do so. In most real-world situations, this assumption works. That is, it doesn't lead us to inaccurate perceptions. Why doesn't it work with this 2-image movie?

With this illusion, with that blank, grey image, this process is disrupted. Usually, when something in the environment changes, it moves and calls your attention to it. During the shift from the photo—the 2nd photo in the movie—to the blank image, everything changes. Then, when the movie shifts from the blank image back to the first photo, everything changes again. In essence, this blocks your usual method for tracking what's changed and what's the same.

Even though the blank gray image flashes for only a few hundred milliseconds, it's plenty of time for your visual system to forget what it's seen before in the very recent past. The result is a perception that every one of those image is different. Only when your attention is called to this fact does the real composition of the movie become apparent.

A related effect is something called motion-induced blindness. This illusion is generated by a display containing 4 colored dots: A green, flashing dot in the center and 3 yellow dots located a short distance away from that green dot. A large grid of blue plus shapes fills most of the display. This grid of these plus-shapes extends beyond the locations of the yellow dots, but it's rendered on the screen as being behind those dots; that is, the light from the yellow, peripheral dots always projects onto your retina, no matter where the grid of plus shapes is located.

The illusion is generated as this display begins to move; specifically as the grid of the blue plus symbols begins to rotate, with the center of the display as its pivot point for that rotation. To view this display, one just keeps the eyes centered on the flashing green fixation dot in the middle of the display. If you keep your eyes still and stare, without blinking, at that green dot, a strange thing will happen after a few seconds: the yellow dots will vanish.

Usually when this happens, especially the first time, people feel an irresistible urge to look at where one of those yellow dots was located. That's okay; you would note that the dot comes back. In fact, all 3 of the dots come back. If you return to staring at the center of the image again, however, the dots will vanish again. They're still there, of course. In fact, you can make them come back very easily just by blinking your eyes or even by moving your eyes a little bit from side to side; making one of those saccadic jumps. If you do any of these things, all of the dots will reappear.

This illusion is so very salient. The yellow dots are completely bright and fully visible all the time. It's hard to imagine that such a bright, clear stimulus could still be projecting onto your retina and yet somehow not be registered as part of your conscious perception. What's going on here? The explanation for this one is very directly related to the story for the motorcycle motion illusion that we talked about a few minutes ago. In that case, that periodic plain gray flash wiped out the motion signals that would be used to link the $2^{nd}$ image in the sequence back to the $1^{st}$ image in the proper way.

Here, the motion—in this particular case, with the induced blindness—is wiping out your perception of something that's actually in the stimulus. The yellow dots are still there; they're still present in the activity of your retinal receptors, as a matter of fact. The motion signals override it, however. Since this big rotating surface, specified by the blue grid, has moved in front of the yellow dots, then they should be blocked by something; and so the visual system's best guess is that you shouldn't be able to see the yellow dots anymore. Voilà: motion induced blindness for the dots.

We've talked a lot about motion as our visual system's preferred source of information. In the domain of depth perception, motion based cues are very dominant. In one of our examples, we saw that Ames room illusion. As salient as that Ames room was, it essentially disappeared if there was even a little bit of relative motion. In terms of our perception and attention, motion's even more powerful. Let's consider a case with a nickel.

Here we have a plain old nickel; it's a regular Jefferson nickel (the most famous alum of the College of William and Mary). Nickels are great—there's nothing wrong with this one—but it would be better if it were a quarter. Given a choice between a nickel and a quarter, most people would choose the quarter, right? With a quick toss in the air, we can make this nickel turn into a quarter. Ready? Ta-da; it turned into a quarter.

Okay, so this demonstration isn't about decision making; I just said that as a cover to distract you for a moment. It's about attention and motion induced blindness. All of magic is, in essence, one big behavioral illusion.

I'm certainly not an expert magician. Many of the really good magic tricks involve well-practiced, very expert sleight of hand. This trick usually works, though, and the beauty of it is that it really isn't much of a magic trick. Of course, the coin didn't change; I have 2 coins here. I held up the nickel so you could see it and tucked the quarter down behind it in my palm. When I threw the coin in the air, it was the quarter I threw and not the nickel that I'd shown you first. As your eyes followed that quarter up in the air, I simply placed the nickel in my other hand, caught the quarter, and voilà! Magic trick. The fact that an audience usually won't see me switching a nickel and a quarter in my hands right in front of them is a real testament to the fact that motion—and the attention capture that goes with it—can blind you to some very large and salient things.

Okay, so I had 2 coins. How did I switch the nickel I was holding to the quarter without it being seen? The key is the diversion of your attention that occurs when I threw the coin up in the air. We just can't resist following it with our eyes, and more importantly following it with our attention. When your attention is focused up in the air on the coin, I can do almost anything down below here without you realizing it.

There's also a bit of an apparent motion effect here. One coin vanished from your view and another appeared at about the same time. It's a natural thing for your visual system to try to connect these 2 events with a motion event, even one that you can't see, with the nickel turning into a quarter. The trick wouldn't have worked nearly as well, for instance, if I tried to change a nickel into a banana.

Most magic tricks work just like this. Your attention is directed away from the place where the method (as magicians would call it) is applied, often by using several techniques at once. If you ever interact with a street magician, for instance, you'll notice that they never stop talking; they never stop asking you where you're from, what you're doing here in town, what your favorite color is, and so on. The magician doesn't really care about your answers— probably not, anyway—it's just that every time you devote some of those finite attention resources to answering one of those questions, you have less attention resource available to notice the real actions behind whatever the trick is. This is also the reason that magicians typically refuse to do a trick more than once. The 1st time you watch an event, you're much easier to manipulate than the 2nd time, especially if you're looking around for the cause of the trick on that 2nd run through.

My coin trick isn't all that spectacular—I'm Professor Vishton, not The Great Visht-one—but this attention manipulation is at the heart of even the most impressive tricks. The famous magician Harry Blackstone tells the story of one of his favorite tricks; it was, in fact, the one he used for many years to start his shows. He could make a goat appear out of thin air right in the middle of the stage. The effect was striking and very entertaining, but the thing he liked best about it was how amazingly simple it was.

Harry Blackstone would always wear a black tuxedo with a big black cape on it. As he was getting ready to walk out on the stage, he would pick his goat up under one of his arms and drape the cape over it. He would take out a white handkerchief for the other hand. He would be introduced by the announcer and then walk out on stage, dramatically waving that white cloth. It's a very eye-catching thing to have this white handkerchief waving around. When he arrived at the center of the stage, he would make a dramatic flourish of some kind and then just put the goat down on the stage. People would "ooh" and "ahh" at this every time. All Blackstone needed to do was keep their attention away from his arm (and the goat) and magic ensued. Magic and illusion based on the inferences made all the time by your sensory systems.

Let's consider an illusion of color, in this case a color adaptation is the thing I want to look at; a color adaptation aftereffect. Stare at this lovely castle image. I'm going to continue speaking, but you should try to keep your eyes as still as possible, fixated on the middle of this image, until I tell you to move them. It's important that as you keep your eyes looking at this that you keep them as stationary as possible, since the adaptation that you're doing is to a retinotopic map of color responsive cells.

We've already discussed one of these color after-effect demonstrations; that was with an American flag that was green, black, and yellow, making the afterimage appear to be red, white, and blue. I also talked about the fact that most colors are perceived as a combination of the inputs received from different color sensitive cells. Given that this is the case, we can adapt your eyes to any color, not just the basic red-green and blue-yellow colors alone.

If you're staring at this image, you may notice that it's a negative of a normal image. Every color in the image is, in a sense, the opposite of the color present in the normal image. Your individual color receptive cells are being adapted. The more green the image is in some location, the more the green receptors in that location are growing fatigued and the more rested the red receptors are becoming. The same is happening for the blue and yellow receptors. Note that these small tug-of-war contests are taking place at every location on your retina, not just in the visual cortex as a whole.

In a moment, you'll notice that the image switches back to its regular coloring; not the negative, but the regular positive colors. That should happen right about now. The regular colors have returned; or have they? If you blink your eyes and move them around a bit—go ahead and do that now—you'll notice that the image is just black and white. The color aftereffect that you've seen has been overlayed onto this black and white image, allowing you to see it not just in color, but in rich, detailed, saturated color tones.

Time is short, but I want to discuss one more quick illusion that you're likely to have encountered in a museum or even in your own home. The illusion is that of a painting with eyes that move to follow you.

This particular example is often called the paper dragon illusion, because you can build one of these yourself out of paper. Instructions can be found online in many places; just use Google or another search engine to look for the key words "paper dragon illusion" and you'll find several. From many different angles, the dragon figure seems to follow you with its eyes and even its head. It seems to be moving. I assure you that it isn't. Any motion that you see in this example is completely illusory.

The key to this illusion is a misperception of the 3D structure of the paper dragon display, sort of like with the Ames room. Based on the shading and the shape of most objects like this, we presume that the nose of the dragon is closer to us than the body; that is, we assume this is a convex object. In fact, the opposite is true: The paper dragon display is, in essence, inside out; it's convex. The closest thing to us is the thing that seems farthest away, and vice versa. As you shift your point of view on the dragon, your visual system is constantly trying to derive that structure from motion relation to determine its shape given the pattern of motion that's present on your retina. The motion information, however, conflicts with the perception of the static form of the dragon. If the dragon is concave in shape—it's not, but if it was—then there's only one way that this pattern of projected images could result: the dragon must be moving. Your visual system reaches this estimate, its best guess of what must be out there, and so that's what you perceive; you perceive the dragon as moving.

A similar effect can happen with many salient pictures of human faces. If the eyes on some painting appear to be fixated on you, then this is what you'll see. If you walk across the room and they still seem to be fixated on you, then there's only one conclusion that can be reached: the eyes are moving.

In this lecture, we've discussed some fun illusions. They look strange, but based on our knowledge of how the human senses work, it's possible to explain why they look the way they do. Illusions can tell us about the nature of human perception, but in most cases they need to be carefully constructed in order to have these surprising effects. Fortunately, under almost all natural, typical circumstances, our visual system delivers accurate and reliable information to us. These illusions don't have so often in the real world just by accident.

In order to rapidly process a tremendous amount of information out there, your visual system—your sensory systems in general—needs to make inferential leaps. What you perceive at any given moment in time is the brain's best guess as to what's going on out there in the world; the thing that's most likely to have produced the sensory inputs that you're currently receiving.

Illusions happen in situations where that guess is inaccurate. As surprising as some of these illusions are, the thing that's really most surprising is just how rarely these inaccurate conclusions are reached. Perception is inferential; we can see that easily here. But that doesn't make perception any less amazing.

In the next lecture, we'll consider the role that emotion plays in human sensation and perception. Humans are very good at picking up on subtle information that tells us about the emotional states of others; and our own emotional state can greatly affect the nature of our own perception of the world around us. I look forward to telling you about it later.

# Perceiving Emotion in Others and Ourselves
## Lecture 19

O nce, on a bus, I sat across from a man wearing a "Life is Good" t-shirt that—in my opinion—showed a stick-figure man running with his stick-figure dog. Next to me on that same bus was a woman in a foul mood. She looked at that same man in that same t-shirt and muttered, "Why would a shirt with a man being chased by a dog say 'Life is Good'?" The funny thing is, both of our perceptions were valid. Where I saw a panting dog, she saw a snarling one. Our perceptions were very much a function of our different emotional states.

- Perception and emotion go hand in hand almost all the time. There are at least 2 main ways in which sensory processing and emotion can interact.

- The first has to do with how we perceive the emotions of others. Humans are remarkably fast and accurate at this, based on a wide range of auditory and visual information. Often, we are unaware that we are perceiving others' emotions.

- Our own internal emotional state also impacts how we perceive the things around us. If I'm sad, happy, or terrified, then the exact same sensory input might be perceived in 3 very different ways.

- Let's start with some very basic measures of visual sensory function. Experimenters placed 4 sets of low-contrast (gray-on-gray) stripes near the corners of a computer screen. Three of the striped patterns were oriented in 1 direction—for instance, vertically—and the fourth in a different direction—say, horizontal.

- The task of the participants was to identify which 1 of these 4 patches was the oddball after a 40-millisecond glimpse of them.

- Prior to showing these patches, participants were presented with a tiny, 50-millisecond cue image of a human face. Some faces had neutral expressions, some fearful.

- Seeing someone in fear sends an important message to us: If that person is afraid, perhaps I should be afraid, too. This is not a conscious decision. Fear is contagious.

- With certain biologically stimuli—not all, but some, like snakes— it is even possible to develop a phobia without ever directly interacting with them.

- The fear faces in this experiment seem to have an impact on a participant's sensory processing. If the participant is cued with brief exposure to a fear face, he or she is more likely to detect the low-contrast stripes and to find the oddball, with faster and more accurate responses.

- The cue works even better if it is placed in same location as the oddball set of stripes. This suggests that the alteration of our sensory processing may be location specific, maybe even retinotopic, in its organization.

- This is a very artificial type of experiment, one an ecological psychologist would not care for, but it is strong evidence that emotion stimuli impact our sensory processing in a basic way.

- There are only 2 synapses between the olfactory sensors in the nose and the amygdala, the brain area largely responsible for emotional processing. There are only 3 synapses between the olfactory receptors and the hippocampus, which makes and recalls memories. Olfaction, memories, and emotion therefore seem closely connected, without much space or time for complex processing of incoming stimuli.

- Recall that transduction occurs in the olfactory system when particular chemicals with particular shapes fit into particular receptors—350 different receptors, such that any given combination of activations may be very rare.

- If you experience a specific aroma in a particular place, you may not experience that same aroma again for years, maybe ever. If certain events and emotions are experienced in the context of a novel aroma, you may file them away using that aroma as the index.

- A variety of research has looked at the facial expressions that go with certain emotions. Facial expressions associated with fear have been the topic of many studies, in part because they seem to be relatively universal.

- The idea of a universal fearful expression as a warning to others is quite sensible from an evolutionary standpoint. Some recent research has suggested that the fear face has important functional consequences for perception.

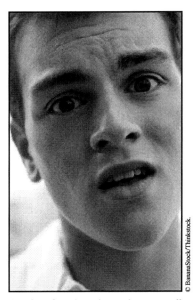

- In a fear face, you open your eyes wide, improving peripheral vision. Grimacing and flaring your nostrils increase your oxygen intake, and the latter makes you more sensitive to nearby aromas. In essence, the fear face seems to ramp up the sensitivity of your sensory systems.

**The fear face is universal among all human beings.**

- The facial expression that goes with disgust seems to work in the opposite way. Scrunching up your face closes your mouth and reduces the openings of the nostrils and eyes. This serves to reduce your exposure to the disgusting stimulus.

- Emotion also influences your perception of time and space. "Time flies when you're having fun" is a cliché, but it is also true. So is the opposite: Boredom seems to slow time down.

- Fear seems to greatly modify perception of both time and space. For example, police officers often report that time seems to slow down during a high-stress conflict with an assailant. In one account, an officer reported several salient changes in depth and size perception; he was shocked when he returned to the scene of a shooting the next day and realized that the space was so small.

- A wide range of studies has demonstrated that everyday changes in emotion do influence everyday perceptions. Psychologist Dennis Proffitt conducted a study where people were asked to judge the steepness of various hills around the University of Virginia campus.

- There is certainly visual information involved in this, but Proffitt found that the internal state of the participant played a role as well. For example, members of the university's cross-country running team who had just run 10 miles judged the hills as steeper than did people who had not run those hills. Proffitt also found that when participants were sad, the hills looked steeper as well.

- An even more salient effect comes from studies of height perception. Most people who climb up to a high diving board at a swimming pool for the first time say it looks higher from that position than it did from the ground. This effect seems to be largely generated by the fear response.

- This study has been performed using a wide range of different spatial situations and tasks. In one example, the participant stands on a box at the top of a hill and makes judgments about the steepness and the distance of the slope. The participant's estimates are usually fairly accurate.

- If the participant stands on top of a skateboard instead of a box, however, so that in principle the participant could roll down the hill at any second, he or she feels that the hill is taller and steeper.

- Some aspects of emotion expression and perception seem to be consistent across cultures; however, there are other ways in which they vary greatly.

- Cultures vary on how much people rely on vision versus hearing to infer the emotions of others. To study this, researchers made video recordings of people saying "Is that so?" in both a happy tone and an angry tone. They then swapped the video and the audio from these recordings and asked people to watch them and to rate how happy or angry the resulting stimuli were.

- They found that relative reliance on vision and hearing varies tremendously across cultures: In the United States, people seemed to be equally influenced by both. In Denmark, people seemed to rely more on vision to judge emotion. In Japan, they seemed to rely more on the sound.

- Poets and artists have been fascinated with love for many centuries—probably as long as there have been poets and artists. Perceptual researchers are interested in love also. More specifically, they are interested in how and why humans judge other humans to be attractive.

- A few perceptual principles seem to apply in this domain. Perhaps the most studied of them is symmetry. The human body is roughly symmetrical, but no one is perfectly so.

- It is possible to objectively measure symmetry as an index of slight differences between the left and right halves of the body or face. According to these objective calculations, the more symmetrical someone is, the more attractive they are judged to be.

- There is some evidence that suggests symmetry is correlated with health and reproductive success as well. This gives us a sensible evolutionary reason why humans are attracted to symmetry. We are attracted to humans who tend to produce more, healthier offspring.

- A similar argument is made for why males and females seem to be attracted to particular waist-to-hip ratios among members of the opposite sex. Males tend to find a waist-to-hip ratio of about 0.9 most attractive; women prefer about a 0.7 ratio. As with symmetry, these body characteristics are related to health and reproductive success.

- Overall, this type of research suggests that when you look across the room and see a beautiful man or woman—when you perceive attractiveness—you are inferring something about that person based at least in part on relative size and symmetry information.

- Bodily symmetry is not only perceived visually. People with symmetrical vocal cords have more resonant voices. We are often attracted to someone's singing or speaking voice; this may well fit with the theory that we are hardwired to find symmetry attractive.

## Suggested Reading

Gladwell, *Blink*.

Wetsman and Marlowe, "How Universal Are Preferences for Female Waist-to-Hip Ratios?"

## Questions to Consider

1. It can be dangerous to send an e-mail to someone with whom I have an ongoing disagreement. Even if I write it with a neutral or generous tone in mind, the recipient may read it and become angry with me. If I just call and say the thing I want to communicate, this is much less likely to occur. Assuming I am not just a bad writer, why might this happen? What is not present in an e-mail that is present in a telephone or face-to-face interaction? Might emoticons help?

**2.** Some evolutionary psychologists have found evidence that attraction to a potential mate can be boiled down to a list of definable characteristics such as waist-to-hip ratio. Could we do the same thing with love? Why or why not?

# Perceiving Emotion in Others and Ourselves
## Lecture 19—Transcript

I was on a bus in Washington, DC a few months ago. I sat on one of those bench seats that's oriented sideways such that you look across the bus at other people who look back at you. I was sitting next to a woman who was in a bad mood. I heard her sigh repeatedly as she shuffled through her papers and her pockets. She yanked roughly on the zipper of her bag as she tried to shut it. When it got stuck, she cursed a bit under her breath and yanked it back and forth until it closed. When I glanced over at her face, the expression was just what you would expect. Her mouth was in a tight grimace, her shoulders were pressed together, her hands were squeezed into fists; she was not having a good day, and anyone who cared to notice could tell.

Sitting across from us was a man with a t-shirt, and it's one that you might have seen; it's produced by a company called "Life is Good." It showed a stick figure of a man in cartoony running shoes. He was out jogging with his dog. In the cartoon logo, the man's slightly in front of his dog and the dog isn't on a leash. The 2 runners are just out, enjoying the day, happy to be alive. As the words on the shirt clearly stated, "Life is Good."

The very unhappy woman in the seat next to me looked over at this shirt and gave a bit of a laugh (sort of; it was more of a snort). She wondered aloud in a not-very-happy voice, "Why would someone wear a shirt like that, with that man running away, being chased by a dog?" I laughed out loud, which made the unhappy woman next to me very unhappy with me. Fortunately, my stop came up just a few moments later, but as I looked at that t-shirt again, I just had to chuckle. There's a cartoon man in a full-on run with his mouth open; there's a dog running right behind him. The dog's mouth is also open, and you can see it's sharp teeth. The dog's almost close enough to bite the man's leg. The unhappy woman's perception was totally consistent with the images on this shirt. My perception of the happy jog outside with the dog was also consistent. Which of these interpretations our perceptual systems chose was very much a function of our 2 very different emotional states. These 2 emotional states formed the context of the perceptual processing for both of us. This phenomenon was especially clear in this setting, but it's far from isolated. Perception and emotion clearly go hand in hand almost all the time.

In this lecture, I'll be talking about how sensory processing relates to emotion. There are at least 2 main ways in which sensory processing and emotion can interact. The first has to do with how we perceive the emotions of others. Humans are remarkably fast and accurate at this, based on a wide range of information sources, both auditory and visual. We're often not even aware of the emotion perception that we're doing, and we're almost never aware of how we're doing it. I'll discuss some of the information sources that we use and how we make connections between that sensory information and particular emotional states.

In addition to discussing how we perceive the emotions of others, I'll be talking a bit about emotion-perception interaction in the other direction as well. Our own internal emotional state can greatly impact how we perceive the things around us. If I'm sad or happy or terrified, then the exact same sensory input might be perceived in 3 very different ways. I'll spend some time talking about emotion and our basic visual sensitivity; specifically, our ability to perceive very small changes in brightness. This is called contrast sensitivity. This basic visual function is influenced by emotion stimuli.

When we feel particular emotions, we tend to make certain facial expressions that correspond to them. There's some evidence to suggest that as we change the posture of our face, we don't just send messages to the people around us, say, on the bus. Those changes in the shape of our face impact our ability to engage in certain types of perceptions that have very functional significance. I'll describe some of those in this lecture as well. I'll also talk about how emotion perception varies across cultures, how it impacts our perception of space and time, and finally how we use sensory inputs to infer how attractive someone is.

Let's start with some very basic measures of sensory function; for the moment, visual function. I talked about measuring infant visual acuity in Lecture 16 using stripe patterns in that case. Remember that infants like stripes and so they look at them, but only if they can see those stripes. To test the limits of infant visual acuity, a researcher can present thinner and thinner stripes until they're invisible.

There's another way to make stripes harder to see, even if they stay exactly the same size: That's by reducing their contrast. A high contrast stripe pattern contains very dark black stripes and very bright white stripes. I could, however, make the black stripes dark gray and the white stripes light gray. If I kept going in this way—making the colors more and more similar— eventually I'd get to the point where they were barely different from one another. I'd have a slightly lighter gray and a slightly darker gray; that would be the only thing that could tell you where the stripes were. If I make those 2 grays similar enough, you won't able to see the stripes anymore.

For the study that I want to describe now, the researchers started by identifying stripe colors that could barely be seen by a participant. These were stripes that were right around those participants' contrast threshold ability. The experimenters placed 4 striped patches near the 4 corners of a computer screen. Three of the striped patterns were oriented in 1 direction, for instance vertically. One of the striped patches was at a different orientation; say, horizontal. The task of the participants was to identify which 1 of these 4 patches was the oddball. The participants weren't allowed to look at these stimuli for very long; in fact, they were flashed in front of their eyes for only about 40 milliseconds. This was a very challenging task.

Prior to showing these patches, participants were very briefly presented with a cue image. Very briefly, again: Only about 50 milliseconds for that cue. The cue images were always small images of human faces. In some cases, the faces had a neutral expression on them. In others, the faces had a fearful expression; a so-called fear face. You probably know what this looks like; you've seen people who were experiencing fear before: The eyebrows were raised, the eyes were wide open, the mouth was wide open in a non-smiling grimace; the faces looked fearful.

Seeing someone in fear sends an important message to us. If that person over there is afraid, there might be something nearby that perhaps I should be afraid of also. We don't consciously decide to feel this way. Fear is contagious, and it spreads according to some very fundamental brain mechanisms.

With certain stimuli—not all, but certain biologically relevant stimuli, like snakes—it's even possible to develop a phobia of those stimuli without ever directly interacting with them. If you just see someone interacting with a snake and you see that person having an extreme fear reaction that may be enough to cause that fear to develop.

This is a pretty tame experimental situation that I'm describing here with the patches of light; there's nothing very frightening about a flickering computer screen. But these fear faces seem to have an impact on a participant's sensory processing. If the participant is cued with the brief exposure to a fear face, he'll be more likely to detect those low contrast stripes, to find that oddball; and he'll be faster and he'll be more accurate in his responses on this task as well.

The cue works even better if those fear face cues are placed in the locations of the targets themselves, rather than just in the center of the screen. This suggests that the alteration of our sensory processing may be very location-specific, maybe even retinotopic, in its organization. This is a very artificial type of experiment; given the things we talked about in Lecture 16, it's the sort of thing that J.J. Gibson and the ecological psychologists would have really just groaned about. My reason for describing this study here is to note that there's good evidence—not just from this study—that emotion stimuli impact our sensory processing in a very basic way; not just for general interpretation of t-shirt logos and what people are thinking about things, but even at this very basic level of just detecting basic aspects of our visual input, something as simple as "Where are the stripes?"

I talked about olfaction and emotion in the lecture on taste and olfaction; I just wanted to remind you of it briefly here. There are only 2 synapses, an almost direct connection, between the olfactory sensors in the nose and the amygdala, a subcortical brain area that seems largely responsible for our emotional processing. The connection between olfaction and emotion is very direct. There are only 3 synapses, still a pretty direct connection, between those olfactory receptors and the hippocampus. This is a subcortical brain structure that's very important for making and recalling memories of things that we've experienced. Olfaction and memories, like emotion, also seem to be very directly connected to one another.

There are only 2 or 3 synapses between where olfaction is sensed and these areas for emotion and memory. Given that, there isn't much space or time for complex processing of these incoming stimuli. But remember how the olfactory system is set up; remember how it accomplishes its transduction. There are very specific stimuli—particular chemicals with particular shapes—whose presence causes the activation of a very specific receptor neuron. There are 350 of those different types of receptors, such that any given combination of activations there may be very rare. It might be that if you experience a very specific aroma in a particular place, you may not experience that same aroma again for years, maybe ever.

If certain experiences occur and certain emotions are experienced in the context of some novel aroma, you may file them away, using that aroma as the index for later looking up those memories in the future. If you smelled a very particular combination of chemicals and a moment later you were attacked by a dog, if you didn't smell that exact combination again for years but then one day smelled it again, it might be sensible to look around and make sure that you're ready to defend yourself or run away. Whether or not that's right—that the smell really does imply some threat—your brain hangs onto that information and seems to make that inference. Your sensory systems maintain that connection between the particular smell and the emotion of fear; and part of getting ready to defend yourself or run away involves a specific change in your emotional state, in this case probably one involving adrenaline and a very racing heartbeat.

A variety of research has looked at the facial expressions that go with certain emotions. Facial expressions associated with fear have been the topic of many studies, in part because they seem to be relatively universal. That is, if you go to almost any place in the world and show someone a picture of a fear face, they'll know what that means; and when people anywhere in the world are afraid, they seem to make the same basic facial expression.

Why do we do this? Why do we make these particular facial expressions for fear? It might be that I want to communicate with the people around me, perhaps by alerting those people of a potential source of danger, the one that I'm afraid of, whatever that is; that if I have this fear face I'll give those people around me a few important seconds of early warning before that danger strikes. That's possible—in fact, that's quite sensible from an evolutionary standpoint—but why this particular face? Wouldn't it be better instead of this fear face to make a little "woop" sound or something that would be easier for other people to pick up when we're afraid if communication is the goal?

Some recent research has suggested that the fear face isn't just an arbitrarily selected facial expression; in fact, the fear face has important functional consequences for perception, and that other expressions might have those consequences as well. For instance, when you make that fear face, as you draw your eyebrows upward, you're opening your eyes very, very wide. This makes it easier to see things in the most extreme parts of your peripheral vision. If you're dealing with some source of danger, that might be very useful. As you make your grimace with the mouth, you increase your ability to breathe in air; to pull in more oxygen. You also open your nostrils to make them more sensitive to aromas that are present there in the air. In essence, the changes associated with the fear face seem to ramp up the sensitivity of your sensory systems. We associate fear with a "fight or flight" response. Regardless of which one of these options is chosen, its effectiveness will be enhanced by the presence of that fear face and the sensory enhancements associated with it.

The facial expression that goes with disgust seems to work in the opposite way in many regards. When you scrunch your face up in the expression associated with sensing something disgusting, you close your mouth tightly and reduce the openings of the nostrils and the eyes. This serves to reduce your exposure to whatever that disgusting stimulus is. Recall from our discussions about olfaction that if you smell something, it's not a remote sensory process. The only way you can smell something is to have a bit of that thing, whatever it is, land on the interior surface of your nose. You have to ingest a little of that stuff. I don't even want to suggest what that disgusting stuff might be; think of something really disgusting. You don't want to ingest any of that, whatever that is, not even a few molecules. It's best to close the nostrils down as much as possible. It's best to make the disgust face.

Facial expressions influence our sensory processing greatly in terms of their sensitivity. Another impact that's often described is the influence of emotion on our perception of time and space. There's an old expression "Time flies when you're having fun" This is a cliché, but it's true. Alternatively, if you're bored, time will not fly; quite the opposite. The emotion that seems to greatly modify our perception of both time and space is fear. Let me give you a few extreme examples and then some more subtle ones.

When police officers are involved in an exchange of gunfire, their lives are on the line. The actions they make in the few minutes or even few seconds of this experience have the capacity to greatly affect or even end their lives and the lives of the people around them. It's not at all uncommon for officers to report experiencing salient sensory illusions during these experiences. Officers often report that time seems to slow down tremendously during a high-stress conflict with some assailant. A gun fight that lasts less than 30 seconds might be recalled as having taken many, many minutes. Often the sense of hearing seems to be attenuated or even tuned out of consciousness by the stress of one of these shootouts. Officers may report that they remember feeling the recoil of their gun firing, but not hearing any noise at all.

In one account that I've read, an officer reported several salient changes in depth and size perception as well. He was really shocked when he returned to the scene of a shooting the next day and realized that the space was so small. He remembered seeing the assailant as being about 40 feet away, at the end of a long dark hallway, when in fact he was in a small space, only about 5 feet long. This same officer reported seeing his partner shooting while—this seemed really strange to him, even at the time—there were beer cans floated slowly through the air. Even stranger was that these beer cans all had the word "Federal" printed on the bottom. The beer cans weren't beer cans; they were the shell casings being ejected from his partner's gun, and each of those shell casings had the word "Federal" on it.

These are extreme changes in perception of time, distance, and size; but these are extremely stressful fear-inducing situations. What about more moderate changes in emotion? Do they result in changes—presumably smaller—in our perception, or is it only in these life-and-death experiences that these shifts are apparent?

A wide range of studies has demonstrated that everyday changes in emotion do influence everyday perceptions. One very famous set of studies was done by a man named Dennis Proffitt. He asked participants to judge the steepness of various hills around the University of Virginia campus. Some hills around that campus are very steep; other hills are less steep. There's certainly visual information involved in this, in judging the slope of the hill, but the internal state of the experimental participant, the person making the judgments, also seems to play a role.

In one version of the experiment—one really good example here, I think—Proffitt studied the cross country team at the University of Virginia. He had the people on that team judge the steepness of hills before or after running 10 miles. After that long run, participants judged the hills to be steeper than they were judged by people who weren't fatigued. When you're tired, hills look steeper.

I've had this experience a lot; this isn't something that's very specific to cross country runners and running 10 miles. The more fatigued you are, the bigger and steeper hills around you look. I have this experience with a staircase at my house. At the end of the day, when I look up those stairs, they seem so much longer and taller than they do in the morning. I know that they must be physically the same size; at some rational level, I know that there wasn't a construction crew that snuck into my house during the day, tore out the old stairs, and put in a new, longer staircase. I know that the stairs are the same, but my visual system looks at them and tells me that they look longer and taller.

The Proffitt study tells us that this sense of the hill being longer when we're tired is not metaphorical. At a fundamental level, visual perception, our internal state of fatigue is rolled into these inferential processes that we keep talking about. Our internal emotional state is considered in this calculation as well. If you feel sad, hills look steeper. If you arrived at the lab to participate in one of these studies, even if you were in a very good mood, if you were given some sad music to listen to for about 30 minutes, and then if you made judgments about the steepness of hills afterwards, they would look steeper. Our perception of distance and surface layout is clearly influenced by our emotional state.

An even more salient effect comes from studies of height perception. Most people who climb up to a high dive at a swimming pool, say to try it out for the first time, have a very relevant experience here. From the ground, the high dive often just doesn't look so high. Then when you get to the top, however—especially if you're preparing to jump off, or alternatively pondering climbing back down the ladder—the water can seem enormously far away. It can seem so much higher from the top than it did from the bottom.

This effect seems to be largely generated by our fear response. The greater one's fear of heights, the farther away things seem in this setting. The measures that are used here are not just general, subjective indicators of height; it's not that the experimenters go to the top of the high dive with someone with a fear of heights and say, "Does this look high to you; or does it look very, very high; or does it look very, very, very high?" It's much more specific than that; it's not that subjective.

The experimental technique involves asking one person to stand on the ground at the bottom of the drop (whatever it is), and another to stand on the horizontal platform with the study participant. The study participant then tells this experimenter on the platform with them to move back and forth until the distance to the person on the platform appears identical to the distance to the person on the ground. These are very basic measures of depth perception that are being used here. Even with this very optical-based measure of depth perception, a fear of heights increases people's perception of how far away someone is, of how high above the ground they are; it seems to change as a function of this fear response.

This study's been performed using a wide range of different spatial situations and tasks. One of my favorite examples is if you stand at the top of a hill on a box and you look out in front of you and make judgments about the steepness and the distance of the slope, you'll get certain estimates; pretty accurate estimates, actually. If you have someone stand in that exact same situation, only instead of being on top of a box they're on top of a skateboard—a skateboard with wheels on it that, in principle, could roll down the hill—even if the skateboard and the box are exactly the same height, so that you have exactly the same view of that hill, the hill seems to get steeper when you step over onto that skateboard. It seems that our fear influences our perception very frequently and as a function of the actions that we are preparing to do or making sure we don't do.

I've emphasized aspects of emotion expression and perception that seem to be consistent across cultures thus far in this lecture. I should note, however, that there are great variations across cultures in terms of how we express and perceive emotions. One example of that comes from a study comparing how people from different cultures rely on vision as opposed to hearing to infer the emotions of others.

To do this for this study, researchers recorded someone expressing a simple statement in both a happy tone and an angry tone; the thing that was stated was, "Is that so?" If my daughter comes home from school and she tells me that she got a 100%, an A+ on her math test, I might say, "Is that so!" On the other hand, if my neighbor tells me that she's really sorry about hitting my mailbox with her car again, I might say, "Is that so." Same words, said in 2 very different ways—"Is that so!" and "Is that so"— 2 very different meanings, same words.

These researchers videotaped a happy "Is that so" and an angry "Is that so" and then switched the audio and video. Researchers asked people to watch these 2 switched videos and rate how happy or angry the 2 resulting stimuli were. Both of these were equally angry and happy, it just depends on whether you rely more on vision or audition to make judgments about the emotion here. The researchers found that the relative reliance on vision and hearing varies tremendously across cultures. In the US, people seem to be about equally influenced by both. In Denmark, it's been found that people rely heavily on vision to judge emotion. If someone's watching the video of someone saying very happily, "Is that so," even if they hear the angry "Is that so" underneath it, they're still going to make a judgment that it sounds very happy. In Japan, the opposite is found; there's a very heavy reliance there on the sound. If you showed that exact same video to the Japanese participants, if they heard the unhappy "Is that so," even if they saw the happy video "Is that so," they would rely very specifically on the sound and ignore the visual stimuli. This factor seems to vary tremendously from culture to culture.

This is just one example of many studies that have found similar differences in emotional expression and perception across cultures. While there's some consistency that applies to the all humans for things like fear and disgust, culture and cultural learning clearly play a big role in how emotion and perception affect one another.

Poets and artists have been fascinated with love for many centuries, probably as long as there have been poets and artists. Perceptual researchers are interested in love also, but in terms of their research topics, if you look at the literature it seems that perceptual scientists have been more interested in lust; specifically in how humans perceive other humans as attractive, some as very attractive, others as less attractive, others not as attractive at all.

There are a few perceptual principles that seem to apply in this domain. Perhaps the most studied of them is symmetry. The human body is roughly symmetrical: We have an arm on one side, a matching arm on the other; we have an eye on one side, and an eye matches it on the other. We look about the same in the left half and right half of our body; but no one is perfectly symmetrical. It's actually possible to very objectively measure symmetry as an index of the difference, those slight differences, between the left and right half of the body or even just of the face, in terms of exactly how similar is the shape of one eye as opposed to the shape of the other; how equal is the distance to one side of the mouth as opposed to the other side of the mouth.

When you measure symmetry, according to these very objective calculations and measures, you find that the more symmetrical someone is, the more attractive they're judged to be. There's some evidence that suggests that symmetry is correlated with health and reproductive success as well. If we see this connection between attraction and reproductive success, now there's a very sensible evolutionary story for why humans are attracted to symmetry. The humans who were attracted to that may have, in the past, tended to produce more offspring than those who were not. We may all be descendants of people who happened to like symmetry.

A similar argument is made for why males and females seem to be attracted to particular waist-hip ratios among members of the opposite sex. To perform these studies, researchers show pictures of many bodies and ask participants to rate all of those many bodies in terms of how attractive they are; say, on a scale from 1 to 10. They then look for factors about those bodies that correlate with those ratings. For males, it turns out one of the best factors to predict those attractiveness ratings is a waist-to-hip size ratio of about 0.9; this is likely to lead to the best attractiveness scores. It's different for females. For females, that same ratio, if it's about 0.7 it seems to be preferred.

As with symmetry, these body characteristics have since been related to health and reproductive success. Men with ratios close to 0.9 tend to live longer and are less likely to suffer from a variety of illnesses including heart disease than men who don't have a waist-hip ration that's close to that 0.9 value. Women with a ratio close to 0.7 are less likely to have problems during childbirth than women with very different ratios. As with symmetry, this perceptual attraction suggests an evolutionary story.

Overall, this type of research suggests that when you look across the room and see a beautiful man or woman, when you feel that emotional attraction, when you perceive attractiveness, you're inferring something about that person, and that, in part, it's based on relative size and symmetry information that you're gathering through your visual senses.

It's not only your eyes that get in on the act. The more symmetrical someone is, the more that their vocal cords tend to be symmetrical, the more they tend to produce a resonant-sounding voice. Some people report that if you hear someone sing with a very beautiful voice that this is something that's attractive; they may feel very attracted to that person with the lovely-sounding resonant voice. That lovely-sounding resonant voice is an indicator of symmetry in that person. Symmetry researchers think this fits very nicely with their theory.

In this lecture, we've considered emotion and perception from a variety of different perspectives. We've considered how emotion influences our perception; for instance, ramping up our sensory sensitivity for fear or reducing that sensitive for disgust. We've seen how an emotional state can even change our perception of space and time. We've also discussed to some extent how we perceive the emotions of others; how we use vision and hearing, how we pick up information about someone's future health and well-being, on the basis of something as simple as symmetry and waist-hip ratio. These are sensory inputs, but they result in emotional responses. In the next lecture, we'll see more detail about how we read the emotions of others as well.

In that next lecture, I'll be telling you about something that's often referred to as "Extra Sensory Perception" or ESP. This is a problematic term, actually, just on the face of it. If we can sense something, then it can't be outside the senses; it can't be extra sensory. Usually when someone talks about ESP, they're intending to communicate the idea of mysterious abilities of some special, gifted people to read the minds of others, for instance; to sense the energy patterns in their brains and somehow know just what they're thinking. In the movies and the world of fiction in general, this mysterious power is typically the gift of a few special people. In reality, however, almost everyone is able to read the minds of the people around them. You read the minds of the people around you every day; you might be doing it right now. It's not based on mystical forces, but the process is quite impressive. We'll discuss this non-extra sensory perception in our next lecture. I know you'll be there.

# Sensing the Thoughts of Others—ESP
## Lecture 20

Through a series of verbal and mathematic tricks that have all the earmarks of the obfuscating magic used by magicians, I can convince you that I have the power of extrasensory perception (ESP). But I have no more planted the word *carrot* in your mind than Harry Blackstone made a goat materialize out of thin air. I am able to create the illusion of ESP because I am aware of how humans think.

- There are many ways in which humans capitalize on sensory information. We pick up tidbits of what people say or of how they say it and then use that to infer what they are likely to be thinking.

- This process is often fast and unconscious, such that we might even experience it as a sort of mind reading. It is impressive and fascinating, but there is nothing magical or paranormal about the process.

- Claims of paranormal phenomena include many different types of things, from mind reading and thought control to contacting the dead, finding underground water, and even predicting the future.

- In almost every case, there is evidence people making these claims are capitalizing on sensory information, tricks just like the ones I demonstrate in this lecture. In a way, we read people's minds and predict the future all the time—just not in a mystical fashion.

- In a sense, even simply catching a ball is a small act of predicting the future. If I reach for the current location of some moving target, I will miss it. I have to reach for some location that it will occupy in the future.

- We will discuss how we infer others' thoughts based on standard perception for most of this lecture. At the end, however, we will examine one particular line of research being conducted by some very reputable researchers that suggests there might be some phenomena that cannot be explained by standard sensory perception.

- One of the most useful sources of information about what is happening in someone else's mind is where that person is looking.

- Humans are exceptionally good at knowing when someone is looking at us. Even in a crowd, among hundreds of pairs of eyes looking in hundreds of slightly different directions, if one of those sets of eyes is looking right at you, your attention will be drawn to those eyes.

- As someone shifts their gaze from place to place, the only thing that changes in that projection is how much of the whites of their eyes are visible. That is what we notice.

- We can also determine the depth of someone's gaze quite accurately. Try this the next time you are in face-to-face conversation with someone: look at a point just behind them. You will not be able to see it, of course, because their head will be in the way, but blur your eyes a little bit and aim your gaze past them.

- Your conversational partner will almost certainly notice something strange is going on within a few seconds; the person may even turn around to see what has captured your attention.

- This ability to track the gaze of others is present within a few months after a child is born. It seems to play a critical role in word learning, which is also a situation in which you need to be able to read someone's mind.

- Children learn new nouns when they and an adult are both attending to some novel object. They both look at the object, and the adult pronounces the object's name. Without gaze tracking, this would be far more difficult, and studies show that in children who lack gaze tracking, language learning tends to be delayed.

- We can infer a lot about what someone is thinking based on where they are looking: a conversation where someone frequently glances at the door and at their watch; a hand of poker where a player sneaks a glance at their stack of chips; 2 criminals engaged in a negotiation and one of them glances at the gun on the table at just the wrong moment.

- As you know from Lecture 14, we need to attend to things to get detailed information about them, and where we look is often where we are focusing our attention. However, we are also able to focus our attention away from the place that we are focusing our gaze. As far as we know, humans are the only species on the planet capable of that particular feat.

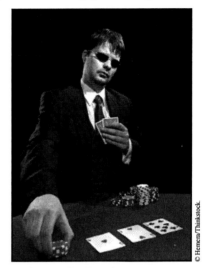

**Professional poker players wear sunglasses to disguise their glances.**

- The emergence of this ability is believed to be related to how much information we give away with our eye movements. In a complex, social society such as our own, there may be a competitive advantage to being able to conceal that information—that is, to lie.

- The best-known, technological method of lie detection is the polygraph machine. It records the heart rate, respiratory rate, and in particular the skin conductance level of the subject. The skin conductance level is a measure of your skin's electric current, a reflection of your rate of perspiration.

- Even small increases in perspiration can increase skin conductance. If you are exerting a little extra mental effort, perhaps through discomfort about telling a lie, that is enough to make this skin conductance response take place.

- An important part of the polygraph process is convincing the subject that the polygraph test is effective. Before hooking you up, the operator might ask you to think of a number between 1 and 9 and write it down on a piece of paper. Once you were hooked up, the operator would slowly count from 1 to 10 and back down again.

- When the operator says the digit you have written down, there would be a detectable tweak in the readouts. This demonstration would magnify your stress and convince you, if you were considering lying, that the machine might work.

- It is actually fairly simple to beat a polygraph machine: Clenching your toes causes similar increases in heart rate, breathing, and skin conductance level to lying. If you clench while telling the truth and relax while lying, the operator cannot tell the difference. A good operator typically asks people to remove their shoes during the test for this very reason.

- There have been recent attempts to assess the brain activity associated with lying directly. If you know you are lying, then should be reflected in the pattern of activity in your brain and an fMRI or other brain-imaging technology could detect it.

- A lot of work has been done in this area, but no simple solution has been found. So far, the best lie detectors in the world are people. Most people can detect lies at a better rate than pure chance, but people from certain professions seem better than most: CIA and FBI interrogators, for instance.

- Some of the best judges of lying are U.S. Secret Service agents. As bodyguards to the U.S. president and other government officials, they spend much of their time watching crowds for suspicious activity.

- None of these experts is good at explaining his or her skills. Clearly, some high-level perceptual learning is essential here. Extensive experience is key.

- Facial expressions tell us a great deal about what people are thinking. You can usually tell when someone is not happy, even when he or she is smiling. We can read the true feelings behind the fake expression.

- One of the best sources for such examples is the domain of politics. Every day, White House press secretaries are grilled by reporters seeking newsworthy and perhaps emotional responses. It's the secretary's job to remain calm, controlled, and polite under all this stress.

- However, no matter how cordial the secretary seems, you can often tell that this official is unhappy about a certain question or topic. Facial movements called microexpressions convey the true feelings in play.

- Microexpressions were discovered and characterized by psychologist Paul Ekman. In essence, when you feel some emotional response, regardless of how socially appropriate it is, your face responds in an unconscious, automatic way. You may consciously mask that response with a more socially appropriate expression, but the true emotion will be briefly visible as a microexpression.

- These microexpressions only last for a few milliseconds, but human vision is fast enough for us to pick up on them. Even if the expressions are not there long enough for us to become consciously aware of them, they enable us to read a person's emotions.

- We also seem to sense information from static facial expressions. A smile of genuine happiness is different from a polite smile with little or no real happiness behind it. The mouth turns upward in both, but there is far more narrowing of the outer corners of the eyes in a real smile than in a false one. This is a difficult muscle movement to master voluntarily.

- As we get better at detecting lies, a sort of evolutionary arms race pushes our species to get better and better at deception. I have suggested that ordinary perception allows us to read minds and predict the future to a certain extent. How can the senses improve on this?

- In the late 1980s, social psychologist Daryl Bem took on an ambitious and risky research project to look for evidence of ESP, telepathy, and clairvoyance—collectively referred to as psi. Many demonstrations seem to suggest the presence of these things, but there have always been more mundane explanations for them.

- Bem, a respected, established researcher, decided to devote his skills to developing a well-designed assessment of telepathy that, if it worked, would be beyond the reach of trick-based explanations.

- He used the Ganzfeld procedure, in which 2 participants sit in 2 different rooms that sealed off from one another, separated by some distance. The "sender" participant watches a 30-second video clip, then meditates on it while wearing white-out goggles and headphones playing static.

- The "receiver" participant, meanwhile, wears a similar but unconnected set of goggles and headphones and meditates for 30 minutes. Then he or she is shown a selection of 5 30-second video clips and is asked to pick which one the sender was sending.

- If the receiver was just guessing, you would expect a correct guess about 20% of the time. Among senders and receivers who are close friends, however, the average performance is consistently around 34%.

- This 14% may not seem large, but the odds of this increased performance being due to chance are in fact vanishingly small. It seems likely that something systematic is enabling some of the receivers to do better than random guessing.

- Just what accounts for this 14% remains a matter of controversy. Many researchers doubt this finding is accurate. We can only say that the experiment and results meets the basic standards of evidence required of all serious research.

## Suggested Reading

Bem and Honorton, "Does Psi Exist?"

Hyman, "Anomaly or Artifact?"

## Questions to Consider

1. I described my ability to read my dog's mind in this lecture. Can you think of times when you have read the mind of your pet, child, spouse, or friend? A time when they confirmed that you were correct?

2. The experiments of Daryl Bem and his colleagues provide evidence for mind reading that is as good as published evidence for many scientific phenomena. He recently published a paper presenting similar evidence for predicting the future of a random event. If Bem is right, then how must our conception of the human senses change?

# Sensing the Thoughts of Others—ESP
## Lecture 20—Transcript

Welcome to our lecture on Extra Sensory Perception (ESP). I'm going to start today by implanting an idea in your head. To get this right, I need you to sit down in a quiet place and relax. Hopefully you're seated now, and you're relaxed. I want you to take a deep breath in, and out. I want you to do this in and out breath again, but this time, when you exhale, say "relax."

Hopefully you're calm and quiet and ready to receive this idea that I'm going to implant into your head. I have this worked out in great detail here. I'm going to read you some math problems, and I need you to say the answer to each one of those problems out loud. For instance, if I say $2 + 9$ you should say … ? Hello? If I say $2 + 9$, you should say … out loud? Thank you. Okay, I'm going to give you these math problems, then I'm going to ask you to say something, and then I'll ask you a question. For all 3 of these kinds of requests, I need you to answer clearly and out loud. I'm not crazy. I know I can't hear you, but it's part of the demo. For your own enjoyment and learning, I strongly encourage you to play along here.

Okay, here we go; for real this time. Ready? $1 + 1$; $2 + 2$; $3 + 3$; $4 + 4$. Now say the number 6 out loud 10 times. Name a vegetable.

If I'm right, you should have said the word "carrot." Pretty good, huh? I hope it was. In case you didn't play along or, if for some reason it didn't work for you, please take my word for it that this usually works. When I run through this set of math problems and speaking exercises, almost everyone who participates says the word "carrot." I have, through my powers of ESP, planted the idea of "carrots" into your heads. Amazing. Amazing? Not really. It turns out that if I'd done the same thing without all of the math problems, without all of the speaking out loud, if I'd just walked up to you and said, "Name a vegetable," you would very likely have said "carrot." The way that the human mind encodes this category of "vegetables" has this structure to it. Carrots are, for a variety of reasons, a prototypical vegetable. They're the first one that comes to mind.

The illusion of ESP is created here—at least I hope it was—because while you weren't aware of that structure to the category vegetables, I was. There's information present in the world—in this case in the structure of how humans think about vegetables—that lets me know something that's happening inside your mind.

There are many examples of this; let's try another on. I want you to think of a country that starts with "D"; any country. Okay, take the last letter of that country name and think of an animal that starts with that letter. Okay? Now take the last letter of that animal name and think of a color that starts with that letter, any color. Okay, now think about those 3 words; focus on them; and now I will read your mind. Are you thinking about an orange kangaroo in Denmark? That's kind of strange.

I'm not reading your mind, of course. Again, I'm using information about you and the world to make an inference. There's only one commonly-known country that starts with "D," Denmark; and only one common animal name that starts with "K," kangaroo. If I ask you for a color that starts with "O," you could have said lots of things—you could have said "onyx" or "olivine"—but you're very unlikely to do so. Orange is a much more common answer.

In this lecture, I'm going to be talking about many ways in which humans capitalize on sensory information in this fashion. We pick up tidbits of what people say or of how they say it, and then use that to infer what they're likely to be thinking. This process is often fast and very unconscious, such that we might even experience it as a sort of mindreading.

This is impressive and fascinating, but there's nothing magical or paranormal about this process. Just like most of our sensory processes, the brain makes its best guess about what's happening around you in the world, and you experience that guess. We've talked about that with color, motion, depth, even tomato soup. In this lecture, we'll be talking about how that functions when the thing you're perceiving is people.

Paranormal phenomena include a lot of different types of things. Mind reading and thought control are 2 I've already touched on in this lecture. There are psychics who claim that they can contact the dead, find water, and even predict the future. In almost every case, there's evidence that capitalizing on tricks just like the ones that I've used here can explain these seemingly mystical phenomena.

For instance, we can read other people's minds. I'll argue that we do that all the time. Can we tell the future? I would argue that the answer is yes, but not in any sort of mystical fashion. By knowing the structure of the world around us, by knowing what events are very likely to follow other events, we can infer what will happen in the future. If that inference is specific and accurate enough, one might perceive it as clairvoyance, but there's no reason to think of it as anything other than regular perception.

In a sense, even the simple example of someone catching a ball is a small act of predicting the future. If I reach for the current location of some moving target, I'll miss it. By the time my hand arrives at that location, the moving ball will have moved to some new location. My hand will have missed the target. If I want to catch a moving target, I have to reach ahead of it along its path of motion, aiming for some location that it will occupy in the future. I can do this, of course; even 4-month-old babies can do this, with a ball that rolls slowly past them anyway. Am I predicting the future? Yes. Am I making use of ESP? Not at all.

I'll talk about how we infer others' thoughts based on standard perception for most of this lecture. At the end, however, I'll tell you about one particular line of research, being conducted by some very reputable researchers, that suggests that there might be something else; something that can't be explained using all of these standard sensory methods that I'll talk about for most of the lecture. Daryl Bem and his colleagues have some hard-to-refute evidence that people can send and receive thoughts even when they're fully isolated from each other in every way that we understand them being isolated from each other anyway.

Let's get back to the more standard reading of minds for the moment. One of the most useful sources of information for what's happening in someone's mind at any given moment is where they're looking. We're really, really good at knowing when someone's looking at us. If you look out at the crowd at a party or the audience even at a sizeable stadium, you might be seeing hundreds and hundreds of eyes, all looking around at slightly different things. If one of those sets of eyes is looking right at you, staring in your direction, your attention will be drawn to just those eyes.

This is an impressive feat in some circumstances, even at a purely optical level. If I'm looking out at hundreds of eyes in the distance, any given eye is only projecting a very tiny retinal image onto my eye. As someone shifts their gaze from place to place, the only thing that changes in that projection is the amount of the whites of the eye that are visible. If I look a little to the left, you see a little more white on one side and a little less on the other. If I look to the right, the opposite happens. Just how much of the white is visible is all we really have to work with to track the eye gaze of others. As I mentioned, we're really accurate in how we use this information, and not just in terms of direction of gaze, but even in terms of 3-dimensional depth, considering where the 2 eyes are looking together to fixate some position that's at a particular distance away from their head. The next time you have a face-to-face conversation with someone, try looking at a point just behind them. You won't be able to see it, of course, because their head will be in the way, but blur your eyes a little bit and aim your eyes past them, sort of through their heads. I can almost guarantee that within a few seconds even the person you're talking to will, first, notice that something strange is going on, and second, they'll turn around and look behind them to see what's caught your eyes.

This ability to track the gaze of others is present within the first few months after a child's born. It's not only available and accurate at this age, but it seems to play a very critical role in word learning, which turns out to be a place where you need to be able to read someone's mind. Kids learn new nouns when they and an adult are both attending to some object; some object that the child doesn't know the name of. When the child and the adult are both fixating on that object with their eyes, the adult then says some new word—"doggy," for instance—and the child files that "doggy" word with that particular object away in their mind for future use. Without the gaze tracking this would be far more difficult, impossible even; and for kids who lack it for some reason, word and language learning in general tend to be delayed.

We can infer a lot about what someone's thinking based on where they're looking. If I glance at the door or at another person when I'm talking to you, you'll know that. If I look at my watch, there's a cue sent to you about my state of mind. If poker player just glances at the stack of chips on the table in front of him, that can give away a lot. Many professional poker players wear sunglasses when they play for this precise reason, so that their opponents can't see their eyes and where they're looking. If 2 criminals are engaged in a tense negotiation and one of them just glances at the gun on the table at the wrong moment, it can lead to a tragic cascade of events.

As you know from Lecture 14, we need to attend to things in order to get certain sources of detailed information about them; and where we look is often where we're focusing our attention. It should be noted, however, that we're able to focus our attention away from the place that we're focusing our gaze. That is, I can look at you, and continue to look at you, while I pay attention to something else over to the side, away from my point of fixation. As far as we know, humans are the only species on the planet that are capable of that particular feat of focusing your gaze and your attention in 2 different places. Some non-human primates might be able to do this, but even there the jury's still out. The emergence of this ability is thought of as very directly related to just how much information we give away with our eye movements.

In a complex, social society such as our own, there may be a tremendous competitive advantage to being able to conceal that information about what we're thinking. There may be even more advantage to presenting other people with a misleading indicator of what we're thinking about. This competitive advantage is typically referred to as the ability to lie.

The lie detector industry is big business. The most well-known, technological method of lie detection makes use of something called a polygraph. It records the heart rate, breathing, some other physiological measures, and, in particular, something called skin conductance level; it's a measure of how much your skin resists the flow of a small electric current. If you do something that causes you to perspire, to sweat even just a little, the amount of water in the top layers of your skin increases. Again, this is all just a small change; it's nothing you could directly see or observe. As that amount of water increases, this skin conductance level drops; the more water is in your skin, the easier it is for it to conduct electricity, and that's something that a polygraph can measure. If you're exerting a little extra mental effort, maybe feeling a little uncomfortable about telling some lie, that's enough to make this skin conductance response take place. The polygraph operator who has you hooked up to this machine sees the meter shift and blammo, you're caught.

In general, this is how polygraphs work. There are certain baseline levels for all of the different things that are being measured—for heart rate, respiration, skin conductance level—and certain changes that occur when you answer basic, verifiably correct questions. (Is your name George Smith? Is your birthday July 15th, 1957? Etc.) If you try to lie in one of these settings, it requires a little more effort than answering one of these truthful questions and it creates a little extra stress. If you weren't in the polygraph, no one would notice this extra stress that you are undergoing, but the physiological changes can often be detected by a polygraph.

Another part of the process is convincing the subject of a polygraph test of its effectiveness. The polygraph operator, if he were hooking you up to his machine, might ask you to think of a number between 1 and 9 and to write it down on a piece of paper without telling or showing him what that number is. He would then, once you were all hooked up, read off the numbers slowly, counting from 1, 2, 3, all the way up to 10; and then in many cases he would start at 10 and count back down to 1. When he says the digit that you've written down on that piece of paper, the digits that you have in mind, there will be a detectable tweak in the readouts, and he'll know the number that you have in your head. Once he's done this, someone who is pondering maybe lying when they're asked a certain question will start to get very worried, because they'll realize that this device seems to really work. This worry will in turn magnify that stress response that the polygraph needs to detect the lying.

There's actually a pretty easy thing that you can do to beat a polygraph test. I don't mean to tell you this to encourage you to actually do it. I just want to make clear how a polygraph works so that I can explain more clearly how the human sensory version of lie detection functions. This trick for beating the polygraph is hard to detect. In fact, I'm doing it right now. Any guess what it is? I'm clenching my toes.

Lying causes changes, very slight changes, in those physiological responses that are measured by the polygraph, but so do a lot of other things. In fact, clenching your toes causes a very similar increase in heart rate, breathing, and skin conductance level. The trick part of this beating a polygraph is to clench your toes whenever you tell the truth and then relax them when you lie. From a polygraph operator's perspective, this will look about the same. (Actually, a very careful polygraph operator typically asks people to remove their shoes for this very reason, to make sure they're not doing something like clenching.)

There have been recent attempts to be more direct in terms of assessing the brain activity associated with lying; rather than just measuring these physiological responses, to measure the activity of the brain while people are lying. In principle, these seem like this approach of measuring the brain during lying as a lie detector seems like it must work. That is, if you're lying, you know you're lying. If you know something, then it has to be due to some pattern of activity up here in your brain. Thus, there should be something that an fMRI or maybe other kind of brain imaging technology, something it could detect. That said, it hasn't been figured out yet. There's been a lot of work done in this area, and whatever it is, it's not going to be really simple. Perfect, automatic lie detection is still very much an inexact science.

The best lie detectors in the world are people. Many studies have been run in which people are specifically instructed to lie about something while being questioned. The test, then, is how well some questioner, some interrogator, can detect when that person's lying. Almost anyone will be better than guessing in this task, but people from certain professions seem to be better than most. It might not be surprising to know that CIA and FBI interrogators are very good at it. Some of the best judges of lying, however—some of the world champs of this—are secret service agents. These are the people who serve as bodyguards to the President and other public officials. It's believed that they're so good at this because they spend so much time watching people, usually in crowds. They may be watching to make sure they don't have a weapon or they're not looking to create some sort of a problem. They're watching people while the crowd isn't watching them; they're watching the speech. Secret service agents are trained, and really their task is, to watch and look for unusual behavior; for any signs that someone's thinking about doing something that might create a problem.

None of these expert lie detectors are very good at saying how they do what they do; how they're able to detect when that unusual behavior is happening. It's clearly a very complex process and based on comparisons of some standard or baseline patterns of behavior with the behavior during the times when a lie might be told. There's some very high level perceptual learning that's essential here. No matter how specifically one of these experts tell you how they're detecting lies, you won't be able to take that information, that lesson they just gave you, and then walk over and be able to perform as well as they do. Extensive experience seems to be essential in this situation.

As I mentioned, however, we're all capable, if not perfect, at knowing when someone's lying to us. How do we do it? To the extent that we can, what's the information that tells us that? It's clear that we're similarly complex in our reasoning about lying, but one of the most important sources of information that we use in general, even without being trained to do it, comes from watching what's happening on someone's face. Facial expressions can tell us a great deal about what people are thinking. There's an obvious level at which this is true. If I'm happy, I typically smile; if I'm sad, I frown. That's sort of mindreading, but it's not very interesting.

What's more impressive is when someone's smiling but you can tell that they aren't actually happy. At the end of the Super Bowl in football, it's common for players and coaches on the losing team to go congratulate the winners. As they do so, they often smile and wish the winners well. It's pretty clear, however, that they're not at all happy about losing. They may return to their locker room and switch to screaming, yelling, even crying about the loss. We often find ourselves in situations in which it's socially appropriate to smile, and so we do, even though we may have no happy feeling behind that smile. Except in the case of very good actors—and one might say very good liars— when we observe someone doing this, putting forward a false front, covering another emotion, we can often tell. We can read their true feelings behind the fake expression.

A great deal of research has gone into trying to figure out how this works, and also into enhancing our ability to detect when these false fronts are being put up. The lie detector industry is big business. The polygraph is a useful piece of technology, but it's easy to beat. What's tougher to beat is a good human visual system.

Let's consider a situation in which we know someone is masking his true emotions about something. One of the best sources of examples of this is, unfortunately, the domain of politics. Almost every day, the White House Press Secretary gives a briefing to the assembled White House press corps. Then the reporters ask questions. Often these questions are very pointed and critical, and frankly aimed at getting a newsworthy, maybe emotional response from this important official. As these zingers come flying at the podium, it's the job of the press secretary to politely, calmly answer these questions with a big smile; and almost every press secretary does this, almost every day. But 2 things are worth noting: First, when we watch these interactions, we know how he's actually feeling about it. No matter how big that smile is or how polite or cordial he seems, you can tell that the press secretary is just not happy about that particular question that he's being asked. Second, there's information in his facial movements that convey that information that we're perceiving about the true feelings. It's this information that we use to "read his mind."

One very rich source of this facial expression information is something called "microexpressions." These were discovered and characterized by a very famous researcher named Paul Ekman. There's been a great deal of very detailed research on how to encode these brief facial movements; it's ultimately resulted in a fairly complex system called the "Facial Action Coding System." If you really want to become expert at this, there are full-length certification courses that you can take. There's a whole lot of expertise in this area.

For the moment, let me just describe the basic concept behind it. The idea is that when you feel some emotional response, regardless of how socially appropriate it is, your face responds in an unconscious, automatic way. You can then mask that response perhaps with the more socially appropriate, consciously chosen facial expression, but that second process is slower than the instant, automatic one. As such, the true emotion leaks out briefly at the onset of some emotional response.

If you look closely at that White House press secretary, particularly with a slow motion video, you can often very clearly see this. For instance, imagine a reporter asks the press secretary about a particular comment made about the President, a very critical comment; a comment in which it was suggested that the President's policies are doing great damage to the US economy. The press secretary will smile and answer that the commentator is mistaken; he's really just playing maybe to that particular program's specific audience. The press secretary might then calmly add that the President's policies are, in fact, making progress and will, given enough time, have all of the desired effects. This all comes out with a big smile, but if you look at the facial expressions as the questions are asked, a very different, much less cordial response is made. Very briefly, just for a few hundred milliseconds, there's a facial expression of disgust; there's another facial expression that's almost like revulsion. There's a moment when great concern and frustration are present right in that facial expression. These expressions are only there for a moment and then they're gone, covered by the intentional choice to smile; but human vision is, as you know, very fast. There's enough there for us to pick up on; there's enough to enable us to do a little mind reading. Even if the expressions aren't there long enough for us to actually be consciously aware of them, they have an impact on our ability to read the emotions of the person behind them.

There's also information that we sense from the posture of static facial expressions. If you see someone making a genuine smile of happiness, they look different than when they're making a polite smile with little or no real happiness behind it. Both real and fake smiles have the same components to them; the mouth turns upward in both, although maybe a little bit more for a real smile. The key to real smiles is the eyes. There's a narrowing of the outer corners of the eyes that happens with real smiles that's far less pronounced for simply polite smiles, even very big polite smiles. It's very difficult to learn to change the position of the eyes in this fashion voluntarily, which makes it in a sense a good tell for when someone's just pretending to be happy.

Before you go around accusing people of fake smiling, however, I should note that the amount of this eye narrowing varies tremendously across individuals, and it's possible to learn to control it; it's difficult, but it's possible. For instance, when a skilled actor needs to pretend to be happy, he or she may think of something happy. Even though there's no happiness about the current situation the actor's in, the other happy thought can generate that eye change associated with a genuine smile.

Lie detection is hard. I mentioned that we seem to have a somewhat unique ability to direct our attention away from our point of fixation, and that this may have evolved, in part, in order to allow us to deceive others. Some research has suggested that this type of adaptation continues today. As we get better at detecting the lies of others, there's a sort of arms race that pushes our species to get better and better at deception.

I've argued up to this point in the lecture that we can read minds and, to some extent, maybe tell the future. I've described this as being due not to any magical powers, but due to standard sensory-based inferential processing; inferences based on the standard 5 senses that we've been talking about throughout this course. We're very smart about perceiving others and their thoughts. We're not perfect, but there's a lot of information that we can and do use to read people's minds. All that said, I'm about to switch gears.

In the late 1980s, a social psychologist at Cornell University, a guy named Daryl Bem, took on a very ambitious and sort of risky research project. He decided to test to see if there was such a thing as ESP, telepathy, or clairvoyance. (He refers to these, by the way, as Psi phenomena. Remember, that extrasensory perception term is problematic since he's suggesting that there is a sense that enables us to take in and process this information; so psi is the word that he tries to use there.) Many demonstrations exist that seem to suggest the presence of these things, but there have always been problems with those demonstrations; there's always been some explanation for the findings that could be explained by other means, the kinds of means that I've been talking about in this lecture.

Bem was already an established, well-known experimenter when he started this project in the domain of social psychology. He was a very accomplished, clever experimenter; he'd run hundreds of studies shedding light on how people reason about themselves and the people around them. Bem decided to devote this experimental skill to developing a well-designed assessment of telepathy that, if it worked, would be beyond the reach of those trick-based explanations. I should mention that in addition to being an experimental psychologist, Darryl Bem is also a rather accomplished magician, so he knows potential tricks very well.

Bem settled on something called the Ganzfeld procedure. For this procedure, you have 2 participants. They sit in 2 different rooms that are sealed apart from one another and then separated by some distance. There is, as far as we can tell, essentially no commonly-understood way that one could send any secret messages between these 2 completely isolated rooms. One of the participants is designated as the sender and the other as the receiver. The sender in these studies watches a randomly selected video clip—a 30-second video clip—and then meditates on that 30-second video clip. As she does, she places white goggles over her eyes and listens to soft static on head phones. This is the Ganzfeld part of the Ganzfeld procedure: By covering your ears and eyes with this kind of stimulation with the goggles and the static, it does as much as possible to remove structured visual and auditory input from the outside world into the brain; those are essentially blocked out. That's the sender.

The receiver, meanwhile, spends some time in this other room. The receiver also wears the goggles and the headphones. I should make a point: They're not connected to the headphones in the other room in any way. The receiver simply sits and for 30 minutes or so mediates while the sender is doing her sending in the other room. At the end, the receiver is shown a selection of 5 30-second video clips and the receiver attempts to pick which ones of those the sender was sending.

If there's no telepathy, then the receiver will still occasionally pick the right video clip; on the average of about 1 out of 5 times. If the person was just guessing, about 20% of the time they'd be correct. If you bring in 2 random people off the street, that's exactly what you find. Among close friends, however, who both spend time each week meditating, the average performance is consistently around 34%. Now 34% is far from perfect, but given the large number of people that have been tested, this is really striking. The odds of getting this extra 14% correct just by chance is vanishingly small. It seems likely that there's something systematic enabling some of the receivers to do better than random guessing.

What is it? What makes these senders and receivers better than chance? The answers to that question remain highly controversial. There are many who still doubt this finding. To be honest, I remain quite skeptical of it myself. That said, the experiment is clearly designed the right way; Bem did set this up in the right way so that there isn't any easy alternative explanation. There's no alternative source of information available to these participants. Remember, the participants don't pick that movie to send; it's picked at random for them. The sender walks in and has a randomly selected clip that's presented to them. It's not clear how this connection happens.

What's also clear is that the standard of evidence that we apply to almost any finding in the sensory sciences for any of the experiments I've talked about to you today or throughout the course—the amount of evidence we require before we, as a field, accept something to be true—that standard of evidence has been achieved by Darryl Bem in his studies of telepathy.

In this lecture, I've talked about different types of paranormal phenomena, such as mind reading and telepathy. I've argued that we're all able to be mind readers, but that we do so via our normal sensory processing combined with our knowledge of how the world works. Here at the end, however, I've noted that there's evidence that beyond these standard methods of mind reading, there may be something more.

In the next lecture, I'll be talking about something called opponent process. We've discussed this in the domain of motion and color perception, the notion that different neurons compete with and inhibit each other in a continual tug-of-war. The winner of those tug-of-wars gets to say what our perception of the world should be. This design principle, however, seems to arise in a wide range of sensory, action, and even decision making contexts. By thinking about the senses, we may be able to understand our minds as a whole better using this opponent process tool. I look forward to telling you about it next time.

# Opponent Process for Perception and Life
## Lecture 21

W̶e have discussed the opponent process in previous lectures as one of many aspects of sensory processing. Now we will look at it in its own right as a fundamental principal by which the whole brain is organized.

- We will review the opponent processes we have already looked at and examine some new ones. Then we will consider how the opponent process is implemented at the level of individual neurons.

- Finally, we will about the opponent process as a theory of behavioral control—how we use it to maintain our internal state of well-being—and argue that opponent process control systems are an efficient way to build a brain or any other robust, adaptive system that operates within widely varying conditions.

- You probably recall from the lecture on color perception the color aftereffect with the reverse-color American flag. In that instance, the light-sensitive cells that prefer green stimuli inhibited the activity of the red-preferring cells while they were themselves active.

- Even without any input, all neurons have a certain baseline level of activity, a baseline frequency of action potentials. If the green cells become active, the red cells action potential frequency falls below this level.

- If the red cells then receive a bit of red light, they will increase their activation and inhibit the activity of the green cells back toward baseline. These inhibitory cross-connections are so strong that if both types of cells receive a lot of stimulation, the outcome is a stalemate. The cells produce about the same level of activity that they would produce if they had no input at all.

- If you walked into a room where there was a greenish light source, the green-preferring cells would become active and would start inhibiting the red-preferring cells. Everything would look green. If you switched the light bulb for a white one a few minutes later, you would see a reddish aftereffect.

- However, if you left the green light bulb on for hours—or forever— the green-preferring cells would grow fatigued as usual. Their level of activation and their ability to inhibit the red-preferring cells would gradually drop. If you waited long enough, the battle would return to a stalemate.

- Therefore, the opponent process is a self-calibrating color-sensing system. No matter the conditions of illumination, the red and green cells keep each other in check, allowing you to gain accurate color information about the world around you.

- The red and green receptors operate this way because of the presence of 2 different light-sensitive chemicals produced in retinal receptor cells. Over the course of your life, the production rate of these chemicals might change. Still, the opponent process can adapt to this.

- This opponent-process organization is not limited to color. In earlier lectures, I described orientation-specific cells in the visual field, which are organized in an opponent fashion as well.

- Vertically oriented edges inhibit the activity of cells that encode other orientations. If I show you a set of stripes that are all tilted left (rotated counterclockwise) by a few degrees, the corresponding cells are very active and are inhibiting the cells that prefer other orientations.

- To see an aftereffect, you would then look at some perfectly vertical edges. The rested rightward-tilt cells would respond substantially more than the fatigued leftward-tilt cells.

- Two different properties of a stimulus can be connected in an opponent fashion. The best demonstration of this is called the McCollough effect. To generate it, you need a pair of stimuli in which color and orientation are related in a consistent fashion, such as a set of vertical stripes that are red and black and a set of horizontal stripes that are green and black.

- Look at each rectangle for about 10 second, then look at the other, back and forth, activating the 2 separate groups of cells and inhibiting the responses of the opposite cells.

- As you kept looking back and forth, there would be a constant correlation between color and orientation: The more vertical something is, the more red it is; the more horizontal something is, the more green it is. The cells that are active at the same time will start to work together to activate each other and to inhibit the opposing sets of cells.

- The McCollough aftereffect would occur when you finally looked away from these 2 triangles to 2 new striped rectangles, 1 with vertical stripes and 1 with horizontal stripes—just black and white, no red or green. But when you looked at the vertically striped rectangle, you would see a green afterimage, and you would see a red afterimage in the horizontally striped rectangle. Yet when you looked at a plain white rectangle, there would be no afterimage at all.

- Perhaps more intriguingly, if you were to come back and look at those black and white stripes a day later, those afterimage colors would still be vaguely apparent. This process has had a lasting effect on your sensory system.

- This McCollough effect is just a laboratory test with no correlate in the real world, but we can imagine some real-world implications. Without consciously pondering any of these things, your sensory systems find these correlations and use them.

- Consider how the patterns of cross-connection among your retinal cells produce illusory brightness differences. They respond to the presence of light and feed their activation to neurons called ganglion cells, which passes that activation on to the next cell in line in the optic nerve.

- Ganglion cells in any particular location in the retina have inhibitory connections to neighboring ganglion cells. When active, they try to keep all the cells around them quiet. This is referred to as lateral inhibition.

- If one area of the retina receives a bright light (let's call it 100 units of light), while an adjacent area receives less (call it 20 units), the illumination results in activity, some of which is passed on to the optic nerve, and some of which is diminished by neighboring cells on the retina.

- In the regions of uniform bright illumination, there is a lot of activation and a lot of inhibition, such that only about 80 units of activation will make it through to the optic nerve. In the regions of uniform dim illumination, there is little activation, but there is correspondingly little inhibition. Perhaps 16 units of activation get to the optic nerve.

- The interesting part is what happens at the boundary between the light and dim illumination: Only the bright-side neurons produce a high level of inhibition. As a result, they pass much more activation on to the optic nerve, about 88 units. On the dark side, there is little activation passed on.

- Ultimately, activity around brightness edges is enhanced. The edges are the most informative areas of any image, so this is a good thing to do. It makes the image input easier for the visual system to process.

- Imagine 2 gray patches near each other in an image. If one patch was surrounded by black and the other by light gray, there will be less lateral inhibition produced by the black background. Therefore, the gray patch on the black background will appear to be much, much brighter, even if the patches are the same color.

- It is worth noting that these oppositional processes do not apply only to the sense of vision. Competitive cross-inhibition shows up in all the senses.

- For the sense of touch, for instance, pressure increases activations for the neurons located in a particular region of the skin and reduces activation in surrounding areas.

- For the sense of hearing, the presence of a tone at one particular frequency reduces the activation of neurons that respond to adjacent positions in the cochlear membrane.

- Opponent processes are so pervasive, they are capable of describing a variety of human behaviors that from an objective perspective seem remarkably odd. When you develop a tolerance to caffeine or any other drug, for example, and its positive effects start to fade, that is due to an opponent process bringing your brain chemistry back to a baseline state.

- The human body likes to maintain a very consistent, controlled internal state. Most people have a consistent internal body temperature of about 98.6°F. It maintains the concentrations of sodiums, sugars, and a wide range of other chemicals. This process of maintaining a consistent internal state is called homeostasis.

- Homeostasis extends to the internal state of your brain, which seeks out and maintains a consistent state of mental arousal. The set point for this is a little different for each person but everyone has one.

- Opponent processes thus not only explain drug tolerances but some very strange human behaviors like jumping out of perfectly good airplanes, saved from imminent death only by the opening of a parachute.

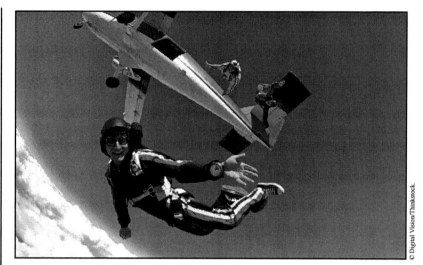

**The pleasure received from risk-taking behavior can be explained as the result of the opponent processes of the brain.**

- These skydivers do not typically receive any reward for doing this; indeed, most of them pay a lot of money to engage in this extremely risky behavior. Why they find such risks pleasurable? The most common theoretical explanation is opponent processing.

- The terror of jumping out of an airplane is a stimulant, just like the caffeine. Your brain registers this terror but immediately sets to work to return to your set level of arousal. When the skydiver returns for the second skydiving experience, the brain anticipates the terror and starts to undo it even before it gets intense. The brain gives the skydiver the opposite of terror—pleasure.

- The opponent process, the pleasure sensation, seems to continue longer than the negative fear response. After the jump has completed, a sense of euphoria may continue for many minutes. This process has been used to explain why people pursue all sorts of behaviors that seem to verge on the irrational: running marathons, climbing mountains, even eating very spicy food.

## Suggested Reading

Iyer and Freeman, "Opponent Motion Interactions."

Solomon, "The Opponent-Process Theory of Acquired Motivation."

## Questions to Consider

1. If you walk or run on a treadmill for 20 minutes and then step off of it, walking feels very strange for a few minutes. It feels as if each stride on the solid ground takes you forward more than one stride's worth of distance? How can this be explained by the opponent-process organization of our brain?

2. Some heroin addicts die of overdoses when they take their usual dose in a novel context. Given your understanding of opponent-process organization of the human brain, why does that make sense?

# Opponent Process for Perception and Life
## Lecture 21—Transcript

Hello again. In this lecture, I'll be describing something called opponent process in detail. We've discussed this concept a bit already as we've considered various aspects of our sensory processing, but I want to step back and consider opponent processing in general in this lecture. Rather than just being a property of certain types of perception, I'll explain that opponent process is actually one of the most fundamental principles by which our whole brains are organized. We see opponent process in our visual perception of motion, color, brightness, and orientation; we see it in our perception of the pitch of different tones; we see it in our perception of touch and texture; we even see it in how our bodies respond to hunger and arousal.

In this lecture, I'll review some examples we've already considered in the course and present you with some others. I'll then consider how opponent process is implemented at the level of individual neurons; how they're wired together to make it happen. We'll consider how the ganglion cells in your retina are wired up in an opponent cross-inhibitory pattern, producing something called lateral inhibition. Next, I'll talk about opponent process as a theory of behavioral control; about how we use opponent process to maintain our internal state of well-being. I'll even use this principle to ponder why people seem to seek out and engage in certain behaviors that, on the surface, seem a little nutty; things like jumping out of an airplane with only a parachute to stop your fall. Ultimately, I'll argue that we see opponent process control systems implemented in our brain so much because it's a good, efficient way to build a brain, or any robust adaptive system that operates within the widely varying conditions of the world around us.

Before we get there, however, let's start by reviewing a few examples of opponent process. You'll probably recall from the lecture on color perception the example of a color aftereffect with the American flag. In that example, I asked you stare at a flag with green and black stripes instead of red and white stripes, and a field of black stars on a yellow background instead of the usual white stars on a blue background. After you stared at this stimulus for a minute or 2, I asked you to blink a few times and then look at a non-chromatic background, something like a white wall. When you did this, you probably saw an afterimage of a red, white, and blue flag. This happens because our brain determines the color of things in the world around us based on the outcomes of several competitions within our brains; that is, opponent processes.

Pardon me for the next few minutes as I anthropomorphize this competition for color. There are visually-receptive cells that like red stimuli; other light-sensitive cells like green stimuli; and these 2 separate sets of cells don't seem to like the other types of cells being active. When they receive some input, they become active and they use that activation to inhibit the activity of the other types of cells. In Lecture 2, you may recall that neurons can influence each other by releasing neurotransmitter chemicals within the tiny synapses that separate them. Some of these neurotransmitters are excitatory and cause the cell on the far side of the synapse to increase its level of activity. Other neurotransmitters are inhibitory and cause the cell on the far side of the synapse to reduce its level of activity. Even without any input, all neurons have a certain standard level of activity; a baseline frequency with which they produce those action potentials. If the green cells become active, the red cells' level of activation is actually pressed below this level; below the level that they exhibit with no input at all. If the red cells then receive a bit of red light, they'll increase their activation and use some of that energy to inhibit the activity of the green cells, reducing the firing rate of those green cells back toward their baseline levels.

These inhibitory cross-connections between the red and green are very strong; so strong that if the red and green cells receive a lot of stimulation, a lot of light—if that light is equal in the amount of green and red light—then the outcome is a stalemate; the cells actually produce about the same level of activity that they would produce if they had no light input at all.

These little green versus red battles take place at every position on the eye, everywhere that there are these color-sensitive cells; almost a million locations within the fovea. Corresponding battles go on at the same time between cells that respond to blue and yellow light. The after-effect occurs because the battles take place between cells that possess a finite amount of energy resources, and as such they get tired. If one cell has extra input for a while, it enables it to win the battle for a while; but when the extra stimulus is removed the well-rested cell now has an advantage, so it wins for a while. After a few minutes, the cells come back into balance—equal inputs and equal fatigue—and the afterimage goes away.

It's worth pondering what would happen if you walked into a room where there was a greenish light source. As you walked into that room, those green cells would become very active. They would start inhibiting the red cells, and everything would look green. If you waited a few minutes and switched to a white light bulb, then there would be a reddish aftereffect. But what if you didn't change to a white bulb? What if you left the green light bulb on for a long time; for many minutes or hours? What if you lived with a green light bulb all the time; what would happen then? The green cells would win the battle for a while, but they would still get tired. As they slowly grew fatigued, their level of activation would gradually drop, as would their ability to inhibit those red cells. As this happens, the room would look less and less green to you. If you waited long enough, the battle would return to that relative stalemate. When you looked at things that were white, you would receive greenish light, but the fatigued green cells wouldn't be able to dominate those red cells anymore. The 2 would fire at approximately equal levels and the white things would look white. In fact, as you looked at everything, it would appear to be the right color.

What we have with this opponent process organization is a self-calibrating color sensing system. No matter the conditions of illumination, the red and green cells keep each other in check, allowing you to accurately gain information about the materials around you based on their relative reflective properties.

The red and green receptors operate this way because of the presence of 2 different light-sensitive chemicals produced in those retinal receptor cells. Over the course of your life, the production of these chemicals might change. As you age or your nutritional intake changes, 1 of these chemicals might be under-produced relative to the other. One might imagine, then, that the color of the world would change as this occurs. Again, the opponent process organization takes care of all of this. If one of the cells becomes overactive, it's always calibrated, kept in check, by the other. Even the best human engineers find the robustness of this system in the face of both internal and external changes remarkably impressive.

This opponent process organization, as I mentioned, isn't limited to color. Consider our perception of how tilted something is. In earlier lectures, I've described how our visual system contains particular receptive cells in the visual cortex that respond best to certain edge orientations and respond less and less as the edge moves away from that orientation. There's a collection of those tilt-specific cells aimed at every location in your visual field; every different location on your retina. Those different cells are connected together in an opponent fashion, much like the cells that encode different colors. If there's a vertically-oriented edge, for instance, the vertical-sensitive cell will become very active and, as the vertical cell becomes active, it inhibits the activity of cells that encode other orientations. Just like the color-sensitive cells, edge-sensitive cells get tired if they're activated for a long time.

Imagine, then, that I show you a set of stripes that are all tilted slightly leftward (more correctly, I would say "rotated counterclockwise by a few degrees"). If you stare at tilted lines, a particular set of orientation-specific cells are very active; they're just going bonkers while you're looking at this. As they are activated, getting their favorite stimulus all over the fovea, they have lots of energy to tell the other cells that encode other orientations to just be quiet. Those inhibitory connections are sending a lot of activity over to the other edge-sensitive cells. If you were to look at lines tilted to the left for a minute or 2, those tilt cells are going to get tired. After the color-sensitive cells were fatigued, I had you shift to looking at a color-neutral stimulus, a white background.

For this aftereffect demonstration, after the left-tilt cells are active, I would ask you to look at some vertical edges. These vertical edges will be our neutral stimulus in this case; they're equally tilted left and right in the sense that they're not tilted left or right at all. This is a stimulus with an equal amount of input for both the left-tilt and the right-tilt cells. If you were to look at some vertical edges, then you would notice they wouldn't seem to be vertical anymore. They are, of course; but because of the fatiguing of the left-tilt cells, that's not how your visual cortex will respond. The rested rightward-tilt cells will respond substantially more than the fatigued leftward-tilt cells. Under normal circumstances, the only way that happens is if the lines are actually tilted to the right; and so your visual system makes this inference and that's what you perceive: rightward-tilting lines.

There are cells that encode color that are wired up in an opponent, cross-inhibitory fashion and there are cells that encode orientation that are wired up in this same opponent fashion. Are the 2 systems connected in this way? Can 2 different properties of a stimulus be connected in an opponent fashion? The answer here is a clear yes. The best demonstration of this is something called the McCollough effect. It's actually one of the longer-lasting adaptation illusion effects ever discovered. To generate it, you need to look at a stimulus in which color and orientation are related in a consistent fashion. For instance, we can look at a set of vertical stripes that are red and black and a set of horizontal stripes that are green and black. As you look at a display like the one I'm describing, you'd look at each of these 2 striped, colored rectangles for about 10 seconds each and then shift your gaze over to the other rectangle. As you'd look back and forth between each one of the rectangles, you'd be activating 2 separate groups of cells, quite a lot; and as you do, of course, those cells are inhibiting the responses of the other cells. The red color-sensitive cells would be very active at the same time the vertical cells would be active. As the green-sensitive cells would become active, the horizontal cells would become active. As you kept looking back and forth between these 2 rectangles, there would be a correlation, a constant relation, between color and orientation. The more vertical something is, the more red it is; the more horizontal something is, the more green it is. As this continues to happen, your visual system somehow notices this correlation between orientation and color. Your sensory systems in general are extremely good at finding these types of correlations. Those groups of cells that are active at the same time start to work together to activate each other and to inhibit the opposing sets of cells.

We're considering this McCollough effect with a stimulus for which there's a correlation between color and orientation; it's a pretty simple relation in this particular case. I'm not envisioning a wide range of orientations—there's just vertical and horizontal—but I certainly could; and I'm only discussing 2 colors, just red and green, but you could certainly imagine a continuous range of colors and orientations for which this correlation might apply. The perceptual linkages that form have a strong effect of the nature of the fatigue that's produced, and the nature of the aftereffect that you would see after staring at these images for a while is affected as well. After a few minutes, I could demonstrate the McCollough aftereffect by showing you 2 new striped rectangles, one with vertical stripes and one with horizontal stripes; only this time, both would only have black or white, no red or green. If you looked at these 2 rectangles, you would see something very strange. When you look at the vertical black and white stripes, the ones that used to be red, you would see a green afterimage. As you move your eyes to look at the horizontal stripes, the ones that used to be green, you would see a red afterimage.

It's worth noting that if you were to look away from the stripes—at a plain white background, for instance—there'd be no afterimage at all. It's almost as if the cells that encode horizontal and green have been fatigued, but not the horizontal or the red cells individually. For vertical and red, the same thing has happened.

The opponent relations between different groups of cells that encode aspects of the visual stimulus are very complex, and they learn very fast. If you were to look at the McCollough effect stimulus for a few minutes—say, 10 minutes or so—a lasting change would be caused in your visual system. If you were to come back and look at those black and white stripes—the horizontal and vertical stripes—a day later, a whole 24 hours later, those afterimage colors would still be vaguely apparent.

For the McCollough effect, an arbitrary relation between color and orientation is formed, but it's just a laboratory relation that's formed between them; there's no correlate of it in the real world. But we can imagine real-world relations that would be functional. As an object moves towards you, its retinal image tends to get bigger; as it moves away, it gets smaller. Size and motion are interlinked ever more strongly than color and orientation. As a stimulus moves toward a light source, it tends to get brighter in color. In some locations—particular rooms in your house, for instance—the lights are brighter and objects thus appear more colorful in those particular rooms. Without consciously pondering any of these things, your sensory systems find these correlations and use them.

How does this work? How could you wire up neurons to enable a cross-inhibitory pattern of connections? The neural networks for effects like the McCollough effect are extraordinarily complex to ponder, but for some simpler effects they're quite straightforward. For the next few minutes, I want to consider how cells at a very basic sensory level are organized in this fashion. Well start with the retina, but then note that the system is applied for other senses as well; for instance, with touch.

Let's consider those cells in your retina and how their patterns of connection produce these illusory brightness differences. The receptors respond to the presence of light and they feed their activation to other neurons called ganglion cells. When a receptor receives some light, it activates its corresponding ganglion cell, which then passes that activation on to the next cell in line in the optic nerve; very straightforward so far. Actually, even at this very basic level of visual processing, that competitive opponent relation begins already. Ganglion cells in any particular location in the retina have inhibitory connections to neighboring ganglion cells. Any time they're active, they try to use that activation to keep all the cells around them quite. This inhibition of the cells all around in a lateral direction on the retina is referred to as lateral inhibition.

Consider what would happen if one area of the retina received a bright light (let's call it 100 units of light), while an adjacent area of the retina received a dimmer amount of light (let's call it 20 units). The illumination results in activity, some of which is passed on to the optic nerve, but some of it's diminished by inhibition neighboring cells on the retina. In the regions of uniform bright illumination, there's a lot of activation, but there's also a lot of inhibition, such that only about 80 units of that activation will be able to make it through to the optic nerve. In the regions of uniform dim illumination, there's not much activation, but there's also correspondingly not as much inhibition. Of the 20 units of illumination that initially hit the retina, about 16 would get through to the optic nerve.

The interesting part is what happens at the boundary between the light and dim illumination regions, at the place where we would see a clear brightness edge. On one side of this boundary, there's a lot of illumination but only a little bit of inhibition, since the cells on the dark side of the boundary don't have much illumination to work with. Only the bright-side neurons—only about half of the surrounding neurons—produce a high level of inhibition. The result is these neurons on the bright side of the edge pass a whole lot of activation onto the optic nerve; about 88 units of activation. On the dark side of the edge, there's extremely little activation passed on. This is because there's a lot inhibition coming from the bright side of the edge and only a little activation from the dim side to start with. Ultimately, this lateral inhibition in the retina results in an input in which the activity around brightness edges is enhanced. The edges are the most informative areas of any image, so this is a good thing to do. It makes the image input easier for the visual system to process.

Imagine 2 gray patches represented near each other in an image. If the background looked the same around these 2 gray patches, they would, of course, look the same. Now consider what would happen if one of these regions was surround by a black background while the other was surrounded by a very light gray background. What should the image look like given our understanding of lateral inhibition? The light gray background neurons will provide a fair amount of lateral inhibition, which will result in a substantial reduction in the amount of activity sent to the optic nerve from that particular gray patch in the middle. For the gray patch that's surrounded by the black background, however, there will be very, very little lateral inhibition because of the dark background. More activity will be passed from that gray patch in the middle of this background onto the optic nerve. The result, which you'll see whenever you look at a figure like this, is a perception of the patch in the middle of the black background appearing much brighter than the patch in the middle of the light gray background. This is true even though the 2 central gray patches are exactly the same color, even though the exact same amount of light is reaching your eye from those 2 patches.

This is all there is to lateral inhibition and to competitive processes for motion, orientation, and color throughout visual system. Neurons are connected to those that encode related features of the sensory input, and through these connections they inhibit their response. It's worth noting that this isn't only true for the sense of vision. For all of the senses, this competitive cross-inhibition shows up. For the sense of touch, for instance, pressure increases activations for the neurons located in a particular region of the skin. Pressure to regions that surround that area will reduce the activation, just like in the retina. For the sense of hearing, there's a similar competition between neurons that encode particular sound frequencies. The presence of a tone at one particular frequency actually reduces the activation of neurons that respond to adjacent positions in the cochlear membrane.

I've presented a variety of evidence that these opponent processes function for almost every aspect of our sensory processes. It's so pervasive, however, that researchers in this field have found that it's capable of describing a variety of human behaviors that from an objective perceptive seem remarkably odd.

Let's start simply here with the activity of drinking coffee. When you have your first cup of coffee, the caffeine contained within that coffee enters your bloodstream through the stomach. Caffeine is a special molecule, one of the few that can pass into the brain and influence its function. What results is a feeling of great energy and alertness. If you have coffee every morning, however, the positive effects of that caffeine begin to fade; indeed, if you don't have a morning coffee, even after plenty of sleep, you'll still feel particularly tired, even groggy. Having the coffee no longer boosts you to a high level of activity; now having the coffee only boosts you to the normal level of activity. This happens with almost any drug or psychoactive chemical that you might consume on a regular basis. The tendency here is to get used to something and need more of it to achieve those same effects over time. It's referred to as tolerance.

How and why does tolerance occur? It occurs because the opponent process organization that we've observed through our sensory processing occurs for all of the control systems throughout the brain. The human body—in fact, all mammalian bodies—likes to maintain a very consistent, controlled internal state. Most people have a very consistent internal body temperature; for instance, about 98.6°F. There are a wide range of chemical reactions that happen in your body that work really well at that temperature, and they break down if you get even a few degrees warmer or colder. Even if you're out on a very cold winter day without a coat, your body will maintain this internal temperature. Your body will modify its blood flow to stay warm, constricting the flow of the blood to your arms and legs, for instance, to reduce the amount of heat that's lost by via radiation there. If you experience even more extreme outer temperatures, you'll start to shiver, rapidly contracting and relaxing your muscles in such a way that they generate some extra heat. Of course the most effective thing that your brain will do is urge you to seek someplace warm, like the inside of your house. Alternatively, if it's very hot instead of very cold, a whole range of other steps will keep your body temperature from rising too high. Perhaps the most obvious one here is sweating, but there are many others as well. Your body doesn't just maintain temperature precisely; it maintains the concentrations of sodiums, sugars, and a wide range of other chemicals.

This process of maintaining a very consistent internal state is called homeostasis. It's very important to your very survival and it doesn't stop with basic properties of physiology; it extends to the internal state of your brain. For instance, your brain seeks out and maintains a consistent state of mental arousal. It doesn't like too much mental activity; it also doesn't like too little. The set point for this is a little different for every person but everyone has one, and your brain does everything it can, really, to keep that level consistent.

The coffee example is very simple here: If you drink coffee every morning, then your brain learns about that. It will learn that morning, especially when the aroma of coffee is perceived, is followed by an infusion of some chemical that ramps up your level of mental arousal. Your brain doesn't know about this the first time you drink coffee, so it has to compensate after the fact; after the level of mental arousal has already been boosted. But over time—and not too much time, actually—if the coffee is consistently administered, your brain will start ramping down its level of motivation before the coffee arrives, so that the caffeine boost just puts things back to where they were before you had any of the coffee.

This compensatory response to the caffeine is very much one of those opponent processes that I've been talking about, much like the ones that operate for the perception of color, tilt, even the pitch of a sound. Opponent processes have even been used to explain some really strange behaviors that humans pursue. For instance, there are people who jump out of perfectly good airplanes. They fall downward at great speed, and they're only saved shortly before an imminent death by the opening of a small sheet of material that slows their descent; people call these things parachutes. These falling people, usually called skydivers, don't typically receive any reward for doing this; no money, no cookies, nothing. Indeed, most of them pay a lot of money for the right to engage in this extremely risky behavior. When people skydive for the first time, almost everyone describes experiencing a tremendous sense of fear, even terror, at the thought of jumping out of an airplane. One might say that millions of years of evolution and many years of developing common sense tell you to not jump. Why would people come back for more? Why would an activity like this be pleasurable? The most common theoretical explanation is opponent processing.

When you jump out of an airplane the first time, your brain is terrified. This terror experience is a result of particular patterns of brain activity. As with the coffee, your brain registers this terror but immediately sets to work undoing that process; to return to that set level of arousal. Eventually, usually after a safe landing, the brain finishes compensating and things get back to normal. The key part is what happens when the person returns for the second skydiving experience. The brain anticipates the terror and starts to undo it even before it gets intense; before it becomes terror at all; before the actual jump. If you've had coffee on a regular basis for many months, then before you drink the coffee in the morning you feel the opposite of arousal; you feel groggy. With skydiving, before the jump occurs, your brain begins to give you the opposite of terror, and most people describe that as a feeling of pleasure.

It's also worth nothing that the opponent process, the pleasure sensation, seems to continue longer than the negative fear response. After the jump has completed, a sense of euphoria may continue for many minutes. This type of explanation has been used to explain why people pursue all sorts of behaviors that seem to verge on the irrational; for instance, running marathons, climbing mountains, even eating very spicy food. There's an old joke about a man seeing a boy hitting himself over and over again in the head with a hammer. "Why are you hitting yourself in the head with a hammer?" the man asked. The boy replied, "Because it feels so good when I stop."

In this lecture, I've talked about opponent process as it relates to a variety of aspects of visual perception. I've also described it as it relates to our other senses and even to our body's general tendency to maintain its internal state of psychological arousal. By studying the senses, researchers have learned not just about perception but about the human mind in general.

In the next lecture, I want to talk to you about a fascinating phenomenon called synesthesia. There are many people—not a high percentage of people, but they aren't all that rare—who have unusual cross-modal sensory experiences with very specific stimuli. There are people that, when they look at a particular letter or number, see it as having a particular color, even if the letter is printed in black ink. Any time there's a letter "a," there's a particular man who sees it as red, regardless of the actual color of the letter. There are people who experience a vivid sensation of a particular taste in their mouth when they hear a certain sound or engage in a certain motor task. There's a man who experiences a vivid bitter taste in his mouth whenever he shapes ground beef into hamburger patties. It's as if the brains of these people are cross-wired in some way, as if there's a connection between the parts of the brain that perceive shape and color, or between the areas that perceive touch and taste. These are fascinating cases to ponder in and of themselves, I think, but studying them has also shed light on how our senses work in general. I'll argue that we all experience synesthesia to some extent, and that this synesthesia has played an important role in the development of our species. I look forward to talking to you about all of these things next time.

# Synesthesia—Tasting Color and Seeing Sound
## Lecture 22

As you are now aware, many distinct sensory subsystems register particular types of information. We assemble different aspects of a stimulus and perceive them that way—most of the time. For some people, however, their perceptual assemblies of certain patterns and objects cross over the usual sensual modality boundaries. Some people report, for instance, that whenever they see a particular letter, it has a certain color to it.

- Many years ago, when I was first starting out as a professor, I had a student with this condition. I had talked in class about how the finding a vertical line among horizontal distracter lines is an easy task but for more complex objects defined on the basis of featured conjunctions, the task is much harder.

- I wanted to make clear to the class that this conjunction could involve 2 aspects of a shape; so you don't need to introduce the notion of color to get this slowed, attention-based search to happen. As a final example, I asked the class to imagine searching the letter *a* among a large number of other letters. This student pointed out that it was quite an easy task; one only had to look for the reddish letter.

- It took me a while to understand what he meant. This student was a synesthete—the first I had ever met in person. For him, the letter *a* always looks reddish, no matter what color ink it is printed in.

- Synesthesia is interesting in its own right, and studying it has revealed some interesting things about normal perception. This type of phenomenon has been found to be quite common. Many people report similar cross-modal or within-modal sensory connections. Some people have reported that certain flavors come with sound. Others report that hearing a certain sound invokes a perception of a certain flavor.

- Studying synesthesia has been somewhat difficult. Nailing down just what synesthetes are perceiving is somewhat hard. For one thing, even though synesthetes have these experiences, for the most part they remain firmly aware of the reality of the situation as well. Perception researchers scratched their heads over this one for a long time.

- Reports of synesthesia date back many, many years. One of the first papers on the topic was published by Francis Galton in 1880. The most common description of synesthesia in old textbooks is a strong association between one type of stimulus and another, not an a multimodal perception.

- Researcher V. S. Ramachandran and his colleagues were the first researchers to develop a method for testing the psychological reality of synesthesia. They spoke to many synesthetes and confirmed that they were not simply experiencing an unusually strong association. Then Ramachandran gave the synesthetes a visual search task like the ones previously described. If the synesthete genuinely, for example, sees a particular color whenever he sees a particular number, then finding a certain number among dozens or hundreds of other numbers will be easier for him than for a nonsynesthete.

- Ramachandran found that this was the case. Analogous tests run with many synesthetes tailored to their particular synesthetic experience have almost always produced this same result. The synesthesia experience is not just a memory or an association with some target. At a fundamental level of perceptual processing, something very different is happening in the brains synesthetes.

- A variety of neuroimaging studies have provided additional evidence for this. For instance, particular areas of the brain become active when you are presented with colorful stimuli. When the man who linked numbers and colors was shown colorful stimuli, the color-sensitive regions of his visual cortex became active. When he was shown black-and-white letter stimuli, this activation dropped.

When he was shown black-and-white numbers stimuli, however, his color-sensitive regions lit up.

- As you know, our perceptions are fast but not instantaneous. We need a few dozen milliseconds or more to perceive things. If I present a number to you for less than about 30 milliseconds, you will have difficulty distinguishing between, say, the number 5 and the number 2. However, a color-number synesthete has a slightly better chance at correctly making the identification at this time threshold. The synesthesia perception seems to happen at the same time, maybe even a bit before, the regular perception of the number's identity.

- A variety of work has been done to explore the nature of these synesthesia experiences and what you need to activate them. The research has been a bit haphazard, since no 2 synesthetes are exactly the same, but some progress has been made. For instance, the Roman numeral 5 or a group of 5 dots is perceived without any color by the color-number synesthete. Cross-modal perception is shape-specific, not linked to the concept of the number.

- Other work has explored synesthesia using more survey- and interview-based methods. One of the findings here is that synesthesia seems to be very haphazard in its linkage between stimuli. For instance, one very typical synesthete associated colors with some calendar-based items but not others. For instance, Monday might always look pink, Wednesday might always look yellow, but there might be no other colors associated with any of the other days. Why some connections and not others?

- Perhaps the most basic question to ask here is, Why does this happen? What is it about the perceptual experience, or the perceptual physiology of the brain, of a synesthete that makes these phenomena occur? Some surveys suggest that it is far from random. Synesthesia is far more common in women than in men, as much as 8 times more frequent. Synesthetes exhibit no apparent neurological deficits or abnormalities. A few studies have suggested that synesthetes tend to be, on average, more intelligent than nonsynesthetes.

- A lot of famous artists and thinkers have reported experiencing synesthesia; many of these famous synesthetes succeeded by finding interesting connections between different types of information. Perhaps synesthete brains grow more and stronger connections between different brain areas average. This theory also fits well with another demographic fact: About 15% of general population is left-handed. As many as 50% of synesthetes describe themselves as lefties.

- The brain has 2 hemispheres; the body has 2 sides. In general, there is a crossover organization: The left motor cortex controls the right side of the body, and vice versa. This applies to the sensory cortices as well.

- Other brain functions seem to be localized to particular hemispheres. For right-handers, language functions are localized to the left hemisphere and face perception takes place in the right hemisphere.

- For left-handed people, language processing seems to take place in both hemispheres; face perception as well. The brains of right-handed people, then, seem to be very lateralized in terms of their organization. For lefties, there is a relative lack of lateralization.

- What does this have to do with synesthesia? It is a little speculative, but the reasoning is that when lefties talk or perceive speech, they are producing a coordinated pattern of activation across a wider range of their brains than righties. The same can be said of recognizing faces. Perhaps the greater use of these connections makes the cross-wiring phenomenon all the more likely.

- It is worth noting that the causation here could run in the other direction as well. Perhaps the presence of a large number of functional, long-range connections is the very thing that causes left-handedness, as well as the thing that causes synesthesia.

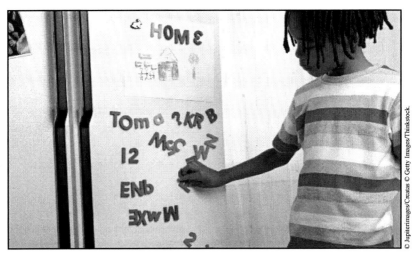
**Some synesthetes may acquire their color-letter associations from early exposure to colorful plastic toys.**

- So where do the colors, tastes, and smells come from? Our best guess, however, is one of simple, strong sensory association. Researchers often discuss what might be around when we first learn letters and numbers. For many children, extensive experience is provided with colorful plastic letters. A child with a wealth of long-range, connected neurons who is learning the alphabet by playing with colorful toys might simply link the colors of the toys to the letters themselves—perhaps inextricably. A similar story can told for any cross-modal connections.

- This is all very speculative, but it is the best theory so far. It is plausible, fits with a variety of other evidence about synesthesia, and is the only story that helps explain the haphazard, highly variable types of cross-modal connections we find among synesthetes.

- On the other hand, several researchers have noted that almost all people say and do some things that, while not truly synesthesia, are synesthesia-like. For example, we accept the notion of a "sharp" cheese even though there is nothing literally sharp about this squishy food, or a "hot" pepper that comes straight out of the refrigerator.

- Perhaps everyone's slight synesthetic tendencies make it possible for us to communicate using language at all. One of the remarkable properties of human language is our ability to use arbitrary sounds to refer to elements of our world. The word *cat* for instance is nothing like a cat itself. We form strong associations between particular sounds and particular objects. To read and write, we form strong, automatically triggered associations between the shapes of letters and words and the objects or features to which they refer.

- When we communicate with each other, we often speak in metaphors. Much of our communication does not involve linking sounds to objects and properties of the world in a literal way. To understand me, you must be able to relate what you are hearing to our shared sensory experiences. Many have suggested that our shared synesthesia is the way that this functions.

## Suggested Reading

Cytowic, *The Man Who Tasted Shapes.*

Ramachandran and Hubbard, "Hearing Colors, Tasting Shapes."

## Questions to Consider

1. In this lecture, I argued that we are all synesthetes—that all of us have cross-wiring between our senses that exerts an influence on what we experience. Some people experience synesthesia dramatically, but perhaps we all experience it a little. If you stare at a photograph of a really delicious looking meal, can you taste them just a little? Do you "feel" the texture of the food on your tongue? If you concentrate, can you tune into your synesthesia? Is this synesthesia?

2. Researchers in this area have suggested that synesthesia has played a role in the development of language in humans. This works for the shape example I presented in the lecture. Can you think of other sound-shape or sound-color labeling that seems to go together in this same way? Does the color blue somehow "sound" blue?

# Synesthesia—Tasting Color and Seeing Sound
## Lecture 22—Transcript

At this point in the course, you know a lot about transduction, sensation, and perception. You know that a lot of the things that we perceive are inferred from the incoming information. Among other things, we have many distinct sensory subsystems that register particular types of information and then assemble those different pieces of information together. For instance, when you view a particular object, you see it as having a certain shape; say, a spherical shape. While some neurons encode that shape, others encode its color; say, red. Still other neurons encode the position of the ball; its direction and its velocity of motion as well. All of this information gets put together and we perceive a single object; for instance a red ball, rolling across the floor in front of us. Sounds primarily have a certain pitch, loudness, and timbre. We combine those factors to perceive something; say, a violin playing a high-pitch note. Taste and olfaction similarly encode the presence of certain chemicals in certain ratios, and give us certain perceptions as we eat; for instance, a nice turkey sandwich on wheat bread with lettuce and peppers.

We assemble different aspects of a stimulus together and perceive them that way; that's how perception works most of the time. For some people, however, their perceptual assemblies of certain patterns and objects cross over the usual sensual modality boundaries. Some people report, for instance, that whenever they see a particular letter, it has a certain color to it.

Many years ago, when I was first starting out as a professor, I had a conversation with a student like this in my office. I'd been discussing some material in class that day about attention and visual search; you might recall this from the lecture on attention and perception. I talked about how certain visual features—for instance, the tilt of a line—seem to pop out at you. If you're searching for a vertical line among horizontal distracter lines, the task is very easy, no matter how many horizontal distracters are there; the vertical just pops right out at you. For more complex objects defined on the basis of featured conjunctions, the task is much harder. For instance, if you search for a red vertical line hidden among green vertical lines and red horizontal lines, you'll need much more time to perform the task; and the more of those distracters are present, the longer it will take you. You need attention, remember, in order to join together the features of the objects, and that's why it takes you longer.

I wanted to make clear to the class that this conjunction could involve 2 aspects of a shape; so you don't need to introduce the notion of color to get this slowed, attention-based search to happen. As a final example, I'd ask the class to imagine searching for a particular letter—the letter "a"—among a large number of other letters taken from the rest of the alphabet. This, I explained, is a hard task; one that requires you to allocate some attention in order to see the letters.

The student came to my office after the class to point out that for him the particular task I'd suggested was really easy because all he had to do was look for the reddish letter. "No," I patiently explained, "all the letters are the same color." The student patiently explained to me that I didn't understand what he was talking about. For him, the letter "a" always looks reddish. I pondered this for a moment and then had to ask him, "What are you talking about?" This student was the first synesthete I'd ever met. He experienced a relatively common form of something called synesthesia. For him, whenever the shape of the letter "a" was present, he didn't just perceive its size, position, and orientation; for him, his brain would overlay a light shade of red on top of that letter "a" shape.

In this lecture, I want to tell you about synesthesia. It's interesting in its own right, and studying it has revealed some interesting things about normal perception as well. This type of phenomenon has been found to be quite common, actually. Many people report similar cross-modal—or even within-modal—sensory connections. Some people have reported that certain flavors come with sound. Others report that hearing a certain sound invokes a perception of a certain flavor. My all-time favorite is a connection between the tactile haptic perception of a motor action and a flavor. Whenever a particular man shapes a ground beef patty, or ground beef into a hamburger patty, he experiences a strong bitter taste in his mouth. There's no sensation of bitter; it's not that the beef emits some trace chemical element that the man's able to smell or taste. Even though there's no sensation of bitter, there's a perception of it. When most people hear this about the nature of synesthesia, it seems almost impossible. Hopefully for you, having learned about how our sensory systems work, it's at least plausible as a possibility to consider.

Studying synesthesia has been somewhat difficult. There's good evidence that these people really do perceive things in this way, and I'll tell you about that in a few minutes; but let me start by saying that nailing down just what they're perceiving is somewhat hard. For one thing, even though synesthetes have these experiences, for the most part they remain firmly aware of the reality of the situation as well. A woman might say that she sees a letter "a" printed in black ink as red, but when describes what she sees, she'll almost always say that she sees a red letter "a" printed in black ink. You might expect that if someone perceived the letter "a" as red than if I projected it onto a computer screen in a yellow color then she should mix those 2 together and perceive it as orange. That's not the case, however. In this example, the woman would report seeing a yellow "a" that was also red. A woman who experiences a certain tone when she smells something will say that she knows there's total silence, but there's also a certain tone. The man with the bitter tastes in his mouth while making hamburgers would say that he knows that there's no bitter substance, but he tastes bitter all the same.

Perception researchers scratched their heads over this one for a long time. Reports of synesthesia date back many, many years. One of the first papers ever published on the topic was by Francis Galton—he's a cousin of Charles Darwin—and that was way back in 1880 when he published that first paper. While people have known about synesthesia reports, then, for many years, the slippery way in which people describe their experiences has led most researchers to just dismiss these as somewhat flimsy in a scientific sense. The most common description offered in old textbooks for synesthesia is that these synesthetes have a strong association between one type of stimulus and another, but that that's not exactly the same thing as perceiving it. For instance, if I tell you about a hot summer day in Georgia, you might think about heat, but that's not the same as actually perceiving an increase in the room's temperature.

That explanation all ended when someone named Ramachandran and his colleagues developed a very clever method for testing the psychological reality of synesthesia. Ramachandran and his colleagues had spoken with many synesthetes and pressed them on what they really perceived. They flat out described this non-perceptual explanation of synesthesia to them and then asked them if that's really what they were talking about. "Maybe you don't perceive colors when you see certain numbers and letters, sir," they might task, "perhaps you just associate the numbers and colors in your memory." The answer for almost all synesthetes was, "No, I understand what you're saying, but this isn't the memory of a color. I see it; clear as day, I see it right there on the paper." Ramachandran set up a challenge for some of the people who gave this explanation. One synesthete in particular indicated that he perceived all of the numbers as having a particular color hue to them, regardless of the actual color in which those numbers were presented.

The challenge that Ramachandran gave the synesthetes was a visual search task, like the ones I've described already. If I ask you to search for a red target among distracters that are another color—say, green—this will be very easy for you. No matter how many distracters are there, you'll find that red target almost instantly; the red target will just pop out at you. This isn't just true for you, by the way; as far as we can tell, every human visual system works this way. If instead of colors I gave you a certain number to search for—say, the number 2—and if I hide that number among a large set of distracter numbers, now the task will get much harder. In general, you'll be slower. In particular, the greater the number of distracters the slower you'll be to find the target. You'll need to allocate at least a little attention to every item in that search display in order to dismiss each distracter until you find the target. Again, this seems to be true for almost every person studied in this way.

Probably you can guess what the test is now, but let me spell it out briefly. If the synesthete genuinely sees the colors whenever he sees the numbers, then the number search task can be a color search task for the synesthete. If I ask him to look for the red number "5," then it shouldn't matter how many other numbers are out there; he should look at the display and the number "5" should just pop out. The amazing thing here is that it does. Analogous tests run with many other synesthetes tailored to their particular synesthetic experience have almost always produced this same result. This synesthesia experience doesn't seem to be just a memory or an association with some target. At a fundamental level of perceptual processing, something very different is happening in the brains of these people with these synesthesia experiences.

A variety of neuroimaging studies have provided additional evidence for this. For instance, particular areas of the brain become active when you're presented with colorful stimuli. When the man who linked numbers and colors was shown colorful stimuli, the color-sensitive regions of the visual cortex became active; nothing surprising there. When he was shown black and white letter stimuli, this activation dropped. Simple again, right? Color, you get a lot of activation in these areas; no color, you don't get activation. When the numbers-to-colors man was shown black and white stimuli that consisted of numbers, those color-sensitive regions lit up, even when the stimuli were just black and white. Again, the synesthesia seems to exert its influence at a very basic, early level of perceptual processing.

As you know, we're able to perceive the identities of objects, and specifically numbers, very fast. But the perceptual process is not instantaneous. We need at least a few dozen milliseconds in order to be able to perceive things. If I present a 5 on the screen to you for 100 milliseconds, you can see that it's a 5. If I present a 2 on the screen for 100 milliseconds, you'll similarly have no problem identifying it. If I reduce the amount of presentation time, however, you'll begin to have trouble making this distinction. Around 30 milliseconds of presentation time, a very brief flash on the screen, you'll be essentially at chance; you won't know whether it was a 2 or a 5.

With the number/color synesthete, a remarkable thing happens at this point. Right around the threshold of time required for perceptual identification, he, like you, would start to say that the stimulus was too fast to really know if it was a 2 or a 5, but he would say that he saw a bit of reddish color, so it was probably a 5. This is a really interesting finding; one that really puts to rest, I think, any remaining thoughts that one might have about the role of memory in this synesthesia experience. The synesthesia perception happens at the same time, maybe even a bit before, the regular perception of the number's identity. Synesthesia seems to function at the very lowest, most basic of perceptual levels.

With these experimental tools in place, a variety of different kinds of work has been done to explore the nature of these synesthesia experiences. What do you need to activate them? The research has been a bit haphazard, since no 2 synesthetes are exactly the same, but some progress has been made. For instance, what happens if you present the number/color synesthete with a Roman numeral 5? Any guess? If you expect that there would be no color experience, then you're right. Similarly, a closely-spaced group of dots—let's say 5 dots—is perceived without any color. There's something very specific about the standard Arabic numeral "5" shape that's required to activate this cross-modal perception. The mere concept of "5" doesn't seem sufficient.

Other work has explored synesthesia using more survey- and interview-based methods. One of the findings here is that synesthesia seems to be very haphazard in its linkage between stimuli. For instance, one very typical synesthete associated colors with some calendar-based items but not others. For instance, Monday might always look pink, Wednesday might always look yellow, but there might be no other colors associated with any of the other days; and yet December might be yellow for this same person. These different targets—Monday, Wednesday, and December—do have something in common; specifically, all are notations to times (times of the week and times of the year). However, they refer to very different ranges of time. The fact that some elements have color connections, but not others—for instance, those other days of the week—is striking; why some connections and not others? Perhaps the most basic question to ask here is why; why does this happen? What is it about the perceptual experience, or perceptual physiology of the brain, of a synesthete that makes these phenomena occur?

Other surveys have suggested that someone who experiences synesthesia, or who experiences that synesthesia, is far from random. For instances, synesthesia is far more common in women than in men. Estimates in various studies have suggested that synesthesia may be as much as 8 times more frequent among women. Synesthetes exhibit no apparent neurological deficits or abnormalities; in almost all respects, they seem to be the same as others except for the presence, of course, of this synesthesia. A few studies have suggested that synesthetes tend to be, on average, more intelligent than non-synesthetes; that is, they score higher on measures of standard intelligence, things like IQ tests. Some of these same studies have noted that there are a lot of famous artists and thinkers who've reported experiencing synesthesia. The famous painter Wassily Kandinsky and the composer Franz Liszt, the poet Arthur Rimbaud, all described regular synesthesia experiences. The list doesn't only include artists. One of the most renowned physicists of the 20th century, someone named Richard Feynman, was a synesthete as well. Many of these famous synesthetes succeeded by finding interesting connections between different types of information. For instance, Kandinsky found fascinating new ways of combining shapes and colors that others found intriguing. Feynman found connections between the domains of mathematics and the physical world that others before him had simply missed.

Most theories about synesthesia suggest that the brains of people who experience it might be especially good at connecting different sources of information. Perhaps there's a biological tendency, for instance, for synesthete brains to grow more and stronger connections between different brain areas than for most people. This cross-wiring, cross-connection idea fits well with the concept of being able to make more remote connections between information that seems unrelated to other people. It also fits well with another demographic discovery about synesthetes: About 15% of people in the general population describe themselves as being primarily left-handed. The proportion among synesthetes is much, much higher. Some estimates indicate that as many as 50% of synesthetes describe themselves as lefties.

Let's talk for a moment about how the 2 hemispheres of the brain and the 2 sides of the body are connected. In general, there's a crossover organization. If I raise and lower my right arm, for instance, it's because of activation patterns produced in my left motor cortex. Conversely, the left side of my body is controlled by the right side of my brain. This applies for sensory inputs as well. If I touch my left leg, it produces activations in the somatosensory cortex in my right hemisphere. Sensations on the right are delivered to the left hemisphere. There are other brain functions that seem to be localized to particular hemispheres. In the lecture on langue perception, for instance, I mentioned the important role that Broca's and Wernicke's areas play in this process of speech perception. For right-handers, these functional areas are localized to the left hemisphere. For right-handers, face perception seems to take place in the right hemisphere. For right-handed people, the left hemisphere is domination in terms of motor control; in terms of mediating actions with the hand and the arm: throwing, writing, kicking, for instance. For left-handed people, the right hemisphere is dominant in terms of motor control for those same throwing, writing, and kicking actions.

Given that this is the case, you might presume that all of the other hemisphere-specific regions would be inverted as well. Lefties, we might be reasonable in guessing, would do language processing in the right hemisphere and face recognition in the left hemisphere. This is a reasonable guess, but it's wrong. The brains of lefties seem to be organized very differently in this regard. For left-handed people, language processing seems to take place in both hemispheres; face perception as well, both hemispheres. The brains of right-handed people, then, seem to be very lateralized in terms of their organization, with certain functions confined to particular sides of the brain. For lefties, there isn't a reverse lateralization but rather a relative lack of that lateralization.

What does this have to do with synesthesia? Why should lefties have such a greater incidence of it? It's a little speculative, but the reasoning goes like the following: Whenever lefties talk or perceive speech, they're producing a coordinated pattern of activation across a wider range of their brains than righties. The same can be said of recognizing faces. Left-handed people aren't just activating short connections within a single region of the brain, they must and do activate much longer-range connections that stretch from one hemisphere into another. This heavier reliance in long-range connections can be quite reasonably associated with the cross-wiring theory of synesthesia. Perhaps the greater use of these connections makes the cross-wiring phenomenon all the more likely. It's worth noting that the causation here, though, could run in the other direction as well. Perhaps the presence of a large number of functional, long-range connections is the very thing that causes left-handedness, as well as the thing that causes synesthesia.

Ok, so we have people with many, perhaps extra, long-range, highly interconnected brain areas. These people are more likely to experience synesthesia than others. That still can't be the whole story. Where do the colors come from? What causes the illusory tastes and smells? The story here can only be guessed at, since no one has been able to—or plans to, for that matter—try to make someone into a synesthete. Our best guess, however, is one of simple, strong sensory association.

Let's think about synesthesia with letters, numbers, and illusory colors. Researchers in this area often discuss what might be around when we first learn letters and numbers. For many kids, extensive experience is provided with colorful plastic letters. Parents might practice naming the letters with their child. The letters are fun toys in their own right. The set I learned with had magnets attached to the back so I could stick them to things, even spell simple words on the refrigerator door. Imagine that you have a child having this experience learning the letters using the plastic toys; say they have a lot of experience with them. Imagine also that the child has a wealth of long-range, connected neurons with a high density of synapses to them. It might be that the colors of those plastic letters would become strongly linked to the letters themselves; perhaps inextricably linked. If the links are strong enough, then perhaps the presence of some letter shapes would spread activation from the form recognition components of the visual system into the color-sensitive regions; and voilà, synesthesis.

A similar story can told for any cross-modal connections. Perhaps a frequent or very salient association might be formed between a very distinct activity (for instance, shaping ground meat into hamburger patties) bitter and a very distinctive taste (for instance, bitter). Maybe that bitter taste was actually present enough times that a neural connection between the burger-making parts of the brain and the bitter taste-sensing parts of the brain. As long as those connections remain, the synesthesia will, too.

This is all very speculative, but it's the best theory that anyone's come up with so far. It's neutrally plausible and it fits with a variety of other evidence about synesthesia, and it's the only story that seems to help explain the haphazard, highly variable types of cross-modal connections that are made; for instance, with particular colors for Monday, Wednesday, and December.

One other theory that's emerged in this synesthesia domain and I think is really interesting is worth considering here. Several researchers in this area have noted that almost all people say and do some things that, while they're not truly synesthesia, they're synesthesia-like. My favorite is the notion of sharp cheese. (I'm a fan of sharp cheeses, so I think about this particular example a lot.) There's nothing even vaguely sharp about even the sharpest of cheeses. Nothing is cutting my tongue when I'm eating a sharp cheese. I'm fully confident that while I'm experiencing this flavor that I describe as sharp that there's nothing literally sharp that's being experienced; yet I'm also experiencing sharpness. This kind of sounds like something that a synesthete would have said to a psychologist 100 years ago; one of those things that caused him to scratch his head in confusion.

You might be thinking, "Well, sharp cheese is causing an irritation in your mouth—a feeling that it's being damaged, for instance—maybe as it would be by something that was sharp, like a knife; so maybe that's why you call it 'sharp.'" OK, if that's the case, then anything that irritates the lining of my mouth should be experienced as extremely sharp. But we usually describe those foods as "hot." No matter how spicy a food is, the temperature in your mouth does not substantially change. Hot and spicy food can, in fact, be quite cold and still be experienced as hot and spicy. I can perceive it as cold, but at the same time say that I'm experiencing it as hot. Again, I sound a little like a synesthete when I say this.

Synesthesia researchers have taken this argument one big step further. Perhaps it's our synesthetic tendencies that make it possible for us to communicate using language at all. One of the remarkable properties of human language is our ability to use arbitrary sounds to refer to elements of our world. The word "cat" for instance is nothing like a cat itself. We don't call cats "meow meows" in any language, at least not beyond the age of 2 years. We're very good at forming strong associations between particular sounds, particular words, and particular objects. For reading, we're particularly good at forming strong, automatically-triggered associations between the shapes of letters and words and the objects or features to which they refer. When we do communicate with each other, we often speak in metaphors: Today it is as hot as Georgia asphalt. That boy is as sharp as a fox. She looked at me with an icy stare. He gave us a warm reception. That job is hard to do. My journal article received a glowing review. This list can go on and on. Much of our communication doesn't involve linking sounds to objects and properties of the world in a literal way. In order for you to understand what I'm talking about, you must be able to relate what you're hearing to our shared sensory experiences. Many have suggested that our shared synesthesia is the way that this functions.

Let's consider some simple evidence for this. Imagine that I show you a rounded, irregular shape next to a pointy, angular polygon; just 2 shapes on the page. I tell you that one of these shapes is called a "kiku" and one of these shapes is called a "bouba"; which one's which? There's no particular reason that you should pick either particular name for either of these shapes. If I ask 100 people, then, in principle I might expect to get about 50 people picking one naming pattern and 50 people choosing the other. That's not what happens; almost everyone says that the pointy, angular shape is the "kiku" and the rounded shape is the "bouba." Why would that be? The best answer that anyone's been able to offer for this kind of finding is synesthesia. Something about the sound "kiku" just goes with our visual sense of corners. Something about "bouba" just matches our visual sense of rounded shapes. If you picked the names in this way—and you almost certainly did—then you're experiencing synesthesia. It may not be as compelling as for some other people, but it's synesthesia just the same.

In this lecture, I've discussed the strange and interesting phenomenon of synesthesia. The brains of synesthetes seem to draw connections between different attributes of their sensory input at a very fundamental level of processing. These connections result in perceptions that are strange but clearly real; experimental evidence provides compelling support for this claim. We've also discussed how synesthesia might relate to our own perception and thinking. We all draw connections between different aspects of our sensory input just like synesthetes do. It may be that synesthesia doesn't represent a qualitatively different kind of brain, just one that's quantitatively a little more interconnected. Finally, I've argued that this interconnection might have been important in the evolution and development of our species. Perhaps the only reason we're able to talk to each other and make sense of it, maybe the only reason language developed so that I can tell you about synesthesia at all, is specifically because of synesthesia; because of the fact that we're all synesthetes.

In the next lecture—our next to last lecture, actually—I want to talk to you about perceptual learning. I discussed the possibility here that synesthesia emerges because of some experience that creates a strong association between 2 different types of stimuli; for instance, the color of plastic letters and the letter shapes themselves. We usually think of associations and pattern recognition as something that occurs at a conscious, high level of our reasoning. In the next lecture, I want to suggest that these types of associations occur all the time. Every time we perceive something, anything, it changes our sensory systems a little bit. If we perceive a particular type of stimulus enough, those small changes can accumulate to become very big ones. If we accumulate enough experience with perceiving some class of stimuli—for instance, wine, faces, or even chess pieces—we often become expert perceivers. After enough experience, our basic visual experience changes. We become able to perceive complex configurations of stimuli as individual units, and we relate those complex configurations to one another in some very impressive ways. I hope you'll join me then and take a little time to learn about how your senses learn.

# How Your Sensory Systems Learn
## Lecture 23

The boundary between perception and cognition is blurry at best. Some things are clearly perceptual and sensory—for instance, the perceiving of colors or aromas. Other things are clearly cognitive—like completing a mathematical proof or a logic puzzle. But many things span these extremes. Walking through a big crowd and searching for the best path to take, I am both perceiving a constantly changing situation and processing my perceptions.

- Our perceptual abilities extend beyond simply transducing energy and making some basic sense of it. We perceive complex configurations of information and use them to plan and execute our actions. This ability is not static and genetically predetermined. In fact, most of it emerges from our ability to learn at a cognitive and a perceptual level.

- Our senses are smart. Every time they are exposed to something, they change just a bit. If we spend a lot of time perceiving a certain class of objects or events, we slowly become perceptual experts in that domain. The pinnacle of this expertise can be very impressive.

- A wine expert, for example, possesses a great deal of knowledge about wines and uses a lot of conscious reasoning to identify and judge them. But this expert also has a lot of experience with seeing, smelling, and tasting wine that is essential to the profession. The wine expert has modified his or her sensory systems.

- Let's start by considering the sensory receptor changes that happen during perceptual learning. One of the ways we get better at perceiving certain types of stimuli occurs at the level of transduction and basic sensory processing. In general, the more we experience a certain class of stimuli, the more our sensory systems modify themselves to receive information associated with those stimuli.

- While some of these perceptual learning changes happen at the level of the receptors themselves, some of the most important changes happen in the cerebral cortex at a more complex information-processing level.

- One of the most useful and important aspects of perceptual learning has to do with your ability to perceive complex sets of sensory inputs as single units or configurations. If I ask you to remember a few individual numbers without writing them down, you would probably be able to remember some of them, but probably not all of them. It is easier to remember them as chunks of numbers that you could associate with specific memories, such as dates.

- This enhancing of mental processing by means of grouping happens with many different types of stimuli. Chess masters are remarkable in their ability to almost instantly size up a game and choose an effective move. The best chess players are remarkably good at reproducing a chessboard configuration from memory—or so it would seem.

- What is remarkable is not the masters' memory but their perception. When chess novices look at a board, they see individual pieces. When chess masters look at the board, they see configurations, groups of pieces: a defensive line of pawns; a queen threatening the bishops and knights; a successful application of the king's Indian defense. Because the chess expert is able to see the pieces as configurations, he actually has much less to remember.

- Learning to instantly, effortlessly perceive complex configurations happens with many types of stimuli. Enough experience seems to even overcome some of the basic attention-based limitations of our sensory systems. In previous lectures, I have talked about visual search tasks—searching for some target among distracter items, and how the more complex the configuration of the target is, the harder it is to find it. This is because attention is a limited mental resource.

- Imagine that instead of colored lines, I asked you to search for several targets—say the letters *t*, *b*, *d*, *l*, or *g*—among a field of other distracter letters. These are hard searches. Some researchers interested in perceptual learning wondered if the human visual system could reorganize itself around such arbitrarily selected targets. They recruited college students to perform this search task for several hours a day, every day for over a month. By the end of the summer, the target letters became pop-out features. Their visual systems had learned to perceive these letters as basic units of input.

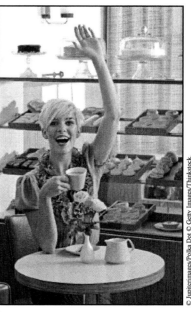

- We do visual searches all the time: Looking for a familiar face in a crowd, looking for your scissors in a cluttered desk drawer, or looking for your car in a large parking lot. In all of these searches, the visual system seems to process configurations as units.

Facial recognition is possible because of the brain's unit-processing capabilities.

- One configuration we each seem to perceive as a unit is our own name, as demonstrated in the cocktail party phenomenon—hearing your own name even over the babble of a large crowd. The sound of your name is a pop-out auditory feature; you have learned through a lifetime of experience to identify the sound of your own name. This is perceptual learning at a very high level of experience and expertise.

- In perceptual learning literature, combining distinct aspects of sensory input into a single unit is referred to as unitization, but perceptual learning is always driven by another process that is in some ways the opposite of unitization, called differentiation. When we perceptually differentiate something, we shift from perceiving a single category of items into 2 or more meaningfully separate categories.

- To study differentiation, psychologist Maggie Shiffrar adapted an area of perceptual expertise of great commercial importance—chicken sexing. Chicks are separated by sex at a few days old, long before they show any obvious-to-laymen signs of being roosters or hens. Expert chicken sexers are extremely efficient; within seconds, the determination can be made, and errors are extremely rare.

- One of the most fascinating things about this process is that if you ask a chicken sexer how they do their job, they will not have much to tell you. They can describe the rules, but they do not consciously apply them. Quite the opposite: They make their determination, then use the rules to explain their decision. Expert chicken sexers have adapted their visual systems to perform this difficult perceptual discrimination test in a very direct fashion.

- Most perceptual learning happens in this unconscious fashion. Just like chicken sexers, we are often able to perceive things expertly without knowing at a conscious level how we accomplished the task. When we recognize a particular face, for instance, we can tell a story about how we have done it, but a lot of evidence suggests the conscious explanation is not how we recognize faces.

- Much of this evidence comes from witness identification of criminal suspects, either in lineups or from photographs. Researchers have found that the best predictor of witness accuracy is very simple: The fewer words a witness uses to explain how he or she identified the suspect, the more likely he or she is to be accurate. The witness who says, "I don't know, I'm just sure of it," is most likely to be correct.

- Perceptual learning, like much of perception, takes place outside of conscious reasoning and awareness. That has led many people to presume that it is a simple, straightforward process. I hope it is clear to you that this is not the case. These are complex information-processing tasks.

- The brain itself changes during the process of perceptual learning. We can see this from studies of how people learn to categorize dots on a computer screen. The dots are very different from what we normally perceive with our visual system, but they have the advantage of being completely novel and completely controllable in an experimental sense.

- To make these patterns of dots, the researchers randomly positioned 7 dots in a particular randomly selected configuration called the prototype. To create each individual experimental stimulus, they shifted each dot in a randomly selected direction by a randomly selected distance. The bigger the shifts in distance, the more different they look from the prototype.

- As with many perceptual-learning experiments, this one starts by showing the participant lots of example stimuli. Often the participants are given some cover task to keep them looking at the images; maybe they are told that they will be asked to recall them later, for instance.

- After they have seen many, many examples of these dot configurations, some interesting changes happen to their visual systems. If you asked the participants to rate, for instance, how pretty a particular pattern of these 7 dots are on a scale from 1 to 10, they will tend prefer the configurations that are more like the prototype. If you ask the participants to press a computer key whenever they see some dots on the screen, they are significantly faster if you present dots in a configuration that is similar to the prototype the more similar it is, the faster they are.

- The really interesting thing that changes is the way their visual cortex processes these dots. As would be expected, their visual cortex increases in activation when presented with visual stimuli. With experienced participants, however, when you present dots similar to the prototype—or the prototype itself—their brains become less active than if you present a random series of 7 dots. It is as if the brain has to do less work to perceive familiar things. This all happens with less than an hour of experience with the stimuli.

- Ongoing research is finding even more dramatic changes in how our sensory systems reorganize themselves as perceptual learning takes place over even a more extended period of time. Almost all of our study of perception has been done with arbitrary, familiar stimuli. Most of our perception occurs in familiar places with familiar people doing familiar, well-learned things. The story we tell about how our brains typically mediate perception may have to change as we delve more deeply into these types of issues.

## Suggested Reading

Gibson and Pick, *An Ecological Approach to Perceptual Learning and Development.*

Goldstone, Landy, and Son, "The Education of Perception."

## Questions to Consider

1. Whenever we perceive something, our sensory systems seem to change a little. If you look at or listen to something thousands of times over the course of many years, your sensory experience of it will gradually change. Can you think of something that your sensory systems have adapted to experience in a richer, more detailed way?

2. Professional athletes are usually evaluated in terms of their behavioral actions on the field of play. One might argue, however, that one of the most important things they do well is "see" the field better. In what ways are athletes you know of expert perceivers—the products of decades of perceptual learning?

# How Your Sensory Systems Learn
## Lecture 23—Transcript

Hello, again. The boundary between perception and cognition, a place where perception ends and cognition begins, is blurry at best. Some things are clearly perceptual and sensory; for instance, the perceiving of colors or aromas. Other things are clearly cognitive; completing a mathematical proof or a logic puzzle, for instance. There are many things, however, that span these extremes. When I'm walking through a big crowd as I'm leaving a baseball game, I look around and perceive the best path to take. Part of that is clearly perceptual; seeing the spaces between the people and the exit that I wish to reach. But my perception of the correct path might also be based on where the people are moving; who's pushing a large stroller while holding another child's hand; the lines at the restrooms; all sorts of things like that.

Our perceptual abilities extend beyond simply transducing energy and making some basic sense of it. We perceive complex configurations of information and use them to plan and execute our actions. This ability isn't static and genetically predetermined. In fact, most of it emerges from our ability to learn; not just learn at a cognitive level but at a perceptual level as well. Our senses are smart. Every time they're exposed to something they change just a little bit. If we spend a lot of time perceiving a certain class of objects or events, we slowly become perceptual experts in that domain. The pinnacle of this expertise can be very impressive. You may have seen depictions on TV or in movies in which a wine connoisseur performs a blind taste test of some wine. He sticks his nose into the tasting glass and deeply inhales. He swirls the glass and looks at color and how the wine clings to the inside of the glass. He takes a sip and he ponders the flavor and swishes the wine in his mouth a bit. Then, sometimes he actually spits it back out. He then confidentially announces that this is a decent burgundy, a chateaux marginale of 1976. This might seem to be a trick or to involve a lot of showmanship—certainly there is some drama to the process—but wine experts really can do this. They can see, smell, and taste a wine and then connect it with their mental representation of some wine that they've tasted before; perhaps many months or years before.

Unless you're also a wine expert, you might taste this wine and many others without being able to tell that there's much of a difference, let alone to use those subtle differences to identify the exact wine that you're tasting. A wine expert possesses a great deal of knowledge about wines—how they're made; what the weather was like in certain growing regions during certain years—there's a lot of conscious reasoning going on here. But there's also a lot of experience with seeing, smelling, and tasting wine that's essential. The wine expert has, through a lot of exposure to different wines, modified his or her sensory systems. This lecture—and perceptual learning in general—is all about those characteristics of those types of changes.

Over the next 30 minutes or so, I'll be telling you about how those changes in our perception occur; how perceptual learning takes place. We'll consider some of the changes that occur at a basic sensory, and others that occur at a more complex level. We'll consider several examples of perceptual learning and how they tell us about this amazing process. I'll talk about how chess masters perceive chessboards, and talk about we all learn to perceive configurations of different, initially discrete sensory inputs as single basic units. I'll talk about how we can learn to perceive almost anything as a basic perceptual unit using an example of visual search experts and an example how you recognize your own name. These are all examples of something called unitization. I'll talk about some research in a very specific agricultural domain—chicken sexing—and how we all learn to differentiate things that initially all look the same. Differentiation is another important component of our perceptual learning process. I'll also mention just how unconscious this complex processing can be, for chicken sexing and face recognition. I'll finish the lecture by talking a bit about the brain changes that are associated with perceptual learning and expertise in general. We often think about the brain as processing things by increasing its activation in certain areas. In this domain, there's some evidence of the opposite. As you develop expertise with some category of items, your brain develops something called perceptual fluency and actually starts exhibiting lowered levels of activation.

Let's start by considering those sensory receptor changes that happen as you perceive with perceptual learning. Actually, we've already discussed this. In the lecture on taste and olfaction, I talked about how you can learn to perceive the odor of androstenone, a pheromone produced by many mammals.

If you're exposed to a lot of androstenone—say, by spending lots of time around a pig farm—your olfactory epithelium, the organ that accomplishes olfactory transduction, changes; you begin to produce new types of sensory cells that are sensitive to this chemical. This happens for other aspects of perceptual learning experience as well. In the unit on touch perception, I talked about how simply stimulating the fingertip of a monkey—stimulating it extensively for several weeks—resulted in an increase in the amount of somatosensory cortex that is devoted to that fingertip. Expert violin players have larger regions of their somatosensory cortex devoted to their fingertips. One of the ways that we get better at perceiving certain types of stimuli occurs at the level of transduction and basic sensory processing. In general, the more we experience a certain class of stimuli, the more our sensory systems modify themselves to receive information associated with those stimuli.

While some of these perceptual learning changes happen at the level of the receptors themselves, some of the most important changes happen in the cerebral cortex at a more complex information processing level. We've talked extensively in this course about how much of your experience of the world is calculated up here. It's only sensible that this would be a place where important perceptual learning would take place. One of the most useful and important aspects of perceptual learning has to do with your ability to perceive complex sets of sensory inputs as single units; as single configurations. Let me ask you to remember a few numbers. I'll say the numbers, then wait and ask you to recall them without writing them down. Ready? One, zero, six, six, one, seven, seven, six, one, nine, eight, four, two, zero, zero, one. Ok, now I'll wait a few seconds for those to sink in. If I now asked you to recall those digits, you'd probably be able to remember some of them, but probably not all of them. Even if your memory for these types of things is very good, it's still a difficult task. Imagine that instead of reading the numbers in this fashion, I said the same numbers in the following manner: 1066, 1776, 1984, 2001. I could wait as long as I wanted. When I ask you to recall as many of those numbers as you can, you'll likely get them all right. When I present the single digits as grouped units—as particular years, some of which you can probably recognize as meaningful dates in history—when I represent them as meaningful chunks of numbers, they're much easier to process.

It's important to note that I presented the same numbers to you in both cases. All I did was present the second time in a fashion that enabled you to process them in groups, in units. This enhancing of mental processing by means of grouping happens with many different types of stimuli. My favorite example of this comes from the study of how chess masters perceive a chessboard. Chess masters are remarkable in their ability to almost instantly size up a game and choose an effective move. Bobby Fischer, one of the great chess masters of the 20th century, used to do demonstrations in which he would play as many as a dozen different opponents at the same time. He would stroll between the different boards, make his move in just a second or 2, and then move to the next board. The opponents would then each have several minutes to make their moves before he returned for his next few seconds of attention to the game.

Even very good chess players—masters, as opposed to grand masters— are very good at remembering and reproducing a chessboard configuration from memory. The task here is straightforward: The experimenter shows the participant a chessboard with some pieces on it, then dumps the pieces off of the board. The study participant attempts to reproduce what he or she just saw. The more pieces in the right place, the higher the score. If you run someone with minimal amounts of chess experience, they can typically place around 7 pieces accurately on the board. Chess masters can not only reproduce a single board with near-perfect accuracy, they can often reproduce many boards at the same time; dozens and dozens of pieces. You show the chess master 5 or 6 chessboards, and then dump the pieces and ask them to reproduce them. The fact that they can do this so accurately is an amazing feat of memory, right? Or so it would seem.

Actually it's not the chess masters' memory that's amazing; it's their perception of the chessboard. When chess novices look at a board, they see individual pieces. When a chess master looks at the same board, they see configurations, groups of pieces: a defensive line of pawns; a queen threatening the bishops and knights; a successful application of the king's Indian defense. Because the chess expert is able to see the pieces as configurations, he actually has much less to remember. When we look at the chessboard, it's like we're hearing individual numbers (1, 7, 7, 6).

When the expert looks at the board, he sees the year in which America declared independence.

Some experimenters in the 1970s ran a very clever experiment to test this particular theory. They ran the same chessboard memory experiment that I just described with one change: In the original study, the chessboard configurations were taken from the middles of actual games. In this second study that was run, the chess pieces were just placed on the board randomly. When the experimenters did this, the perceptual expertise of the chess masters couldn't help them any longer and suddenly they performed no better than the average chess novice, getting 6 or 7 pieces right, and that's about it. It's not the memory that's amazing here, it's the perception; more specifically, the perceptional learning and expertise acquired over many, many years of looking at and reasoning about chess boards. The exposure to this type of perception over time has changed the way this particular category of stimuli is processed.

This learning to instantly, effortlessly perceive complex configurations happens with many types of stimuli. Enough experience seems to even overcome some of the basic attention-based limitations of our sensory systems. In a few of the lectures in this course, I've talked about visual search tasks; tasks in which you search for some target that's hidden among distracter items. I've explained about how we can search for a target that's defined on the basis of a single characteristic—say, its color or its orientation—with relative ease. If I search for a green target among red distracters, it doesn't matter how many distracters there are, the green target just pops out at me. If I search for a more complex configuration—say, a target defined by 2 features—then this task gets much harder. If I ask you to search for a red vertical line among distracters consisting of green vertical lines and red and green horizontal lines, then you'll be slower. What's more, the greater the number of distracter items, the slower you'll be to find that red vertical target. The standard theory here is that you require attention in order to combine the color and the orientation of the targets. Our attention is a limited mental resource such that you have to apply it to perceive and dismiss each distracter until you come to the target.

Imagine that I asked you to search for several targets; say, letters: the letters "t," "b," "d," "l," or "g." In this experimental task, I would hide one of these targets within a field of other distracter letters; letters that were not "t," "b," "d," "l," or "g." Do you think this would be one of those fast, pop-out searches or slow, attention-based searches? Trust me; this is one of those hard searches. Each of these target letters—and any letter, for that matter— is defined by a spatial configuration of particular line and curve elements placed in particular spatial relations to one another. For instance, "t" is 2 lines, 1 horizontal and 1 vertical, with the horizontal approximately centered on top of the vertical. The letter "d" is a vertical line and a curved line, with the curve projecting out to the right of the vertical. Note that my description of a "d" here is actually the same as the description for the letter "p." To differentiate between "p" and "d" I have to consider the relative sizes and positions of the line and the curve. When you do this visual search task for these letters, that's exactly what your visual system is doing. That said, it requires attentional resources to accomplish it and so the search functions relatively slowly.

This is a basic visual search task that I'm describing here; no perceptual learning here yet. Some researchers interested in perceptual learning wondered if the human visual system could reorganize itself around some arbitrarily selected targets, like these letters. Could these letters become automatically processed configurations that would just pop out of a stream like a single feature, like color? The researchers understood that perceptual learning can be powerful, but they understood that it can be slow as well; so they recruited a few college students and gave them a really strange summer job: doing this visual search task. For several hours a day, every day, all week for over a month, the students searched for a set of target letters among non-target distracters; thousands and thousands and thousands of these trials. By the end of the summer, an amazing thing happened: For these students, the letters—the ones they were searching for—became pop-out features. If they looked for the letter "d" among the set of distracters, no matter how many distracters, it just popped off the screen at them. Over the course of just a few months, their visual systems had learned to perceive these letters, these configurations, as basic units of input; as basic as color or orientation would be for you or me.

We don't typically do this type of visual search for letters, so most of us never develop this particular perceptual expertise, but we do visual search all the time. Looking for the face of your wife in a crowd; looking for your scissors in a cluttered desk drawer; looking for your car in a large parking lot; with all of these searches, our visual system seems able to learn to process configurations as units. One of the configurations that we all seem to perceive this way is the sound of our own name. Most people have had the experience of being in a room in which many different conversations are taking place simultaneously. The thing I'm describing to you is often called the cocktail party phenomenon. Let's consider a cocktail party where there are lots of people talking.

In this situation you might be having a conversation with a small group of people about something in particular. Other groups are talking about completely different things. You can hear the sounds of their voices, of course, but you tune them out as you focus on the conversation that you're having. It might seem as if you aren't listening to those other conversations, but there's a part of your auditory system that is. It's always listening for one very specific, very familiar stimulus: the sound of your name. If one of those other groups says your name, it sounds as if it's much louder than the other sounds, much clearer. The sound of your name is like a pop-out auditory feature that cuts through all the other sounds. Just as those very practiced college students had altered their perceptual systems to encode letters at a very basic pre-attentive level of processing, so you have learned through a lifetime of experience to identify the sound of your own name. This is perceptual learning at a very high level of experience and expertise.

Up until now, I've described perceptual learning as a process of learning to perceive configurations; to put together distinct aspects of the sensory input into a single unit. In the perceptual learning literature, this is often referred to as unitization. Perceptual learning is always driven by another process that is in some ways the opposite of this: differentiation. When we perceptually differentiate something, we shift from perceiving a single category of items into 2 or more meaningfully separate categories. This is a big part of becoming a wine expert, for instance. Even the first time that you taste wine, you can probably differentiate the flavor of red and white categories, but most reds will taste about the same. As you're exposed to many reds, the categories of Bordeaux and cabernet will become differentiated. With enough time, these categories will be further differentiated; for instance, into California cabernet and French cabernet.

To study this process of differentiation, a brilliant young researcher named Maggie Shiffrar adapted an area of perceptual expertise that's of great commercial importance, but one that only a few people know about: chicken sexing. If you run a chicken farm, you probably have a hatchery where eggs are incubated until the chicks break through their shells. These chicks spend a little time as a mixed group, but after a few days it's important to separate the males from the females. The females may go on to be egg layers themselves; the males obviously not. For a variety of reasons, it's important to accurately separate male and female chicks. To do this, you need expert chicken sexers to pick up the chicks and check out their genitalia. Male and female chicks are not very developed in their first days of life, such that chicken sexing is actually a quite challenging perceptual task. There's no automated system available for doing this, by the way; this is one of those many situations where the amazing human perceptual system is really essential.

Expert chicken sexers are extremely efficient; they're really good at this. Within seconds, the determination can be made and errors are extremely rare. There are rules that have been determined to define the genitalia for male and female chicks, but there's a tremendous amount of variability. For instance, the male chick genitalia tend to be round and bulb-like whereas the female chick genitalia tend to be more extended to the sides. That said, they are all somewhat bulblike and all somewhat extended to the sides. The real determination has to take into account the relative sizes of the parts, their spatial positions relative to one another, and even the relative shapes of the parts. Only by considering the full configuration of the chick genitalia can the sex determination be made.

One of the most fascinating things about this is that if you ask the chicken sexer how they do it, they won't have much to tell you. They can describe some of the rules involved, but they don't consciously apply those rules in order to make their determinations. Actually, it works in the opposite direction: They make their determination of male or female and then use the rules to explain to you how they made their decision, or at least how they think they made their decision. Expert chicken sexers just perceive the genitalia as male or female. By practicing this task a lot, and receiving feedback when they make mistakes (usually from other, more expert chicken sexers), they've adapted their visual systems to perform this difficult perceptual discrimination test in a very direct fashion.

Most of perceptual learning happens in this unconscious fashion. Just like chicken sexers, we're often able to perceive things in an expert fashion without really knowing at a conscious level just how we accomplished the task. When we recognize a particular face, for instance, we can tell a story about how we've done it, but there's a lot of evidence to suggest that the conscious explanation that we come up with isn't really how we recognize faces. For instance, it's very common for police to ask a witness of some crime to try to identify the perpetrator among a lineup of other people. Sometimes this is done with a lineup of actual people; more often a lineup is done with a set of photographs. The witness looks at 5 or 6 pictures and tries to pick out that man they saw running from the bank after the robbery, for instance.

Investigators have done a lot of research in which they've tried to figure out when people are accurate in these lineup situations and when they're not. Ideally, they want to do this so that we can know when we should trust their identifications and when we should doubt them and look for other evidence. This research has often involved showing people a lineup and allowing them to make a selection and then asking them how they know they've selected the right person. There are a lot of answers that can be given to this question: "I remember that he had a beard and he has those wide-set eyes; I think he had a big nose and the man in this picture has a big nose." Researchers in this area presumed at first that you could collect a lot of data like this and then analyze these answers to find clues to the accuracy of the witness. For instance, maybe people who focus on the eyes are more accurate than people who focus on the shape of the head, or vice versa. Maybe people who describe the internal features of the face in general are more accurate. There are a lot of hypotheses that can and have been tested here. The best predictor, however, turns out to be really simple: The fewer words a witness uses in their answer, the more likely they are to be accurate. If you ask the witness how they know they've selected the right face, the best answer—the one that suggests most strongly that this person is correct—is: "I don't know; it's because it's him, I just know it."

Perceptual learning, like much of perception, takes place outside of our conscious reasoning, outside of our awareness. That facet of our perception has led many people to presume that it must be a simple, straightforward process. Twenty-three lectures into this course, I hope it's clear to you that this isn't the case. These are complex information processing tasks that your brain is solving, and it solves many of them at this very unconscious level of perception.

The last idea I want to introduce here in this lecture has to do with how our brain itself changes during this process of unconscious perceptual learning. My favorite example of this effect comes from studies of how people learn to categorize some very odd stimuli; they're just dots on a computer screen. The ecological psychologists that we've talked about wouldn't like this experiment very much. The dots are very different from what we normally perceive with our visual system, but they have the advantage here for this experiment of being completely novel and completely controllable from an experimental sense.

To make these patterns of dots, the researchers start by randomly positioning 7 dots in 1 particular randomly-selected configuration. We'll call this the prototype. To create each individual stimulus that's used in the experiment, you shift each of these dots in a randomly-selected direction by a randomly-selected distance. The individual stimuli all look kind of like the prototype, but they all look different. The bigger the shifts in distance, the more different they look. As with many perceptual learning experiments, this particular one starts by showing the participant lots and lots of example stimuli. Often the participants are given some cover task to keep them looking at the images; maybe they're told that they'll be asked to recall them later, for instance. After they've looked at the dots for a while—after they've seen lots and lots of examples of these configurations—some interesting changes happen to their visual systems. If you asked the participants to rate, for instance, how pretty a particular pattern of these 7 dots are—say, on a scale from 1 to 10—they might think that sounds strange when you ask them the first time but they will tend to say that they like the dots that are more similar to the prototype; they'll say they look prettier. The more similar it is to the prototype, the more they like it. Also, if you just ask one of these participants to press a computer key whenever they see some dots on the screen, they're significantly faster if you present dots in a configuration that's similar to that prototype; and the more similar it is, the faster they are.

The really interesting thing that changes is the way their visual cortex processes these dots. In general, when you present a visual stimulus to someone, their visual cortex increases in activation; that happens here, of course, as well. With these experienced participants, however, when you present dots that are very similar to the prototype—or especially with the prototype itself—their brains become less active than if you present a random series of 7 dots. It's as if the brain has to do less work to perceive things when those things are familiar than when those things are novel.

This all happens with less than an hour of experience with the stimuli. Ongoing research is finding even more dramatic changes in how our sensory systems reorganize themselves as perceptual learning takes place over even a more extended period of time. Almost all of our study of perception has been done with arbitrary, familiar stimuli. It's interesting to ponder that most of our perception occurs in familiar places with familiar people doing familiar, well-learned things. It might be that the story we tell about how our brains typically mediate perception will have to change a lot as we delve more deeply into these types of issues.

In this lecture, I've talked about many examples of human perceptual learning. I started by briefly reviewing some ideas from our earlier lectures about how our sensory systems change at a basic receptor level as a result of just mere repeated exposure to a particular kind of stimulus; for instance, when we learn to smell androstenone. I then presented several examples of what researchers call unitization, in which different discrete aspects of a stimulus come to be treated as a single complex unit. We talked in a particular about examples of chess, visual search, and recognizing the sound of your own name. I then considered some examples where differentiation was key; where some class of stimulus that was initially perceived as all the same came to be seen at a very perceptual level as 2 or more different things. I presented some examples of chicken sexing and talked a bit about recognizing faces.

It should be noted that almost all perceptual learning involves all 3 of these things, not any 1 of them. As you acquire experience with some type of stimulus, your sensory transduction systems get better at encoding them. Your perceptual systems also get better at making sense of those inputs, learning to unitize certain configurations and also learning to differentiate important categories of stimuli. With all 3 of these mechanisms functioning together, our perceptual learning can be quite powerful.

I finished by talking about how our brain changes as this perceptual learning takes place; in particular, the levels of sensory activation seemed to decrease, not increase. This perceptual fluency effect seems to be a very important aspect of perceptual learning. It may also be why perceiving things with which we're very familiar seem so easy. Our brains just don't have to work very hard to do so.

In the next lecture, our final lecture of the course, I want to discuss a topic that I find fascinating and one that also enables us to pull together many of the different things that we've covered in this course: repairing and replacing damaged sensory systems. As you'll see, some remarkable technologies have been developed to aid people who are blind, deaf, or paralyzed. These systems have been designed and built on the foundation of our understanding of the human senses, an understanding that you now possess. By exploring these different types of interventions, we can review some of the key concepts of your knowledge. The successes of these systems, and their failures, have taught us even more about the senses; not just damaged or missing senses, but normally-functioning sensation and perception as well. I look forward to talking to you about all of this next time.

# Fixing, Replacing, and Enhancing the Senses
## Lecture 24

It has often been said that if you really understand a system, you should be able to build one. I started the first lecture of this course discussing early forays into computational vision and how those early efforts were met with great frustration, but the field has continued to make progress as our understanding of human perception has increased. If we truly understand some aspect of the human senses, then we should be able to fix, replace, or even enhance its normal function.

- Let's begin by considering one of the most successful sensory substitution systems ever developed: the cochlear. Recall that sympathetic vibration causes different portions of the cochlear membrane to vibrate. The cochlea takes all of the sounds delivered to the ear and performs a Fourier transform on them, decoding a complex sound into its component frequencies.

- Many forms of deafness result from damage to the parts of the ear that convey the sound to the cochlea or to the cochlear membrane itself but the auditory nerves are still there and capable of delivering signals to the brain. In these situations, a cochlear implant can restore hearing.

- One of these devices consists of an external electronic system that performs that Fourier transform surgically implanted into the cochlea. Small electric charges are delivered via tiny electrodes, causing action potentials in just the right locations and, voilà, hearing is restored.

- The way a number of patients describe the experience of having a cochlear implant turned on for the first time is not unlike the much more common experience of, say, a nearsighted person putting on that first pair of glasses—trepidation or doubt, followed by wonderment at the richness of the sensory experience.

- Researchers thought that the development of the cochlear implant meant many types of deafness had been cured. However, even the best cochlear implants only a few dozen of locations within the cochlea. The resulting sound inputs are thus much rougher than they would be for normal hearing.

- Patients can hear something right after the cochlear implant is switched on, but it takes time to learn how to use this information effectively. Perceptual learning takes time. Indeed, the best results come from cochlear implants given to young children.

- It is worth noting that deaf people do not need cochlear implants to communicate effectively. Some deaf communities have argued strongly against these imperfect hearing devices. Some believe that the combination of vision and sign language offers better communication than a cochlear implant.

- Analogous work is being done to try to replace the transduction process for vision. This research is much more exploratory but is progressing rapidly. Some researchers are working to develop materials and methods for producing implants; other labs are working to develop surgical techniques; and still others are working patient rehabilitation and training systems.

- The basic idea of a retinal implant is directly analogous to that of a cochlear implant. Many cases of blindness result from damage to the retina, while the optic nerve and the brain remain intact. All that is needed is an artificial transduction system.

- Most systems involve an external video camera, often attached to glasses for ease of use. Signals from this camera are conveyed to a miniature array of electrodes attached to the retinal surface, which in turn activate the intact neurons that connect to the optic nerve and the rest of the visual system.

- A smart engineer came up with a way to provide power to this system by imbedding a tiny solar cell within the stimulator array.

The incoming light itself can be used to generate enough electricity to power those electrodes, and it never runs out of energy.

- As with the cochlear implant, the temporal and spatial resolution of these systems are low compared to normal human vision. The prototype systems have at most a $10 \times 10$ array—a 100-pixel image. Even a bad phone camera produces much higher resolution images than that. But the human brain is able to integrate several 100-pixel saccades into a more complete image, just as it integrates several saccades from the normal fovea.

- Perceptual learning is gradual with artificial retinal implants as well. When the system is first activated, participants sense light but they cannot make much of it. With time and experience, people start perceiving objects in space, an inference of the state of the world that produced the sensory input.

- This artificial retina system presumes that the optic nerve is still intact. Other systems are being developed that deliver electrical signals directly to the visual cortex.

- It is worth noting that the notion of providing artificial vision to the blind has been around much longer, using much lower-tech methods, since at least the early 1970s. Early researchers produced "tactile television," where light was converted into a pattern of vibration produced by a set of piezoelectric metal plates embedded into the back of a chair.

- Remember Müller's doctrine of specific nerve energies. As participants learned to use this system, they began to perceive objects with it. As with the other senses, participants got better and better at seeing with the skin the more they used the chair, and their visual cortices showed activation from this vibratory stimulus. Results such as this suggest that the brain is an extremely plastic and adaptable organ.

- The original tactile television system was built into a dentist chair—hardly portable or convenient. More recent systems are using more portable systems and more tactile-sensitive regions of the body, including the surface of the tongue. One tongue-based television device helps soldiers see in infrared wavelengths, like night-vision goggles.

- Other vision-replacement systems make use of auditory input. One early version sensed the distance to a surface in front of the user and made a particular sound. The closer the surface, the louder the sound; the harder the surface, the higher the pitch. More modern systems scan the environment every second or so and produce a sound pattern that is a more complex function of the nearby surfaces.

- Some early studies with sound-based vision-substitution systems were unsuccessful with children. Young children would grow frustrated with the systems and simply refuse to wear them. The key problem was that the sense of hearing is blocked or at least interfered with by all of these devices, and sound perception is a very effective source of information about the world all by itself.

- One might argue that normal auditory perception provides better spatial information about the world than even the best sound-based vision substitution system. Even more interesting is the periodic emergence of a new skill among blind children: echolocation. This is truly perceptual learning in its highest form. The lack of sight clearly does not mean the lack of spatial perception.

- Although people lose their senses of smell, taste, and touch, little work has been done in terms of replacing these senses. Damage to the particular sets of nerves involved in transduction as well as to the parts of the brain that process them can and do remove these senses completely, but there are some reasons for the lack of research that may occur to you from your study of the human senses.

- For touch, we could try to replace the inputs with something visual, but many of those connections are already there. You can usually tell how a surface is going to feel based on how it looks.

- As for smell and taste, the reasons probably have more to do with the limits of our understanding. Some attempts have been made to develop artificial noses, not for sensory replacement but to replace bomb-sniffing or drug-sniffing dogs, for example, or to detect rotten ingredients in food factories.

- With vision and hearing, transduction is an important first step, but a great deal of inference happens after transduction. With smell and taste, the connection between transduction and perception is very direct. The best electronic systems are still readily outperformed by humans, let alone dogs.

- In many of the lectures in this course, we have considered the strong link between perception and action control. It is worth noting that some of the same methods used to replace sensory transduction are being used to replace damaged action-control systems, slowly enabling victims of paralysis to control their world again.

- Most of these systems involve implanting a set of recording electrodes into the motor cortex. A computer reads the signals in these electrodes and relates them to a different control system. For instance, several patients have learned to use their brain to control the movement of a cursor on a computer screen. Learning to use these systems is slow and difficult, but with practice, somehow the brain figures it out.

- Some systems have been developed that might connect to more complex devices, such as an artificial limb. It would not be at all surprising to see these implants controlling reaching and grasping in the next few years. The hardest work for this will be done not by the artificial system or the implants or even the control system but by the brain itself.

- The brain has its own methods for compensating for loss of motor function as well. One program of research, conducted by Jennifer Stevens and others, has explored how people recover from strokes. For many strokes, only one side of the body is affected, and over time motor function improves as the patient's brain figures out how to make use of undamaged brain tissues. Stevens and her colleagues developed a technique that enhances the rate and eventual amount of this recovery using mirrors and mental imagery.

- The systems described in this lecture could not have been built without a foundation of knowledge about the human senses. Their success and their failures have taught us even more about the senses—not just damaged or missing senses, but normally functioning sensation and perception.

- We have considered the senses from a wide range of different perspectives. As you wander the world, I hope that you will not just perceive things but take a few moments every once in a while to ponder why you perceive them as you do. You may understand, then, why many individuals can look at the same thing but perceive it very differently.

## Suggested Reading

Abbott, "Neuroprosthetics: In Search of the Sixth Sense."

Blume, *The Artificial Ear.*

## Questions to Consider

1. Sensory-replacement systems have almost always been targeted at replacing the loss of the transduction part of the perceptual process. Why do you suppose that is? Why would a replacement of higher sensory functions be so much harder?

Neural prosthetics have great promise for replacing the human ability to control movement. In principle, however, they could also be used to enhance normal human abilities. Can you think of a control ability that would be nice to have directly connected to your brain function? Hands-free driving? Hands-free, no-carpal-tunnel-syndrome typing?

# Fixing, Replacing, and Enhancing the Senses
## Lecture 24—Transcript

Hello, again. Over the first 23 lectures of this course, we've discussed the senses extensively. Hopefully you already feel somewhat comfortable in your knowledge of what the human senses can do and how they function. It's often been said that if you really understand something—if you really understand some system, any system—then you should be able to build one. I started the first lecture of this course discussing early forays into computational vision, in which researchers hooked a video camera up to a computer and then tried to program it to see like a person does. I talked about how those early efforts were met with great frustration; but the field has continued to make progress as our understanding of human perception has increased. In this final lecture, I want to consider similar approaches to building sensory devices; specifically, replacing damaged sensory systems. If we truly understand some aspect of the human senses, then we should be able to fix, replace, or even enhance its normal function. As you'll see, we can.

Thinking about replacing damaged systems is a good place to finish our discussions of the human senses. You'll see how the sensory substitution systems relate to our understanding of the secret life of the senses. You'll also see where some of the boundaries of our understanding are. In particular, we'll discuss cochlear implants, artificial retina projects, and something called tactile television. We'll also discuss the possibility of replacing visual information with sound. We'll next ponder why, even as there's been great progress in replacing lost sight and hearing, there's been no real progress toward replacing the senses of touch, taste, and smell for those who've lost them. On several occasions now, we've discussed how perception and action are inherently linked. I'll describe some recent attempts to replace the ability to control actions via neural prostheses; devices that make artificial connections between the brain and a computer control system that can then cause actions. Finally, we'll ponder the human brain's own preexisting, very natural methods for compensating for sensory loss. As you'll see, some of those processes are even better than the best that modern technology has to offer.

Let's begin by considering one of the most successful sensory substitution systems ever developed: the cochlear. Let's quickly review how the normally-functioning cochlea works to transduce sound into patterns of neural impulses. Recall that the cochlea sits coiled up within the inner ear, where sound vibration is conveyed to it. If we were able to uncoil the cochlea, we would see a set of movement-sensitive neurons located along a triangular sheet of flexible membrane. Sympathetic vibration causes different portions of that membrane to vibrate. High-pitched tones cause the thin areas to vibrate, whereas lower tones cause the wider areas to vibrate. The cochlea essentially takes all of the sounds that ear delivered to the ear and performs that Fourier transform on it, decoding a complex sound into its subcomponent frequencies.

Many forms of deafness result from damage to the parts of the ear that convey the sound to the cochlea, or to the cochlear membrane itself. In many cases, the auditory nerves are still there and still capable of delivering signals to the brain. In these situations, a cochlear implant can restore hearing. One of these devices consists of an external electronic system that performs that Fourier transform. It calculates how much of each different frequency is present in the ambient sound of the environment. It also consists of an internal part that's surgically implanted into the cochlea itself. Small electric charges are delivered via tiny electrodes within this implant inside the ear. Neurons, remember, communicate and process information via electrical action potentials. The implant stimulation causes these action potentials to occur in just the right locations and, voilà, hearing is restored.

Somewhere around the 7th grade, I began to become nearsighted. At first, when my teachers started sending home notes talking about my defective vision, I was horrified. The thought of wearing glasses and maybe being teased, called 4-eyes; these were things that I found very upsetting. For about 2 years, I managed to find a way to sit in the front row of all my classes and just make do with the vision that I had. I can still recite the "EVSPO" letters at the 20/20 vision line of the eye testing chart; by reciting them from memory, I passed that basic vision screening for years. Somewhere around the 9th grade, however, I finally had to give in and consent to getting glasses.

I've heard a number of patients talk about their experience of having a cochlear implant turned on for the first time. I've always been able to hear so I can't know exactly what that's like, but I think my first experience of wearing corrective glasses was probably a little similar; not the same, for sure, but similar. As horrified as I was to put those frames on the first time, when I did I found that I couldn't stop smiling. I turned around and looked out the window of the optometrist's shop at the stores that were across the street. The people and things in those store windows rushed into my eyes with such clarity, I felt like I could touch them; I felt oddly as if I was touching them. Many new recipients of a cochlear implant describe a similar wonderment of hearing sound for the first time. The idea that falling things make a noise when they impact the ground is, in most cases, already understood by a deaf person at a rational level, but experiencing that new sense for the first time is somehow much richer, much different. There's actually a story of a little girl who received a cochlear implant flushing a toilet over and over and just laughing in fascination. The emotion that these well-learned, very familiar visual events—like a flushing toilet—have another dimension of existence, an auditory dimension, is just fascinating to the human brain; it just gets a kick out of it.

Researchers in this area figured that with the development of the cochlear implant that many types of deafness had been cured. There's a bit more to it than that, however. For one thing, humans are able to encode thousands of different sound frequencies. Even the best cochlear implants only stimulate dozens of locations within the cochlea. The resulting sound inputs are thus much rougher, much more approximate, than they would be for normal hearing. The temporal resolution of normal hearing is also much more precise in normal hearing than even the fastest electronic Fourier transform process. As such, the sound is blockier than it would normally be. Patients can hear something right after the cochlear implant is switched on, but it takes some time to learn how to use this information effectively. It's clear that a great deal of perceptual learning that we've discussed takes place with patients with these cochlear implants after they're implanted the first time. Indeed, the best results with cochlear implants are often obtained when they're given not to adults, but to young children. Recall that our language learning abilities seem to be best in childhood. Beyond puberty, the learning is much more difficult. Learning to use a cochlear implant seems to tap into some of these same brain mechanisms that function for normal language perception.

It's also worth nothing that deaf children and deaf adults don't need a cochlear implant at all to communicate. Some deaf communities have argued strongly against installing these imperfect hearing devices into deaf children. With vision and sign language, some people believe that the communication is actually better than with a cochlear implant.

Replacing damaged hearing transduction systems has become commonplace. Analogous work is also being done to try to replace the transduction process for vision as well. This research is much more exploratory, but it's progressing quite rapidly. Among the leading candidates is a device being developed by a coalition of dozens of laboratories under the direction of the U.S. Department of Energy. Some researchers are working to develop the materials and methods for producing these implants; other labs are working to develop surgical techniques for actually implanting them; still others are working on systems to help with the rehabilitation involved in learning to use these systems. By working together and dividing and conquering the problem, this very interdisciplinary team of researchers is moving quickly towards a workable, usable device.

The basic idea of a retinal implant is directly analogous to that of a cochlear implant for hearing. Normally, energy from the environment—in this case, light energy—impinges on a receptor surface on the backs of our eyes and causes a resulting pattern of neural responses. Many cases of blindness result from damage to the retina, either from injury or illness. In many of these cases, the optic nerve and the brain areas involved in processing visual information remain fully intact. All that's needed to restore vision is a new, artificial transduction system. Usually this involves an external video camera, often attached to glasses for ease of use. Signals from this external camera area are then conveyed to a miniature array of electrodes attached to the retinal surface. Those electrical stimulations activate the intact neurons that connect to the optic nerve and the rest of the visual system.

One of my favorite innovations in this artificial retina domain has to do with how to provide electrical power to this tiny electrode within the eye. It would be really awkward to have a power cord, even a tiny one, entering the eyeball. The eye needs to move, and dragging a wire around would be very difficult. Similarly, imbedding a battery in the eye would be a problem as well; how would you change it when it ran out of power? A very smart engineer came up with the idea of imbedding a tiny solar cell within the stimulator array. The light itself can then be used to generate enough electricity to power those electrodes, and it never runs out of energy. This is pretty cool, I think.

As with the cochlear implant, the temporal and spatial resolution of these systems are especially low compared to normal human vision. The prototype systems that have been implanted in test participants have been at most a 10 by 10 array; essentially 100 pixels of an image. Even a bad phone camera has many thousands of pixels to it. How can you see with only 100 pixels of input? The secret here is the same as how we accomplish normal vision, even with that tiny fovea in the center of our visual field. Remember, we can only see with enough resolution to read in the middle $2°$ of our visual field. The rest of our view—most of our visual field, actually—is much lower resolution, and with relatively little sense of color. What do we do? We move our eyes; we scan the environment, moving our sensitive fovea around the visual field to collect information. These retinal implant patients do the same thing. By moving their eyes across a visual stimulus and then integrating the different inputs—the different inputs that they receive over time—they can see what's out there; they can perceive the environment that's around them.

Imagine a barrier between you and some object or display that you wanted to see. Imagine also that there's just a tiny vertical slit in the middle of that barrier. If the object moves past the slit, you can only ever see a tiny vertical slice of the object at a time. Our visual system, however, is remarkably good at putting all of those individual slices together, integrating them so that you can perceive the object, even though you never really sense much of it all at the same time.

With artificial retinal implants, as with the cochlear implant, there's a gradual process of perceptual learning that takes place. When the system is first activated, participants sense light but they can't make much sense of it. I've heard the experience described as "figuring out what's out there," kind of like maybe how you'd figure out what letter someone's tracing on your back with a fingertip. After time and experience, however, participants stop sensing light at the receptor surface; they start perceiving objects in space. They're sensing the light that's projected onto the retinal surface, of course, but they stop perceiving that; they start perceiving an inference of the state of the world that produced those sensory inputs. This is just like normal vision.

This artificial retina system presumes that the optic nerve is still intact. Other systems are being developed that deliver those electrical signals directly to the visual cortex. These systems have progressed much more slowly. In principle, they should work the same way, but it's a much harder thing to install anything under the skull in the brain itself.

It's worth noting that this notion of providing artificial vision to the blind has been around much longer, using much lower-tech methods, since at least the early 1970s. Early researchers in this area produced something that they called tactile television. Light was sampled by a video camera and converted into a pattern of vibration produced by a set of piezoelectric metal plates that were embedded into the back of a chair. A blind participant would sit down in this chair, and as they leaned back on the vibrating plates they would feel the light information as it was conveyed to the back.

You may remember our discussion about Müller's doctrine of specific nerve energies, and the notion that what you sense is a direct function of where your brain is activated. In that segment of the course, we discussed a thought experiment. What would happen if you could unplug the inputs of one sense and plug it into a different part of the brain? Could you hear taste? Could you see sound? Here we have this experiment: Can we feel light? In short, we can. As participants learn to use the system over time, they begin to perceive objects in space. It turns out to be important to let the person move the camera around themselves to enable them to actively explore the environment with the camera. That sound familiar? Action and perception are not just tightly, inseparably linked for normal perceptual processes, they seem to be linked for artificial substitution systems as well.

As with the other senses, participants get better and better at seeing with the skin when they're in this tactile television system. At least one study suggests something really fascinating that happens as they do this. Once participants can see—once they're perceiving objects in the environment rather than just sensing the vibration on the skin—the parts of their brain that become activated by this stimulus are not just in the somatosensory cortex, but in the visual cortex as well. This is fascinating, I think; this is worth taking a moment to think about. The touch stimuli are still connected to the somatosensory cortex; there's still activation there. But somehow the visual cortex seemed to recognize this input as familiar; as the type of information that it's well-suited to process. It somehow reaches out and begins helping with the processing that takes place.

Results such as this suggest that the brain is an extremely plastic and adaptable organ; maybe more plastic and adaptable than we ever really thought. Most theories—essentially all major theories—of perceptual development presume that the neurons in the eye project to the back of the brain according to a very specific set of genetically encoded instructions. A similar process is presumed to take place for connecting the neurons of the cochlea to the auditory cortex and the sense of touch to the somatosensory cortex. The connections that seem to occur between touch inputs for tactile television and the visual cortex suggest an alternative: Perhaps the visual brain area finds the spatial, visual input and not the other way around. Additional research into sensory replacement systems has the potential to really radically change how we think about typical sensation and perception in this domain.

If you see a picture of the original tactile television system, you'll probably marvel at how big and clunky it looks. It was originally built into a large chair; it's actually a dentist chair. This isn't a very easy thing to carry around the world with you. More recent systems have moved away from this vibro-tactile methodology to an electrical stimulation method in order to make it more portable. Researchers in this area have also moved away from using the back as an input surface. You might remember from our discussion of the somatosensory cortex and the sense of touch that the back is actually one of the least sensitive regions of the skin. One of the most precisely encoded is the surface of the tongue.

Using some of the newest vision substitution systems, you can see with your tongue. The light is encoded by a small video camera and processed into a grid of electrical stimulation. Rather than connect this electrical output to the back, the eye, or even the brain, a grid of electrodes is held in the mouth in direct physical contact with the tongue. Just like the tactile television systems, after some experience is acquired, a basic ability to see objects in the environment emerges. In addition to helping the blind, the military has actually been working with these tongue-based television devices to help soldiers see in infrared wavelengths—using their tongues, that is—while still being able to see regular light using their eyes in the normal way. Up to this point I've talked about how these sensory substitution systems can be used to replace missing sensory abilities; here we have something else. It might be that some of these technologies can be used to augment normal perception as well as replacing damaged systems.

Other vision replacement systems have been developed that make use of auditory inputs, rather than the skin. One early version was developed for blind children. A range-finder would sense the distance to a surface in front of the child and make a particular sound. The closer the surface, the louder the sound. The harder the surface was, the higher the pitch of the sound that would be produced. The hope was that children would be able to learn to scan the environment with this device and gather information about their surroundings. Even if they were unable to see it, they could gather information by just listening to the sounds. The device produced some initial successes, but kids tended not to like to wear these devices for very long. The vast majority of them, after being given to study participants, would just end up in a drawer somewhere, sometimes within a few weeks or months (more on that in a moment about why that was).

More modern systems scan the environment every second or so and produce a pattern of sound that's a more complex function of the nearby surfaces. Volume, the loudness of the sound, indicates the brightness of the light. The pitch of the sound conveys the angles and elevation of the surfaces. This pattern of sound is presented to the ears every few seconds, providing information about the surroundings. The sounds are based on 2 different scans of the environment made from 2 different locations. If you wear headphones while listening to one of these recordings, you can get a sense of the space derived from this binaural recording. Recall from the lecture on sound localization that our brains are very good at using slight differences in the timing of different sounds to derive the 3-D structure of the surrounding environment.

With enough practice and perceptual learning, the makers of this device have found that participants can encode enough information about the environment to guide walking navigation; to actually walk around in the environment without being able to see. You might not be able to get that much from hearing these sounds. For one thing, you're only hearing them for a few seconds, and you're also only hearing them from one particular environment. In order for good perceptual learning to take place, much more time and a much greater variety of inputs is necessary. Also, you aren't moving around, actively causing the sounds to change as you do so. If you had the luxury of both of these things—time and action control—you would gradually develop the ability to pick up on the spatial and the visual information that's present in these sounds.

I mentioned that some early studies with sound-based vision substitution systems were unsuccessful with children. Young children would grow frustrated with the systems and simply refuse to wear them. That seemed odd to the researchers at the time. Why wouldn't blind children love the opportunity to see the world around them? The key problem here is that the sense of hearing is blocked—or at least interfered with—by all of these sound-based, vision replacement devices, and sound perception is a very effective source of information about the world around you, all by itself. Indeed, one might argue that normal auditory perception provides better spatial information about the world than even the best sound-based vision substitution system. Blind children can perceive the world around them quite well, even without any artificial vision system. As you know from the lectures on hearing, when a sound is made, our auditory system is exquisitely good at figuring out the location of the sound source relative to our bodies. Blind kinds, who focus on this information a lot, tend to be even better than normally-sighted kids.

Even more interesting, however, is the periodic emergence of a new skill among blind children; a skill that we associate with bats, whales, and submarines, but not usually humans: the skill of echolocation. The best example of this is a blind teenager who's completely blind and has been for many, many years. If you saw him walking down the street, however, especially if you watched him from a distance, you wouldn't be able to tell that he's blind. As he moves around, he makes frequent clicking noises with his tongue and mouth. As these click sounds propagate away from him, they sometimes impact surfaces and some of the sound bounces back. You can experience this by putting your head very close to something—say, a solid wall—and making these click noises. You can hear the sound reflections. If you move further away and make them, you'll notice that it sounds very different. This boy has become well-attuned to this, however; so well attuned that he can hear those reflections at a distance of over a dozen feet. He can walk, run, even—although watching it still makes me cringe whenever I see this video—ride a bike down the street.

This is truly perceptual learning in its highest form. Not all children are quite as good as this boy at using sound to replace vision, but the lack of sight clearly doesn't mean the lack of spatial perception. It also makes very clear why some children might not want to give up on their sense of hearing in order to gain some approximate information about nearby surfaces from an artificial system. They may do better with their natural compensation systems.

I've talked about sensory replacement systems for hearing and seeing. It's interesting to note that there really hasn't been much of anything for smell, taste, or touch, and people do lose those senses. Damage to the particular sets of nerves involved in transduction will remove these senses completely. Damage to the parts of the brains that process them can also eliminate these important senses. Why do you suppose there haven't been attempts to replace them? I don't have a good answer here, but there are some reasons that may occur to you from your study of the human senses.

For touch, we could try to replace the inputs with something visual, but many of those connections are already there. You can usually tell how a surface is going to feel based on how it looks. Rough surfaces and smooth surfaces look very different from one another. To make a device that conveyed that information would, in a sense, be redundant. As for smell and taste, the reasons probably have more to do with the limits of our understanding. Some attempts have been made to develop artificial noses, but those haven't been for sensory replacement; instead, those systems have been aimed at detecting explosives in airports like dogs, or rotten ingredients in food factories. With vision and hearing, transduction is an important first step, but there's a great deal of inference that happens after the transduction. With smell and taste, the connections between transduction and our perceptions are very direct. That is, the subtlety of the process is very much in the transduction process itself, and the best electronic systems available are still readily outperformed by humans, let alone dogs.

In many of the lectures in this course, we've considered the strong link between perception and action control. It's worth noting here that some of the same methods used to replace sensory transduction are being used to replace damaged action control systems. This work is very exploratory, but it's slowly enabling victims of paralysis to control their world again. Most of these systems involve implanting a set of recording electrodes into the motor cortex. When you choose to perform some action, any action, it's accomplished by creating a pattern of activity in this region of your brain. If I lift my arm or turn my head, it starts with activity in these brain regions. For the action control substitution system, a computer reads the signals in these electrodes that are implanted and relates them in some systematic way to a different control system. For instance, several patients have learned to use their brain to control the movement of a cursor on a computer screen. The learning that takes place is slow and difficult; at first it feels to participants in these studies as if the cursor's just moving randomly. But with practice, somehow the brain figures it out.

The experience is usually compared to learning to drive a car. At first, when you get behind the wheel you have to think about every little thing you do: To go faster, I need to press the pedal on the right with my foot; to turn right, I need to rotate this steering wheel; to turn right more quickly, I have to turn it more. Eventually, however, you don't think about driving, except at the level of maybe thinking of where you want to go. The rest of it—how you implement the action—just happens automatically, and that's the end-state of one of these systems as well, the artificial implant systems. The participant thinks about moving the cursor to a particular place and, voilà, it moves.

Some systems have been developed that might connect to more complex devices, such as an artificial limb. It wouldn't be at all surprising to see these implants controlling reaching and grasping in the next few years. The hardest work for this will be done not by the artificial system or the implants or even the control system, but by the brain itself. As long as there's some consistent relation between the pattern of brain activity and the movements of the artificial arm and hand, the brain of the participant will figure out how to map them onto one another. This makes total sense in principle, but we'll have to wait for researchers to finish more work in this area before it comes to fruition.

The brain has its own methods for compensating for loss of motor function as well. One program of research, conducted by Jennifer Stevens and others, has explored how people recover from strokes. For many such strokes, one side of the body is affected—that is, one arm or leg might be almost paralyzed—but even in extreme cases, some motor function is usually spared on that side. Over time, this motor function will improve as the patient's brain figures out how to make use of the brain tissues that haven't been damaged by the stroke. What Stevens and her colleagues have developed is a technique that enhances the rate and eventual amount of this recovery using mental imagery. In one of her tasks, patients sit with a mirror placed at their midline. It's placed such that when the participant looks into the mirror, the reflection of the unaffected limb looks like the affected limb. If participants perform some tasks with their good arm, they will see their injured arm performing as it used to before the stroke. Giving the brain this type of input seems to activate the brain regions near the damaged areas and to facilitate recovery. Even imagining performing a task with the injured arm seems to have a similar effect.

In this lecture, we've considered a variety of different sensory substitution systems, some that have been developed and many that are still being studied. These systems couldn't have been built without the foundation of knowledge that we have about the human senses. Their success and their failures have taught us even more about the senses; not just damaged or missing senses, but normally functioning sensation and perception as well. In this course, we've considered the senses from a wide range of different perspectives. We've considered how the brain processes different sensory information, and how you use that information to infer the nature of the world around you. We've considered how seeing, hearing, touching, tasting, and smelling—doing all of those with the world—combine to provide the rich sensory experiences that we have. We've talked about how that information works within the ecological, real-world context of the environment around us; how we use sensory information to control our actions and to understand what the people around us are saying. Above all, we've considered how our senses connect us to the world around us and to each other. As you wander the world after learning this material, I hope that you'll not just perceive things but take a few moments every once in a while to ponder why you perceive them as you do. How you focus your attention greatly influences your perception. You may understand, then, why many individuals can look at the same thing but perceive it very differently. Everything we ever know or experience comes to us through our senses.

I hope what you've learned increases not only your understanding of the world, but helps you to enjoy and appreciate it more. Thank you for joining me on these first steps of this journey. Don't hesitate to contact me by email if you ever have questions or thoughts about any of this material; I'd love to hear from you. For now, goodbye.

# Bibliography

Abbott, Alison. "Neuroprosthetics: In Search of the Sixth Sense." *Nature* 442 (2006): 125–127. The sixth sense that this title refers to is proprioception, the combination of skin, tendon, and muscle receptors that enable us to perceive where our body parts are located. This author argues that, as researchers develop new robotic systems that enable paralyzed individuals to control their movements in new ways, a lack of proprioception is limiting their progress. The article summarizes recent research on this topic and suggests some important areas in which progress is likely to be made.

Aglioti, Salvatore, Joseph DeSouza, and Melvyn A. Goodale. "Size-Contrast Illusions Deceive the Eyes but Not the Hand." *Current Biology* 5 (1995): 679–685. This original-source journal article presents a simple experiment that has been tremendously influential since its publication in 1995. For over a century, pictorial illusions have been assessed by asking study participants to make overt, conscious judgments about stimuli. In this experiment, participants made judgments but also reached to grasp an element of the display. The illusion affected the judgments as expected; the grasping actions, however, seemed remarkably resistant to the illusion.

Bem, Daryl J., and Charles Honorton. "Does Psi Exist? Replicable Evidence for an Anomalous Process of Information Transfer." *Psychological Bulletin* 115 (1995): 4–18. The field of paranormal psychology has long been considered a secondary science or even pseudoscience. Time and again, claims of mind reading have been debunked, explained away as tricks or implicit biases in the designs of studies. Bem and Honorton—2 senior, highly respected, extremely careful psychological scientists—have invested many years conducting a careful investigation of a particular type of telepathy. This paper reports some of those results. They are highly controversial even now, but they suggest that at least some component of telepathy is real. (Also see the Hyman article below for a response to this study.)

Bermeitinger, Christina, Ruben Goelz, Nadine Johr, Manfred Neumann, Ullrich K. H. Ecker, and Robert Doerr. "The Hidden Persuaders Break into the Tired Brain." *Journal of Experimental Social Psychology* 45, no. 2 (2009): 320–326. This original-source journal article explores the extent to which subliminal advertising changes people's choosing behaviors. It reviews prior evidence that subliminal suggestion can be effective if a participant craves something (e.g., subliminal suggestion of a particular brand of beverage is effective if the participant is thirsty). The authors also report new evidence that subliminal advertising (embedded into a video game) is effective when participants are tired.

Birren, Faber. *Color Perception in Art*. West Chester, PA: Schiffer Publishing, 1986. This book describes how humans perceive color in the context of works of art. The book contains a wide range of different examples of interesting artworks. By describing how the colors on the canvas produce perceptions of color in the mind, the author fosters a better understanding of both the visual system and a better appreciation of the artistic craft.

Blume, Stuart. *The Artificial Ear: Cochlear Implants and the Culture of Deafness*. New Brunswick, NJ: Rutgers University Press, 2009. When scientists developed the first cochlear implants, there was a sense that they had "cured" a broad class of deafness. It was surprising to many that most deaf adults were not interested in using them. Even as many deaf children receive these implants, many others claim that using these implants is not the obvious, best course of action. The author describes the nature of deaf communication and culture and how this controversial area has evolved over the years.

Chabris, Christopher, and Daniel Simons. *The Invisible Gorilla: And Other Ways Our Intuitions Deceive Us*. New York: Crown, 2010. This very readable book presents the case that humans often fail to perceive things that are right in front of them—objects, people, even events. The title is drawn from one famous study in which participants watched a video and counted the number of times a group of people bounced a ball back and forth to each other while a person in a gorilla suit walked across the video screen—unnoticed by most viewers. The book considers this type of phenomenon across a wide range of different, real-world contexts.

Cutting, James E., and Peter M. Vishton. "Perceiving Layout and Knowing Distances: The Integration, Relative Potency, and Contextual Use of Different Information about Depth." In *Handbook of Perception and Cognition*, edited by William Epstein and Sheena Rogers. Vol. 5, *Perception of Space and Motion*. San Diego, CA: Academic Press, 1995. Hundreds of studies have explored how humans perceive the layout of surfaces and objects in the world around us. Our sensory systems make use of literally dozens of different sources of information. This paper presents a theory about how we combine these different, sometimes conflicting sources of information to produce a single perception of the world around us.

Cytowic, Richard E. *The Man Who Tasted Shapes*. Cambridge, MA: MIT Press, 2003. Synesthesia is the phenomenon in which a sensation in one modality (such as visual perception of a square shape) causes a sensation to arise in another (such as the taste of tomato soup). This book on synesthesia considers the history of these phenomena and the exploration of them. The author presents a variety of fascinating case studies and considers, in some detail, how the brains of people who experience synesthesia might be different from the brains of people who do not.

Doesburg, Sam, Lauren Emberson, Alan Rahi, David Cameron, and Lawrence Ward. "Asynchrony from Synchrony: Long-Range Gamma-Band Neural Synchrony Accompanies Perception of Audiovisual Speech Asynchrony." *Experimental Brain Research* 185 (2008): 11–20. Much research has made it clear that we rely on both visual and auditory information for perceiving speech. Anyone who has ever watched a poorly dubbed movie will tell you it can be disconcerting if sound and video are not well synchronized. This study identifies particular brain circuits that are activated when sounds and images are not synchronized and describes how they may function to bring them into register.

Dolins, Francine L., and Robert W. Mitchell. *Spatial Cognition, Spatial Perception: Mapping the Self and Space*. Cambridge, UK: Cambridge University Press, 2010.

Drewing, Knut, and Marc O. Ernst. "Integration of Force and Position Cues for Shape Perception through Active Touch." *Brain Research* 1078 (2006): 92–100. Even if you cannot see an object, you can accurately perceive its shape by holding and exploring it with your hands. This study considers the information available during an active touch experience and how the human brain makes sense of it to accurately perceive shape.

Dworkin, Robert H., Alec B. O'Connor, Miroslav Backonja, John T. Farrar, Nanna B. Finnerup, Troels S. Jensen, Eija A. Kalso, et al. "Pharmacologic Management of Neuropathic Pain: Evidence-Based Recommendations." *Pain* 132 (2007): 237–251. Under normal circumstances, pain conveys important information to us about when our body is being damaged. In some cases, however, the pain system gets broken and sends continuous, illusory pain signals to the brain. The resulting neuropathic pain can be extremely debilitating. This article considers research on the best ways to deal with the disorder using drugs that alter the function of sensory systems.

Gegenfurtner, Karl R., and Lindsay T. Sharpe, eds. *Color Vision: From Genes to Perception.* Cambridge: Cambridge University Press, 2001. This book includes 20 review articles written by 35 experts in the field of color perception. Some papers consider how human genes influence the formation of rod and cone receptors; others consider how those receptors are connected to networks of neurons in the retina and the visual cortex. The book is written at a very high level but contains a wealth of information.

Gibson, Eleanor J., and Anne D. Pick. *An Ecological Approach to Perceptual Learning and Development.* Oxford: Oxford University Press, 2000. Most people think of learning as something that we engage in at a cognitive, intentional level. Many who study learning, however, have found that important aspects of learning take place at a basic, perceptual level. Human sensory systems continuously adapt themselves to better pick up information that is relevant to the individual. This book considers a range of theoretical and experimental approaches that have been taken toward perceptual learning in children and adults.

Gilbert, Avery. *What the Nose Knows: The Science of Scent in Everyday Life.* New York: Crown Publishers, 2008. This clearly written book by a leading olfaction researcher summarizes a state-of-the-art understanding of how human smell functions. In addition to describing the anatomy, physiology, and functional neuroanatomy of olfaction, she relates it to a wide range of everyday phenomena, ranging from how perfumes are developed to how some restaurants market their foods by pumping aromas into shopping malls.

Gladwell, Malcolm. *Blink: The Power of Thinking without Thinking.* New York: Back Bay Books, 2007. This *New York Times* best-selling book considers how human gut reactions—rapid, automatic perceptions of things and situations—strongly influence our behavior. The author conveys several compelling examples of situations in which these rapid responses function, sometimes leading to very good outcomes and at other times leading to disaster. The author considers a range of studies on the topic and presents good advice about when to follow your initial responses and when to proceed with caution.

Goldin-Meadow, Susan. *The Resilience of Language: What Gesture Creation in Deaf Children Can Tell Us about How All Children Learn Language.* Essays in Developmental Psychology, edited by Janet F. Werker and Henry Wellman. New York: Psychology Press, 2003. Most people presume that children who are born without the ability to hear do not naturally develop language and are thus relatively socially isolated from their families, peers, and community. This book makes it quite clear that this is not true. Deaf children naturally develop alternative methods to communicate and interact with the people around them. The book describes these coping strategies and suggests things that parents can do to nurture deaf children's development.

Goldstein, E. Bruce. *Sensation and Perception.* 8th ed. Belmont, CA: Wadsworth Cengage Learning, 2009. This excellent textbook has been under continuous revision and development for more than 20 years. It is primarily used as a college-level textbook, but it provides an excellent, readable overview of our understanding of human sensation and perception. Good coverage is provided of both the historical, philosophical foundations of the field and of modern, state-of-the-art research paradigms.

Goldstone, Robert L., David H. Landy, and Ji Y. Son. "The Education of Perception." *Topics in Cognitive Science* 2 (2009): 1–20. This article reviews recent advances in the area of perceptual learning. How is it that human sensory systems adapt to better encode information and relate it to appropriate actions? What are the mechanisms of this change, and what activates them? What can we do to enhance the rate and quality of perceptual learning? The paper describes many particular studies and provides answers to these and other questions.

Gopnik, Alison, Andrew N. Meltzoff, and Patricia K. Kuhl. *The Scientist in the Crib: What Early Learning Tells Us about the Mind.* New York: HarperCollins, 2000. Three leaders in the field of cognitive development collaborated on this book, which summarizes our modern understanding of the infant mind. They summarize many of the innovative methods and experiments that have led to this knowledge and couch it all within the idea that babies think and act, in many ways, like scientists: They collect sensory data, develop expectations about how the world works, and then collect additional data to test and refine those expectations. Even adult humans function this way, of course, but it is surprising to many just how early this complex level of thinking emerges.

Gregory, Richard. *Eye and Brain.* 5th ed. Princeton, NJ: Princeton University Press, 1997. This book explores the nature of visual perception, with a particular focus on how optical illusions provide insight into the general workings of our sensory systems. Gregory has spent many years developing the notion of perceptual intelligence—the idea that our visual system proceeds in a manner that is analogous to more general problem solving. What state of reality could be responsible for what the senses are currently encoding? Gregory argues that the answer to such a question is what we actually perceive. The first edition of this book was published in 1966; this updated edition considers new brain-imaging methodologies and how they shed light on the questions raised in prior versions of the book.

Hubel, David H., and Torsten N. Wiesel. *Brain and Visual Perception: The Story of a 25-Year Collaboration.* Oxford: Oxford University Press, 2004. Hubel and Wiesel shared the 1981 Nobel Prize in Physiology or Medicine for their groundbreaking, field-transforming work on how the cells of the mammalian visual cortex encode information. We take for granted so many of the things they discovered that it is hard to imagine how we conceived of the brain's sensory systems before they began their work in the 1950s. The book describes their many discoveries, couching it within the story of these 2 genuinely interesting people.

Hurley, Robin A., and Katherine H. Taber. *Windows to the Brain: Insights from Neuroimaging.* Washington, DC: American Psychiatric Publishing, 2008. The development of techniques to record the activity of the brain of an awake, active, perceiving, thinking human has dramatically influenced our understanding of human thought and behavior. It has rendered at least some aspects of the secret life of the senses somewhat less secret. This book explores how neuroanatomy and neuroimaging are able to shed light on a variety of disorders. The book is relevant for learning more about human sensation and perception but also a wide range of other topics, such as post-traumatic stress disorder, anxiety, and dementia.

Hyman, Ray. "Anomaly or Artifact? Comments on Bem and Honorton." *Psychological Bulletin* 115 (1994): 25–27. The author, a highly respected psychological scientist, presents a critique of the findings reported by Bem and Honorton (1995; see above). His review provides a glimpse into how modern science progresses, with some papers making new assertions while others carefully dissect those claims to glean what has been satisfactorily proven and what should still be subjected to additional study.

Iyer, Padma B., and Alan W. Freeman. "Opponent Motion Interactions in the Perception of Structure from Motion." *Journal of Vision* 9, no. 2 (2009): 1–11. Many sets of self-calibrating, self-regulating, opposing cells exist within human sensory systems. Cells that encode a certain motion are self-calibrated by cells that encode motion in the opposite direction. This paper considers how these opponent motion interactions can influence our perception of the shape of moving objects.

Joyce, Kelly A. *Magnetic Appeal: MRI and the Myth of Transparency.* Ithaca, NY: Cornell University Press, 2008. Magnetic resonance imagery (MRI) has become an extremely common tool in our medical offices and laboratories. It is used to assess tissue damage, explore the inner workings of the human mind, find tumors, and myriad other activities. The author explores this from sociological, medical, and scientific perspectives. Based on interviews with doctors, scientists, and technicians, she ponders our great faith in the outcomes of these tests and how they are likely to influence our understanding of the world around us in the decades to come.

Kellman, Philip J., and Martha E. Arterberry. *The Cradle of Knowledge: Development of Perception in Infancy.* Cambridge, MA: MIT Press, 1998. This book provides a detailed review of research on infants' perceptual development. Various chapters consider infant perceptual abilities within various domains (e.g., object, space, motion, intermodal, and speech perception). The book identifies which sensory and perceptual abilities newborns seem to possess at the beginning of their lives as well as describing how they progress from these foundations to adultlike perception. The book takes care to describe particular studies in detail.

Livingstone, Margaret S. *Vision and Art: The Biology of Seeing.* New York: Harry N. Abrams, 2002. The author describes the nature of visual perception based on how great painters and other artists fool the brain. These art-based techniques implicitly contain much information about how the visual system, even its individual cells, functions to encode and interpret the surrounding environment. This entertaining book provides a better understanding of how the human visual sense functions both at the art gallery and in the outside world.

Macknik, Stephen L., Susana Martinez-Conde, and Sandra Blakeslee. *Sleights of Mind: What the Neuroscience of Magic Reveals about Our Everyday Deceptions.* New York: Henry Holt and Company, 2011. These leading neuroscientists turn their attention to a group of other experts on how the mind works (and sometimes does not work) to perceive the events around us. For centuries, magicians have developed techniques to fool the normal processes of perception and memory and in so doing produce seemingly impossible results. The book explores how magic works, how it can be explained by our knowledge of human perception, and what magic suggests about how we should approach the study of the human senses in general.

McMurray, Bob, and Richard N. Aslin. "Infants Are Sensitive to Within-Category Variation in Speech Perception." *Cognition* 95 (2005): B15–B26. Infants who participated in the study reported in this original-source journal article were presented with a sequence of computer-simulated speech sounds. When they heard a change in the sounds, they tended to respond by turning their heads. The experimenters capitalized on this to explore the extent to which children are sensitive to changes in speech that are difficult for adults to consciously identify. Clear evidence is presented that infants are capable of differentiating these sounds at 8 months of age.

Milner, David, and Melvyn Goodale. *The Visual Brain in Action.* Oxford Psychology Series. Oxford: Oxford University Press, 1995. This book has been remarkably influential among vision researchers since its publication in 1995. The authors describe a theory, based on research with animals and brain-injured humans, that the mammalian brain contains 2 largely independent visual systems, one for our conscious perception and a second for controlling visually guided actions. The book then presents a broad collection of studies of humans with normally functioning, uninjured brains that support this 2-visual-system theory.

Moore, Brian, Lorraine Tyler, and William Marslen-Wilson. *The Perception of Speech: From Sound to Meaning.* Oxford: Oxford University Press, 2010. One of the most amazing abilities of humans is to convert ideas within their minds into sounds. Those sounds are then conveyed through the air, to the ears, and ultimately into the minds of others. This process has been the subject of much research over the past century. This book summarizes our understanding of speech perception based on careful studies of human behavior and on assessments of the patterns of brain activity that arise during speech perception.

Nijhawan, Romi. "Motion Extrapolation in Catching." *Nature* 370 (1994): 256–257. The visual system, like all sensory systems, requires time to process incoming stimulus information. This paper presents a clever experiment that demonstrates how the human visual system compensates for these delays by making implicit, short-term predictions about what will happen in the immediate future. The paper argues that these predictions are what we actually perceive.

Pinker, Steven. *How the Mind Works.* New York: W. W. Norton & Company, 1999. This *New York Times* best seller pulls together a wide range of very different sources of evidence to describe, in laymen's terms, our modern understanding of how the human mind functions. A central part of that, of course, is how our brains gather and make sense of the continuous stream of available incoming sensory information.

Pratkanis, Anthony R. "The Cargo-Cult Science of Subliminal Persuasion.' *Skeptical Inquirer* 16, no. 3 (Spring 1992): 260–272. http://www.csicop. org/si/show/cargo-cult_science_of_subliminal_persuasion. This article presents a skeptical, historical account of the history of research on subliminal persuasion. It summarizes some early studies that produced a strong public (and even political) response. The paper puts the phenomenon into an appropriate context, debunking some extreme claims while leaving the door open for things that might yet be demonstrated by future research. In addition to providing a fascinating exploration of this topic, the article provides an interesting example of how science and society interact.

Ramachandran, Vilayanur S., and Edward M. Hubbard. "Hearing Colors, Tasting Shapes." *Scientific American* 288 (2003): 52–59. The authors of this paper consider the scientific meaning of people who report unusual connections between stimuli in one sensory modality and another, a phenomenon known as synesthesia. The authors present experimental evidence that these effects are real and then describe a theory of cross-modal brain connections that explains why they occur. Finally, the article suggests that we are all synesthetes to some extent and that this may have been the origin of our species' tremendous ability to communicate with complex, symbolic language.

Repp, Bruno H., and Günther Knoblich. "Action Can Affect Auditory Perception." *Psychological Science* 18, no. 1 (2007): 6–7. It is commonly understood that we use our sensory inputs to intelligently guide our actions. Less well known is that, as we engage in particular actions, our perceptual systems change, often in fundamental ways. This paper, published in one of the leading journals in the field, describes a study in which pianists touched a sequence of keys and heard several tones. (The keys looked like piano keys but were not connected to a piano.) The job of these participants was to judge whether the notes were increasing or decreasing in pitch. When the pianists played keys corresponding to ascending notes, they tended to hear ascending notes even if the notes were not ascending. In general, the pianists tended to hear what they were playing, even when the sound itself did not correspond to it.

Sacks, Oliver. *The Man Who Mistook His Wife for a Hat and Other Clinical Tales.* London: Duckworth, 1985. A casual look at the human brain itself suggests a homogeneous, unified organ. It is folded and bent in predictable, consistent places, but other than a large fissure in the middle, it can seem undifferentiated. Our understanding that the brain consists of separate, functional pieces is based on case studies in which particular brain injuries have resulted in remarkably consistent and specific losses of function. Sacks is a neurologist who has studied many such cases. He is also a master of compellingly describing those cases and their meaning to the general public. This book is just one of many such examples from this author. The title of the book refers to a man who, while retaining seemingly all other perceptual abilities, lost the ability to recognize or even identify faces, suggesting that a particular part of the brain is responsible for this specific task.

Schnupp, Jan, Israel Nelke, and Andrew King. *Auditory Neuroscience: Making Sense of Sound.* Cambridge, MA: MIT Press, 2010. The authors of this book consider how human hearing functions, converting complex, ever-changing patterns of vibration into our richly detailed experience of speech, music, and the surrounding environment. They consider the acoustics of how sound is produced, how the ears process that sound into neural impulses, and then how the brain uses that information to infer what produced those sounds.

Seckel, Al. *Optical Illusions: The Science of Visual Perception (Illusion Works).* Buffalo, NY: Firefly Books, 2009. The author presents almost 300 different optical illusions along with explanations of how and why they work. Not only are these illusions fun to look at; understanding the illusions leads to a better understanding of how the human senses function normally in everyday situations.

**Bibliography**

Solomon, Richard L. "The Opponent-Process Theory of Acquired Motivation: The Costs of Pleasure and the Benefits of Pain." *American Psychologist* 35, no. 8 (1980): 691–712. This classic paper presents a theory about why humans engage in certain types of seemingly strange, stress-inducing behaviors such as skydiving, watching scary movies, running marathons, and riding roller coasters. The author argues that the inherent nature of how the human body maintains its internal, homeostatic state is responsible. When something impacts our body, it responds to counteract that influence. Solomon argues that thrill seekers are motivated by the pleasure of activating these opponent processes.

Stewart, John, Olivier Gapenne, and Ezequiel A. Di Paolo, eds. *Enaction: Toward a New Paradigm for Cognitive Science.* Cambridge, MA: Bradford Books/MIT Press, 2010.

Thernstrom, Melanie. *The Pain Chronicles: Cures, Myths, Mysteries, Prayers, Diaries, Brain Scans, Healing, and the Science of Suffering.* New York: Farrar, Straus and Giroux, 2010. This book addresses a little-understood and little-appreciated disorder in which people exist in a nearly constant state of chronic pain. Some estimates suggest that approximately 10% of the United States population suffers from this disorder to some extent. The story considers how chronic pain impacts the lives of sufferers, as well as how pain perception functions in both normal and pathological states.

Tipper, Steven P., and Marlene Behrmann. "Object-Centered Not Scene-Based Visual Neglect." *Journal of Experimental Psychology: Human Perception and Performance* 22, no. 5 (1996): 1261–1278. These researchers studied brain-injured patients who exhibit something called visual neglect, in which they ignore one side of their visual world. This research suggests that it is not one side of the patients' field of view that is neglected but one side of the object to which they are attending. This paper sheds light on how human attention and perception function in the uninjured brain as well.

Tsuchiya, Sho, Masashi Konyo, Hiroshi Yamada, Takahiro Yamauchi, Shogo Okamoto, and Satoshi Tadokoro. "Vib-Touch: Virtual Active Touch Interface for Handheld Devices." *The 18$^{th}$ IEEE International Symposium on Robot and Human Interactive Communication* (2009): 12–17. http://ieeexplore.

ieee.org/xpls/abs_all.jsp?arnumber=5326160&tag=1. If we fully understand how touch information is integrated to result in a perception of shape, then we should be able to simulate a perceived shape, creating a virtual object. These researchers describe their attempt to do so, developing a virtual, active touch experience for human perceivers. All information in this system would be delivered via slight vibrations, delivered from a handheld device, based on recordings of where the hand makes contact with it.

Uttal, William R. *The New Phrenology: The Limits of Localizing Cognitive Processes in the Brain.* Life and Mind: Philosophical Issues in Biology and Psychology. Cambridge, MA: MIT Press, 2003. The field of sensory neuroscience progresses from an assumption that the brain consists of a vast collection of separable, largely independent subsystems. There is much evidence suggesting that, but an important alternative perspective exists and is presented in a fascinating way by Uttal. This book considers the limitations of this approach—both the evidence for it and the eventual usefulness of a theory based on it. Uttal argues that a better understanding of the human brain would be based on a more Gestalt approach to its function.

Vishton, Peter M. *What Babies Can Do: An Activity-Based Guide to Infant Development.* DVD. Williamsburg, VA: Power Babies and TNT Media, 2009. This DVD presents a sequence of simple, in-home activities that can be used to test the perceptual processing of young infants and children. By repeating the tests every few weeks, it is possible to track a child's perceptual, cognitive, and motor development.

Vishton, Peter M., and James E. Cutting. "Wayfinding, Displacements, and Mental Maps: Velocity Fields Are Not Typically Used to Determine One's Aimpoint." *Journal of Experimental Psychology: Human Perception and Performance* 21, no. 5 (1995): 978–995. How do we use visual information to sense the direction of our motion? This paper provides a review of several theories about the nature of heading perception and provides evidence that humans make use of a particular source of information known as differential motion parallax in conjunction with our perception of the relative distance to objects to determine where we are going.

Vishton, Peter M., Nicolette J. Stephens, Lauren A. Nelson, Sarah E. Morra, Kaitlin L. Brunick, and Jennifer A. Stevens. "Planning to Reach for an Object Changes How the Reacher Perceives It." *Psychological Science* 18, no. 8 (2007): 713–719. This paper reports a series of studies demonstrating that, when we prepare to reach for a target, the way in which we perceive the target changes. The effect of a visual-size illusion on people's perceptual judgments is reduced just prior to reaching, or even if the reaching is imagined. The paper makes clear that our action control systems can exert a strong influence on our sensory processes.

Watanabe, Takeo. *High-Level Motion Processing: Computational, Neurobiological, and Psychophysical Perspectives.* Cambridge, MA: MIT Press, 1998. The human visual system heavily emphasizes motion information not just for perceiving motion but for identifying and recognizing objects, people, and events. This book provides a detailed, state-of-the-art account of recent research on how the human brain makes sense of visual motion stimuli.

Wetsman, Adam, and Frank Marlowe. "How Universal Are Preferences for Female Waist-to-Hip Ratios? Evidence from the Hadza of Tanzania." *Evolution and Human Behavior* 20, no. 4 (1999): 219–228. Evolutionary psychologists have argued that the hip-to-waist ratio is an important determinant of why some female bodies appear more attractive than others to males from the perspective of a potential mate. This study presents at least one example in which this factor did not influence a particular cultural group. The authors clearly present their methodology and consider why their results seem so different from those of other studies. The article provides a good understanding of the strengths, but also the limitations, of the evolutionary approach to understanding human perception of attractiveness and perception in general.

Zald, David H., and Jose V. Pardo. "Emotion, Olfaction, and the Human Amygdala: Amygdala Activation during Aversive Olfactory Stimulation." *Proceedings of the National Academy of Sciences of the United States of America* 94, no. 8 (1997): 4119–4124. The authors describe how emotion and smell work together in the human amygdala, a part of the human brain associated with emotional processing. They describe a range of studies of animals and humans and a particular new study in which they recorded patterns of brain activity produced by exposure to different odorants. They consider the meaning of their findings in terms of how olfaction has evolved to support human memory, cognition, and behavior.

**Notes**

# Notes

# Notes

# Notes

# Notes

# Notes